Lippincott's
Review Series

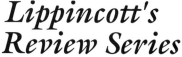

Pediatric
Nursing

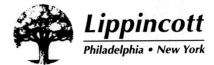

Lippincott
Philadelphia • New York

Lippincott's Review Series

SECOND EDITION

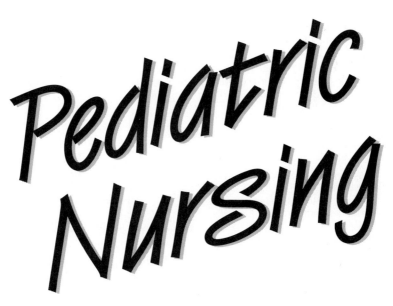

Pediatric Nursing

Mary E. Muscari, RN, PhD, CRNP, CS
Assistant Professor, Department of Nursing
University of Scranton
Scranton, Pennsylvania

Pediatric Nurse Practitioner
Psychiatric Clinical Specialist
Pediatric Practices, Northeastern Pennsylvania
Honesdale, Pennsylvania

Acquisitions Editor: **Susan Glover**
Sponsoring Editor: **Deedie McMahon**
Project Editor: **Tom Gibbons**
Production Manager: **Helen Ewan**
Design Coordinator: **Doug Smock**
Indexer: **Maria Coughlin**

2nd Edition

Library of Congress Cataloging in Publication Data
Pediatric nursing / [edited by] Mary Muscari.—2nd ed.
        p.   cm.—(Lippincott's review series)
    Includes bibliographical references and index.
    ISBN 0–397–55195–9 (pbk. : alk. paper)
    1. Pediatric nursing—Examinations, questions, etc.   2. Pediatric
nursing—Outlines, syllabi, etc.   I. Muscari, Mary.   II. Series.
    [DNLM: 1. Pediatric Nursing—examination questions.   2. Pediatric
Nursing—outlines.   WY 18.2 P3714 1996]
RJ245.L57   1996
610.7362076—dc20
DNLM/DLC
for Library of Congress   95–39932
                                                                CIP

The material contained in this volume was submitted as previously unpublished material, except in
the instances in which credit has been given to the source from which some of the illustrative material
was derived.

Any procedure or practice described in this book should be applied by the health-care practitioner
under appropriate supervision in accordance with professional standards of care used with regard to the
unique circumstances that apply in each practice situation. Care has been taken to confirm the accuracy
of information presented and to describe generally accepted practices. However, the authors, editors, and
publisher cannot accept any responsibility for errors or omissions or for any consequences from application of the information in this book and make no warranty, express or implied, with respect to the contents of the book.

The authors and publisher have exerted every effort to ensure that drug selection and dosage set forth
in this text are in accordance with current recommendations and practice at the time of publication.
However, in view of ongoing research, changes in government regulations, and the constant flow of information relating to drug therapy and drug reactions, the reader is urged to check the package insert for
each drug for any change in indications and dosage and for added warnings and precautions. This is particularly important when the recommended agent is a new or infrequently employed drug.

Materials appearing in this book prepared by individuals as part of their official duties as U.S.
Government employees are not covered by the above-mentioned copyright.

9 8 7 6 5 4 3 2 1

REVIEWERS

Ruth Bindler, RN, MS
Associate Professor
Intercollegiate Center for Nursing Education
Eastern Washington University, Washington State University, and Whitworth College
Spokane, Washington

Vicki Christenson, RN, C, MN
Pediatric Instructor
Intercollegiate Center for Nursing Education
Eastern Washington University, Washington State University, and Whitworth College
Spokane, Washington

Victoria Dianne Sandin, RN, MSN
Instructor
Intercollegiate Center for Nursing Education
Eastern Washington University, Washington State University, and Whitworth College
Spokane, Washington

Jo Trilling, RN, BSN, MSN
Nursing Instructor
Intercollegiate Center for Nursing Education
Eastern Washington University, Washington State University, and Whitworth College
Spokane, Washington

INTRODUCTION

Lippincott's Review Series is designed to help you in your study of the key subject areas in nursing. The series consists of six books, one in each core nursing subject area:

Medical-Surgical Nursing *Mental Health and Psychiatric Nursing*
Pediatric Nursing   *Pathophysiology*
Maternal-Newborn Nursing *Fluids and Electrolytes*

Each book contains a comprehensive outline content review, chapter study questions and answer keys with rationales for correct and incorrect responses, and a comprehensive examination and answer key with rationales for correct and incorrect responses.

Lippincott's Review Series was planned and developed in response to your requests for outline review books that address each major subject area and also contain a self-test mechanism. These books meet the need for comprehensive subject review books that will also assist you in identifying your strong and weak areas of knowledge. Each book is a complete source for review and self-assessment of a single core subject—all six together provide an excellent comprehensive review of entry-level nursing.

Each book is all-inclusive of the content addressed in major textbooks. The content outline review uses a consistent nursing process format throughout and addresses nursing care for well and ill clients. Also included are such necessary additional concepts as growth and development, nutrition, pharmacology, and body structures, functions, and pathophysiology. Special features of each book are key concepts and nursing alerts, which are identified by distinctive icons. Key concepts ☀▲ are basic facts the nurse needs to know to perform with ease and efficiency. Nursing alerts ⚑ are fundamental guidelines the nurse can follow to ensure safe and effective care.

You can use the books in this series in several different ways. Overall, you can use them as subject reviews to augment general study throughout your basic nursing program and as a review to prepare for the National Council Licensure Examination (NCLEX-RN). How you use each book depends on your individual needs and preferences and on whether you review each chapter systematically or concentrate only on those chapters whose subject areas are particularly problematic or challenging.

You may instead choose to use the comprehensive examination as a self-assessment opportunity to evaluate your knowledge base before you review the content outline. Likewise, you can use the study questions for pre- or post-testing after study, followed by the comprehensive examination as a means of evaluating your knowledge and competencies of an entire subject area.

Regardless of how you use the books, one of the strengths of the series is the self-assessment opportunity it offers in addition to guidance in studying and reviewing content. The chapter study questions and comprehensive examination questions have been carefully developed to cover all topics in the outline review. Most importantly, each question is categorized according to the components of the National Council of State Boards of Nursing Licensing Examination (NCLEX).

▶ Cognitive Level: Knowledge, Comprehension, Application, or Analysis
▶ Client Need: Safe, Effective Care Environment (Safe Care); Physiological Integrity (Physiologic); Psychosocial Integrity (Psychosocial); and Health Promotion and Maintenance (Health Promotion)
▶ Phase of the Nursing Process: Assessment, Analysis (Dx), Planning, Implementation, Evaluation

For those questions not related to a client need or to a phase of the nursing process, NA (not applicable) will be used, as in questions that test knowledge of a basic science.

Unlike the NCLEX examination that tests the cumulative knowledge needed for safe practice by an entry-level nurse, these practice tests systematically evaluate the knowledge base that serves as the building block for the entire nursing educational process. In this way, you can prepare for the NCLEX examination throughout your course of study. Good study habits throughout your educational program are not only the best way to ensure ongoing success, but also will prove the most beneficial way to prepare for the licensing examination.

Keep in mind that these books are not intended to replace formal learning. They cannot substitute for textbook reading, discussion with instructors, or class attendance. Every effort has been made to provide accurate and current information, but class attendance and interaction with an instructor will provide invaluable information not found in books. Used correctly, these books will help you increase understanding, improve comprehension, evaluate strengths and weaknesses in areas of knowledge, increase productive study time, and as a result help you improve your grades.

MONEY BACK GUARANTEE—Lippincott's Review Series will help you study more effectively during coursework throughout your educational program, and help you prepare for quizzes and tests, including the NCLEX exam. If you buy and use any of the six volumes in Lipincott's Review Series and fail the NCLEX exam, simply send us verification of your exam results and your copy of the review book to the address below. We will promptly send you a check for our suggested list price.

Lippincott's Review Series
Lippincott-Raven Publishers
Marketing Department
227 East Washington Square
Philadelphia, PA 19106-3780

CONTENTS

Contents

Lippincott's
Review Series

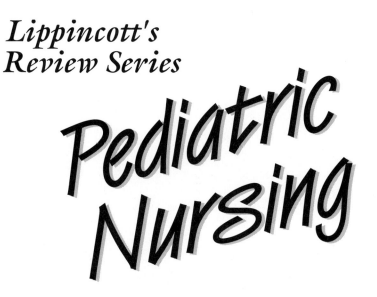

Pediatric Nursing

Overview

I. **Influences on pediatric health**
  A. Family
  B. Culture, religion, and socio-economic factors
  C. Environment
  D. Growth and development
II. **Influences on pediatric mortality and morbidity**
  A. Leading causes of death in children by age
  B. Leading causes of morbidity in children
III. **Roles of pediatric nurses**
  A. Family advocate
  B. Health promoter

  C. Health teacher
  D. Counselor
  E. Collaborator
  F. Researcher
IV. **Pediatric nursing health assessment**
  A. General considerations
  B. Health history
  C. Developmental assessment
  D. Physical assessment
Bibliography
Study questions

I. Influences on pediatric health
A. Family
1. Family functions
   a. Childbearing and child rearing
   b. Providing basic needs: food, safety, clothing, shelter, and health care .
   c. Providing communication and emotional support
   d. Enabling enculturation and socialization
   e. Preparing children to become citizens in society
2. Family structures
   a. Nuclear or conjugal: husband, wife, and children (natural or adopted) living in the same household
   b. Single parent: created by death, divorce, desertion, illegitimacy, or adoption

      c. Reconstituted or step family: one or both married adults with children from previous marriages

      d. Extended: nuclear family plus lineal or collateral relatives

      e. Same sex: common-law arrangement between two men or two women with children

      f. Two career: both parents with jobs

      g. Commuter families: parents living and working apart for professional or financial reasons

      h. Return to nest: family members returning home to live for financial, social, or cultural reasons

3. Family reactions to child's illness or hospitalization

      a. Possible impaired coping: increased fears and anxieties about a child's illness or hospitalization leading to family's decreased ability to cope and to help the child cope

      b. Decreased sense of control over the situation resulting from stressors such as seriousness of the illness, previous hospitalizations, medical procedures involved and lack of information, support systems, ego strengths, other family problems, cultural and religious beliefs, family communications, previous coping abilities

      c. Possible parental manifestations of stress: including anxiety, denial, guilt, anger, fear, frustration, depression, and such defense mechanisms as displacement and projection

4. Implications for nursing process

      a. Assess parents' energy levels, physical health, and developmental levels; each parent's parenting as child, if appropriate; stressors; family support systems; cultural and religious beliefs; and education and experience in child rearing.

      b. Develop nursing diagnoses based on assessment findings (*e.g.*, altered parenting, role performance, and family processes).

      c. Identify goals and outcomes (*e.g.*, strengthen parenting role).

      d. Plan and carry out interventions: (*e.g.*, help parents accept child's individuality; encourage warm, nurturing behaviors, and support participation by all family members; help parents develop realistic goals; allow parents to verbalize concerns; facilitate support groups; explain child's growth and development; provide anticipatory guidance and explain child's anticipated reactions; identify effective role models; identify family and community resources; facilitate bonding [positive comments about child, touch, role model, praise for positive parenting behaviors]; be empathetic; include parents in child's care; accept family's cultural and religious beliefs; encourage parents to eat and sleep; avoid making parents dependent on the nurse; encourage sibling visits; utilize other caregivers).

♬ e. **Keep parents informed.**

5. Evaluate outcomes (*e.g.*, parents can perform their parenting role).

B. Culture, religion, and socioeconomic status

1. Cultural and religious influences
   a. Beliefs influence kinship bonds, parenting practices, dietary customs, communication patterns, interpersonal relationships, and health beliefs and practices.
   b. Folk healers are considered powerful in their communities.
   c. All cultures use home remedies; some remedies are compatible with medical treatment, many have no scientific basis, and some actually may be harmful.
   d. Some cultural practices, such as coining, are considered abusive by the dominant culture.
   e. Nursing implications
      (1) Nurses need to understand their own beliefs and values, be sensitive to the beliefs and values of families, and avoid imposing personal beliefs and values on clients.
      (2) Nurses need to consider clients' cultural and religious beliefs when developing and implementing a plan of care.

☀ 2. **Socioeconomic influences: Low socioeconomic status has the greatest adverse influence on health.**

C. Environment

1. Safety hazards in the home and community may contribute to falls, burns, drownings, and to motor vehicle and other accidents.

☀ 2. **Passive smoking is a recognized serious health hazard for children and adolescents. Other pollution (*e.g.*, from radiation, chemicals, and water, air, or food contamination) poses significant health hazards as well.**

3. Miscellaneous hazards
   a. Children may identify with and mimic characters or criminals portrayed in the mass media (TV, videos, movies, magazine, newspapers), which may lead to violence and harm to self and others.
   b. Excessive TV viewing also has been linked to obesity and high blood cholesterol levels in children. (Researchers have not established how TV viewing affects overweight and cholesterol levels; they have established only the relationship.)

4. Nursing implications
   a. Nurses need to assess the effect of environmental factors on individual clients and families.
   b. Nurses can contribute to community health by becoming involved in education and policy making.

D. Growth and development
   1. Definitions
      a. Growth refers to an increase in body size (*i.e.*, height and weight).
      b. Development refers to a gradually increasing capacity to function at more advanced levels.
   2. Stages (approximate age ranges)
      a. Prenatal: from conception to birth
      b. Infancy: from birth to about 12 months (neonatal, birth to 28 days; infancy, 29 days to about 12 months)
      c. Early childhood: 1 to 6 years (toddlerhood, 1 to 3 years; preschool, 3 to 6 years)
      d. Middle childhood (schoolage): 6 to 12 years
      e. Later childhood: 11 to 18 (up to 21) years (prepubertal period, 11 to 13 years; adolescence, 13 to 18 [up to 21] years)
   3. Patterns (trends) of growth and development (definite and predictable)
      a. Directional patterns
         (1) **Cephalocaudal (head-to-tail) development occurs along the body's long axis.** Control over the head, mouth, and eye movements precedes control over the upper body, torso, and legs.
         (2) **Proximodistal (midline-to-peripheral) development progresses from the center of the body to the extremities.** The child develops arm movement before fine motor finger ability. Development is symmetric with each side developing in the same direction at the same time.
         (3) **Mass-to-specific (differentiation) development occurs as a child masters simple operations before complex ones.**
      b. Sequential patterns involve a predictable sequence of growth and development stages through which a child normally proceeds. Sequential patterns have been identified for motor skills, such as locomotion (*e.g.*, a child starts crawling before walking), and for behaviors, such as language and social skills (*e.g.*, first a child plays alone, then with others).

c. Secular patterns are universal trends in the rate and age of maturation. In general, children mature earlier and grow larger than their counterparts in preceding generations.

4. Theories of growth and development: in general, theorists consider that emotional, social, cognitive, and moral skills develop in stages. Table 1-1 lists the stages defined by well-known theorists. Chapters 2 through 6 explain each of the stages.

a. Psychosocial: Erikson's theory of psychosocial development is the most widely used. At each stage, children are confronted with a crisis that requires the integration of personal needs and skills with social and cultural expectations. Each stage has two possible components, favorable and unfavorable.

b. Psychosexual: Freud considered sexual instincts to be significant in the development of personality. At each stage, regions of the body assume prominent psychologic significance as sources of pleasure, and conflicts gradually shift through each stage.

c. Cognitive: Piaget proposed four major stages of development for logical thinking. Each stage comes from and builds on the previous stage in an orderly fashion.

d. Moral: Kohlberg's theory of moral development is based on cognitive development and consists of three major levels, each containing two stages.

TABLE 1-1.
Developmental Theories

STAGE	ERIKSON	FREUD	PIAGET	KOHLBERG
Infancy (birth to 1 year)	Trust vs mistrust	Oral	Sensorimotor (birth to 2 years)	
Toddlerhood (1 to 3 years)	Autonomy vs shame and doubt	Anal	Sensorimotor (1 to 2 years); preoperational or preconceptual (2 to 4 years)	Preconventional
Preschool (3 to 6 years)	Initiative vs guilt	Phallic	Preoperational or preconceptual (2 to 4 years); preoperational or intuitive (4 to 7 years)	Preconventional
Schoolage (6 to 12 yrs)	Industry vs inferiority	Latency	Concrete operations (7 to 11 yrs)	Conventional
Adolescence (12 to 19 yrs)	Identity vs role diffusion (confusion)	Genital	Formal operations (11 to 15 yrs)	Postconventional

5. Nursing implications

    a. **The nurse must understand that the maturation pattern varies with the individual child.**

    b. The nurse provides parents with the information needed to promote normal growth and development of children.

    c. The nurse provides health education for families within the constraints imposed by illness, disease, or disability.

    d. Developmental assessment involves consideration of physiologic, neuromotor, cognitive, and psychosocial parameters using a systematic approach to ensure coverage of all significant areas.

II. Influences on pediatric mortality and morbidity

    A. Leading causes of death in children by age

        1. Under 1 year: congenital anomalies

        2. Ages 1 to 24 years: injuries (Table 1-2)

        3. Unintentional injuries account for more death and disability in children than all combined causes of diseases.

    B. Leading causes of morbidity in children

        1. Acute conditions that contribute to morbidity in children are respiratory illness (50%), with the common cold being the most prevalent; injuries (15%); infections and parasitic diseases (11%).

            a. Factors contributing to morbidity involve low birth weight, poverty, homelessness, chronic illness, foreign-born adopted children, and day care.

TABLE 1-2.
Leading Causes of Death in Children by Age Group

RANK	UNDER 1 YEAR	1–4 YEARS	5–14 YEARS	14–24 YEARS
		AGE GROUP		
1	Congenital anomalies	Accidents	Accidents	Accidents
2	Sudden infant death syndrome (SIDS)	Congenital anomalies	Cancer	Homicide
3	Low birth weight and short gestation disorders	Cancer	Congenital anomalies	Suicide
4	Respiratory distress syndrome	Homicide	Homicide	Cancer
5	Maternal complications of pregnancy	Heart disease	Heart disease	Heart disease

(Adapted from National Center for Health Statistics: Advance report of final mortality statistics, 1991. Monthly Vital Statistics Report 42 (Suppl 21):21 DHHS Pub. no. PHS 93-1120. September 28, 1993.)

     ☀   b.   **Low socioeconomic status has the most overwhelming adverse influence on health.**

    2.   "Pediatric social illnesses" that adversely affect health include violence, aggression, noncompliance, school failures, and adjustment to divorce and bereavement.

III. Roles of pediatric nurses

  A. **Family advocate: The primary responsibility of the nurse is to the child and the family. The nurse assists in identifying their needs and goals and in developing appropriate nursing interventions.**

  B. **Health promoter: The nurse assists in maintaining health and preventing disease by fostering growth and development, proper nutrition, immunizations, and early identification of health problems.**

  C. **Health teacher: The nurse provides the family with information on topics such as anticipatory guidance, parenting, and disease processes.**

  D. **Counselor: The nurse supports the family through active listening and a therapeutic relationship that includes caring as well as carefully defined boundaries between the nurse and the child and family.**

  E. **Collaborator: As a key member of the interdependent healthcare team, the nurse collaborates with and coordinates nursing services with other healthcare services.**

  F. **Researcher: The nurse uses and contributes to research that enhances the nursing care of children and adolescents and their families.**

IV. Pediatric nursing health assessment

  A. **General considerations**

    1. For the child:

        a. Maintain eye contact (if culturally appropriate); bend to the child's level as needed.

        b. Use language appropriate for the child's cognitive level; involve the child in the assessment interview by asking appropriate questions.

        c. Keep in mind that a child is aware of caregiver's nonverbal communication and body language.

        d. Allow the child some warm-up time to become acquainted with the caregivers and the environment; introduce yourself and explain your purposes.

        e. Respect the child's responses and need for privacy as appropriate for age.

        f. Incorporate play into the assessment as appropriate.

    2. For the family:

        a. Develop a family-oriented approach that encourages parents to participate in the child's assessment.

    b.   Choose a quiet environment for the assessment and for any teaching sessions.

    c.   Ask open-ended questions to elicit responses other than "yes" or "no."

    d.   Focus on the information needed or problem to be solved.

    e.   Communicate the importance of parental roles with the healthcare team in planning and providing care for the child.

    f.   Listen attentively, respect responses, and provide appropriate feedback. Use silence judiciously.

    g.   Encourage parents to express concerns and ask questions.

B. Health history

1. Purpose: to collect subjective data about the child's health status and provide insights into actual or potential health problems

2. Interview techniques

    a.   Infants: Speak softly; allow the child to identify you with a parent; use touch.

    b.   Toddlers: Allow child to stay close to parent; acknowledge a favorite toy or a unique characteristic about the child.

    c.   Preschoolers: Use simple questions and simple words without double meanings; allow child to manipulate equipment; use toys, puppets, and play.

    d.   Schoolagers: Offer explanations; teach about health; provide demonstrations.

    e.   Adolescents: **Maintain confidentiality.** Also, facilitate trust; ask to speak to adolescent alone; encourage open and honest communication; be nonjudgmental; use open-ended questions.

3. Components of the history

    a.   Biographic data

    b.   Chief complaint

    c.   Current health or illness status

    d.   Past health status

    e.   Review of systems

    f.   Family health history

    g.   Nutritional history

    h.   Sleep history

    i.   Psychosocial data

4. Biographic data: name, address, telephone number, parents' or guardians' names, date and place of birth, gender, race, religion, and nationality or cultural background

5. Chief complaint: the client's reason for seeking health care or the parent's (informant's) reason for seeking health care for the child

6. Current health or illness status: the sequence of events leading up to the chief complaint and related information, including:

       a. Symptom analysis of chief compliant
       b. Other current or recurrent illnesses or problems
       c. Current medications
       d. Any other health concerns

7. Past health: information concerning past health status, previous problems, and health promotion activities, including:
   a. Birth history (pregnancy, labor and delivery, perinatal history)
   b. Previous illnesses, injuries, or surgeries
   c. Allergies (identify and describe manifestations)
   d. Immunization status
   e. Growth and developmental milestones
   f. Habits

8. Review of systems
   a. General: overall health status
   b. Integumentary: lesions, bruising, skin care habits
   c. Head: trauma, headaches
   d. Eyes: visual acuity, last eye examination, drainage, infections
   e. Ears: hearing acuity, last hearing examination, drainage, infections
   f. Nose: bleeding, congestion, discharge
   g. Mouth: lesions, soreness, tooth eruption, patterns of dental care, last dental examination
   h. Throat: sore throat frequency, hoarseness, difficulty swallowing
   i. Neck: stiffness, tenderness
   j. Chest (respiratory): pain, cough, wheezing, shortness of breath, asthma, infections
   k. Breasts: thelarche, lesions, discharge, performance of breast self-examination (BSE)
   l. Cardiovascular: history of murmurs, exercise tolerance, dizziness, palpitations, congenital defects
   m. Gastrointestinal: appetite, bowel habits, food intolerances, nausea, vomiting, pain, history of parasites
   n. Genitourinary: urgency, frequency, discharge, urinary tract infections, sexually transmitted diseases, enuresis, sexual problems or dysfunctions (male); performance of testicular self-examination
   o. Gynecologic: menarche, menstrual history, sexual problems or dysfunctions
   p. Musculoskeletal: pain, swelling, fractures, mobility problems, scoliosis
   q. Neurologic: ataxia, tremors, unusual movements, seizures
   r. Lymphatic: pain, swelling or tenderness, enlargement of spleen or liver

      s.   Endocrine or metabolic: growth patterns, polyuria, poly-dypsia, polyphagia

      t.   Psychiatric history: any psychiatric, developmental, substance abuse, or eating disorders

9. Family history: identification of any family genetic traits or diseases with familial tendencies, communicable diseases, psychiatric disorders, substance abuse

10. Nutritional history

    a.   Quantity and kind of food or formula ingested daily (use 24-hour recall; food diary for 3 days: 2 weekdays and 1 weekend day; or food-frequency record)

    b.   Problems with feeding

    c.   Use of vitamin supplements

    d.   Description of any special diets

    e.   Cultural or religious food practices, preferences, or restrictions

    f.   Assessment of dieting behaviors including body image, types of diets, frequency of weighing, or use of self-induced vomiting, laxatives and diuretics

11. Sleep history

    a.   Time child goes to bed and awakens

    b.   Quality of sleep

    c.   Nap history

    d.   Sleep aids (blanket, toy)

12. Psychosocial history

    a.   Home and family: *structure,* including composition of family members, occupation and education of members, culture and religion; *function,* including communication patterns, family roles and relationships, financial status

    b.   School: grades, behavior, relationship with teachers and peers

    c.   Activities: types of play, number of hours of TV viewing daily, amount of nonschool-related reading, hobbies

    d.   Discipline: type and frequency at home

    e.   Sex: child's or adolescent's concerns, abuse history, sexual activity patterns, number of partners, use of condoms and contraceptives, AIDS awareness

    f.   Substance use: amount, frequency, and circumstances of use for tobacco, alcohol, prescribed or illicit drugs, steroids, and substances such as inhalants

    g.   Violence: domestic violence, self-abusive behaviors, suicidal ideation and attempts, violence perpetrated on others by child or adolescent client

C. **Developmental assessment**

1. **Purpose: to identify any problems or possible concerns and to confirm normal achievement of growth and developmental milestones in the following areas:**

    a. Gross motor skills
    b. Fine motor skills
    c. Language development
    d. Cognitive development
    e. Social and affective development
2. Observe the child's behavior before structured interaction for spontaneous activity; observe the child's responses to the environment.
3. Administer developmental tests as appropriate for age (*e.g.*, Denver Developmental Screening Test, Brazelton Neonatal Behavior Assessment Scale, Goodenough-Harris Draw-A-Person Test, temperament questionnaires).

D. Physical assessment
1. Purpose: to obtain objective data on body systems functioning and overall health status
2. General guidelines
    a. In most cases, physical assessment involves a head-to-toe examination that covers each body system.
    b. Complete less threatening and least intrusive procedures first to secure child's trust.
    c. Explain what you will be doing and what the child can expect to feel; allow the child to manipulate equipment before it is used.
3. Developmental approaches
    a. Infants: Allow infant to sit in parent's lap; encourage parents to hold infant; use distraction; enlist parent's assistance.
    b. Toddlers: Allow toddler to sit on parent's lap; enlist parent's aid; use play; praise cooperation.
    c. Preschoolers: Use storytelling and doll and puppet play; offer choices when possible.
    d. Schoolagers: Maintain privacy; provide gown; explain procedures and equipment; teach schoolage clients about their bodies.
    e. Adolescents: Provide privacy and confidentiality; provide option of having parent present or not; emphasize normality; include health teaching.
4. Vital signs assessment

    a. Blood pressure: Measure blood pressure annually in children 3 years and older. **Select appropriate cuff width, so that cuff covers three fourths of the upper arm.**
        (1) Normal systolic ranges:
            Systolic: 1 to 7 years = age in years + 90
            8 to 18 years = (2 × age in years) + 83
            Diastolic: 1 to 5 years = 56
            6 to 18 years = age in years + 52

b. Pulse rate: Radial pulses may be taken in children over age 2.
    (1) Normal resting and awake rates:
        Newborn: 100 to 180
        1 week to 3 months: 100 to 220
        3 months to 2 years: 80 to 150
        2 years to 10 years: 70 to 110
        10 years to adult: 55 to 90

c. Respiratory rate: Monitor infants by observing abdominal movements; monitor older children the same as adults.
    (1) Normal respiratory rate ranges:
        Birth to 6 months: 30 to 50
        6 months to 2 years: 20 to 30
        3 to 10 years: 20 to 28
        10 to 18 years: 12 to 20

d. Temperature: Use rectal, axillary, skin, tympanic thermometer in children under age 4; do not use oral thermometer until children are over age 4. Normal temperature ranges are the same as in adults.

5. Head-to-toe assessment

    a. Measurements: height and weight, and head circumference in infants

    b. General appearance: physical appearance, nutritional state, hygiene, behavior, interactions with parents and nurse, overall development and speech

    c. Skin: color, texture, turgor, temperature, lesions, scars, edema, tattoos

    d. Hair: distribution, characteristics

    e. Nails: texture, shape, color, condition

    f. Lymph nodes: swelling, mobility, temperature, tenderness

    g. Head: symmetry, condition of fontanels

    h. Eyes: visual acuity, external and internal (ophthalmoscopic) examinations

    i. Ears: hearing acuity, external and internal (otoscopic) examination

    j. Nose and sinuses: discharge, tenderness, turbinates (color, swelling)

    k. Mouth: tooth eruption, condition of gums, lips, teeth, palates, tonsils, tongue, and buccal mucosa

    l. Neck: suppleness

    m. Chest: shape, breasts (sexual development stage), discharge, lesions

    n. Lungs: breath sounds, adventitious sounds

    o. Heart: heart sounds, murmurs, rubs

    p. Abdomen: appearance of umbilicus, shape, bowel sounds, inguinal area for hernias, liver, spleen, kidneys, masses, tenderness

q. Genitalia
  (1) Female: sexual developmental stage (pubic hair), vulva, meatus, external genitalia examination
  (2) Male: sexual development stage (penis, scrotum, and pubic hair), penis, scrotum, testes, urinary meatus
r. Anus: external examination
s. Musculoskeletal: muscle size and strength, posture and body alignment, symmetry, range of motion, gait
t. Neurologic: cerebral function (language, memory, cognition), cranial nerve function, deep tendon and superficial reflexes, balance and coordination, sensory function, motor function, and infantile reflexes

Bibliography

Castiglia, P.T. & Harbin, R.B. (1993). *Child Health Care: Process and Practice*. Philadelphia: J.B. Lippincott.

Engel, J. (1993). *Pocket Guide to Pediatric Assessment*, 2nd ed. St. Louis: C.V. Mosby.

Jackson, D.B. & Saunders, R.B. (1993). *Child Health Nursing: A Comprehensive Approach to the Care of Children and Their Families*. Philadelphia: J.B. Lippincott.

Malloy, C. (1992). Children and poverty: America's future at risk. *Pediatric Nursing, 18,* 553.

Skale, N. (1992). *Manual of Pediatric Nursing Procedures*. Philadelphia: J.B. Lippincott.

Wong, D.L. (1993). *Whaley and Wong's Essentials of Pediatric Nursing*, 4th ed. St. Louis: C.V. Mosby.

Wong, D.L. (1995). *Whaley and Wong's Nursing Care of Infants and Children*, 5th ed. St. Louis: C.V. Mosby.

STUDY QUESTIONS

1. Which of the following has the most adverse effect on the health of children?
   a. Cultural background
   b. Religious influences
   c. Environmental influences
   d. Low socioeconomic status

2. Infants are able to lift their heads before their trunks. Which universal principle of development is this related to?
   a. Development proceeds in a cephalocaudal direction.
   b. Development proceeds in a proximodistal direction.
   c. Development proceeds from the simple to the complex.
   d. Development proceeds from the general to the specific.

3. What is the primary cause of death and disability in children over the age of 1 year?
   a. Cancer
   b. Injuries
   c. AIDS
   d. Anomalies

4. When assisting families in identifying their needs and goals, what role does the nurse perform?
   a. Health advocate
   b. Health promoter

   c. Health teacher
   d. Health counselor

5. The sequence of events that leads parents to seek health care for their child is called:
   a. Chief complaint
   b. Present illness (health)
   c. Past history
   d. Review of systems

6. When examining a 2-year-old, what should the nurse perform first?
   a. Chest auscultation
   b. Abdominal palpation
   c. Otoscopic examination
   d. Oral examination

7. Assessment of family structure includes all of the following, except:
   a. Composition of family and community environment
   b. Occupation and education of family members
   c. Cultural and religious background
   d. Intrafamily communication patterns

8. When interviewing a 4-year-old, the nurse should:
   a. Ask detailed questions
   b. Maintain confidentiality
   c. Disallow the use of equipment.
   d. Avoid words with double meaning.

For additional questions, see
Lippincott's Self-Study Series Software
Available at your bookstore

ANSWER KEY

1. *Correct response: d*
   Low socioeconomic status has the most overwhelmingly adverse influence on health.
   a, b, and c. All have adverse influences on health, especially environment; however, none of these has the most adverse influence on health.
   Comprehension/Health promotion/NA

2. *Correct response: a*
   Cephalocaudal development occurs along the body's long axis, in which control over the head precedes control over the upper body, torso, and legs.
   b. Proximodistal development progresses from the center of the body to the extremities.
   c. The child learns to perform simple tasks before complex ones.
   d. The child learns general before the specific.
   Knowledge/Health promotion/NA

3. *Correct response: b*
   Injuries cause more death and disability in this age group than all combined causes of disease.
   a. Cancer is a leading cause, but not the leading cause, of death in children over 1 year of age.
   c. AIDS is becoming a leading cause of death.
   d. Congenital anomalies are the leading cause of death in children under 1 year of age.
   Comprehension/Health promotion/NA

4. *Correct response: a*
   The advocate assists in identifying needs and goals.
   b. The promoter fosters health practices that facilitate positive growth and development.
   c. The teacher provides information.

   d. The counselor develops a therapeutic alliance.
   Application/Health promotion/Implementation

5. *Correct response: b*
   The sequence of the present illness (or present health) leads to the chief complaint.
   a. The chief complaint is the actual reason for seeking health care.
   c. The history is information regarding past health status.
   d. The review of systems leads to identifying specific problems in each of the body systems.
   Knowledge/Physiologic/Assessment

6. *Correct response: a*
   Chest auscultation is the least intrusive choice here, and the nurse should always proceed from the least to the most intrusive when examining a toddler.
   b. Abdominal palpation is somewhat intrusive and should be performed after chest auscultation.
   c and d. The otoscopic and oral examinations are very intrusive and should not be performed until the end of the examination.
   Application/Physiologic/Assessment

7. *Correct response: d*
   Evaluation of communication patterns among family members is part of the assessment of family function.
   a, b, and c. These are all components of family structure assessment.
   Application/Psychosocial/Assessment

8. *Correct response: d*
   Preschoolers are prelogical and understand only one meaning of a word, words with more than one meaning will create confusion and possible apprehension.

a. The prelogical thought patterns are too immature to allow for understanding of detailed questions.

b. Although important, this is more appropriate for older children and adolescents.

c. Equipment handling should be encouraged to alleviate fears that are common to the preschooler.

Application/Psychosocial/All

Infant Growth and Development (Age 1 Month to 1 Year)

I. Physical growth and development
A. Growth parameters
1. General characteristics
   a. The best indicator of good overall health in an infant is steadily increasing size, specifically height (length), weight, and chest and head circumference, with normal fontanel changes.
   b. Growth and development is monitored by plotting measurements on a standardized growth chart, specific for boys and girls, from birth to 3 years, and from 3 to 18 years.
2. Length
   a. From 0 to 6 months an infant grows 1 inch (2.5 cm) per month.

   b. Average 6-month-old infant is 25.5 inches (63.8 cm).
   c. Average 12-month-old child is 29 inches (72.5 cm).
   d. Birth length increases 50% by 12 months.

 3. Weight
   a. From 0 to 5 months child gains 1.5 lb (682 g) per month.
   b. Birth weight doubles by 5 months.
   c. Average 6-month weight is 16 lb (727 g).
   d. Birth weight triples by 12 months.
   e. Average 12-month weight is 21.5 lb (977 g).

 4. Head circumference (HC) or occipital frontal circumference (OFC) and chest circumference
   a. From 0 to 6 months HC increases 0.6 inches (1.32 cm) per month.
   b. Average HC by 6 months is 17 inches (37.4 cm).
   c. From 6 to 12 months HC increases 0.2 inches (0.44 cm) per month.
   d. Average HC by 12 months is 18 inches (45 cm).
   e. By 12 months, HC increases by one third and brain weight increases 2.5 times from birth measurement.
   f. Chest circumference is normally about 1 inch (2 cm) less than HC; it is measured at the level of the nipples.

 5. Fontanel changes
   a. Anterior: diamond-shaped; at birth measures about 2 inches (4 to 5 cm) at widest part; closes between 12 and 18 months.
   b. Posterior: triangular, at birth measures about 0.5 inch (0.5 to 1 cm) at widest part; closes by 2 months.

B. **Nutrition**
 1. Breast milk is the most desirable complete food source for the first 6 months.
 2. Commercially prepared iron-fortified formula is an acceptable alternative.
 3. Formula intake varies per infant but averages 4 oz six times per day at 1 month to 4.2 oz five times per day at 6 months when solid foods are introduced.

 4. **Solids are not recommended before 4 to 6 months largely because of the protrusion or sucking reflexes and the immaturity of the gastrointestinal tract and the immune system.**
 5. Breast milk or formula is the primary source of nutrition for 6 to 12 months, although solid foods should be added.
 6. **Infant rice cereal is usually the infant's initial solid food.** It is easy to digest, contains iron, and rarely causes an allergic reaction.
 7. Additional foods usually include other cereals, then fruits and vegetables, and finally meats.

8.   Finger foods are introduced at 8 or 9 months.

   9.   Weaning from breast or bottle to a cup should be gradual. The infant's desire to imitate (between 8 and 9 months) increases the success of weaning.

   10. **Honey should be discouraged because it may be a source of infant botulism.**

C.   Sleep patterns

   1.   Sleep patterns vary among infants.

   2.   During the first month, most infants sleep when not eating.

   3.   Between 3 and 4 months, most infants sleep between 9 and 11 hours at night.

   4.   By 12 months, most infants take morning and afternoon naps.

   5.   Bedtime rituals should begin in infancy to prepare the infant for sleep and prevent future sleep problems.

D.   Dental health

   1.   **Fluoride supplements are needed for exclusively breast-fed infants, those receiving ready-to-feed formula, and those infants age 2 weeks and older in areas where the local water is inadequately fluorinated.**

   2.   Primary tooth eruption usually begins by 6 months.

   3.   Teeth should be cleaned with a damp cloth.

   4.   Breast and bottle feeding should be discouraged during sleep to prevent dental caries that may result from prolonged contact with milk.

II.   Cognitive development

A.   Overview (Piaget)

   1.   In the *sensorimotor stage*, between birth and 18 months, intellect develops and the infant gains knowledge of the environment through the senses. Development progresses from reflexive activity to purposeful acts in five substages:

      a.   Substage 1 (birth to 1 month): *use of reflexes* characterized by innate and predictable survival reflexes (infantile reflexes such as sucking and grasp)

      b.   Substage 2 (1 to 4 months): *primary circular reactions* marked by stereotyped repetition and the infant's focus on his or her own body as the center of interest (discovers own body parts)

      c.   Substage 3 (4 to 8 months): *secondary circular reactions* characterized by acquired adaptation and a shifting of infant's attention to objects and the environment (searches for objects that have fallen)

      d.   Substage 4 (8 to 12 months): *coordination of secondary schemes* marked by intentionality and consolidation and coordination of schemes (actively searches for hidden object)

e. Substage 5 (12 to 18 months): *tertiary circular reactions* characterized by interest in novelty, creativity, and discovery of new means through active experimentation; stage completed when infant achieves a sense of *object permanence* (infant senses self as separate from others and retains mental image of an absent object or person)

2. An emerging sense of body image parallels sensorimotor development.

B. Language

1. Crying is the first means of communication.
2. Parents usually can differentiate cries.
3. **Cooing begins between 1 and 2 months.**
4. **Laughing, babbling, and consonant sounds begin between 3 and 4 months.**
5. Imitative sounds begin by 6 months.
7. Combined syllables (ma-ma) begin by 8 months.
8. Infant understands no-no by 9 months.
9. Infant says and understands "ma-ma" and "da-da" in correct context by 10 months.
10. Infant can say between 4 and 10 words in correct context by 12 months.

III. Psychosocial development

A. Overview (Erikson)

1. **Erikson terms the crisis faced by an infant (birth to 1 year) "trust versus mistrust." The sense of trust developed in the first year forms the foundation for all future psychosocial tasks.**

a. In this stage, developing a sense of trust in caregivers and the environment is a central focus for an infant. The significant other in this process is the "caregiving" person, and the quality of the caregiver-child relationship is a crucial factor in the infant's development of trust.

b. An infant who receives attentive care learns that life is predictable and that his or her needs will be met promptly; this fosters trust.

2. **An infant who experiences consistently delayed needs gratification will develop a sense of uncertainty, leading to mistrust of caregivers and the environment.**

B. Fears

1. Infants exhibit a reflexive startle (Moro) response to loud noises, falling, and sudden movements in the environment.

2. **Stranger anxiety typically begins around age 6 months.**
3. A caregiver's cuddling and warmth can ease fears.
4. An infant commonly seeks comfort from a security object (a blanket or a favorite toy) during times of uncertainty or stress.

C. Socialization

1. Attachment to significant others begins at birth and is increasingly evident after 6 months.
2. Signs of socialization progress almost monthly:

   a. **Age 2 months: social smile**
   b. Age 3 months: recognizes familiar faces
   c. Age 4 months: enjoys social interactions
   d. Age 5 months: smiles at mirror image
   e. Age 6 months: begins to fear strangers

   f. **Age 8 months: consistently manifests "stranger anxiety"**
   g. Age 12 months: shows emotions such as jealousy and affection

D. Play and toys

1. **Play is the work of children.**
2. Play reflects the infant's development and awareness of the environment.

3. **From age 1 month to 1 year, play is basically solitary (non-interactive).**
4. The infant develops sensory and motor skills by manipulating toys and other objects. Toys serve several purposes. They:
   a. Stimulate psychological development
   b. Offer diversion from boredom, pain, and discomfort
   c. Provide a means of communicating and expressing feelings
   d. Aid in developing sensorimotor skills
5. Infant toys should be safe and age appropriate. Safety considerations include:
   a. No sharp parts or edges
   b. No small or detachable parts
6. Age-appropriate toys take into account an infant's short attention span with such features as bright colors to provide stimulation.

7. **Examples of safe, age-appropriate infant toys are:**
   a. Age 1 to 3 months: mobile, mirror, music box, stuffed animal without detachable parts, and a rattle
   b. Age 4 to 6 months: squeeze toys, busy boxes, play gym
   c. Age 7 to 9 months: various cloth-textured toys, splashing bath toys, large blocks, and large balls

           d.   Age 10 to 12 months: durable books with large pictures, large building blocks, nesting cups, and push-pull toys

  E. **Discipline**

    1. Spoiling an infant with too much attention is difficult; meeting the infant's needs always takes precedence over promoting discipline (training that molds behavior).

    2. An infant has no ability to accept delayed gratification; learning to wait develops progressively after infancy. Therefore, disciplinary actions for an infant often seem fruitless.

    3. Nevertheless, discipline and limit setting should begin in infancy; the earlier effective disciplinary measures are started, the easier they are to continue.

    4. Effective disciplinary measures may include negative voice, stern eye contact, and time-out.

    5. Corporal punishment is not recommended.

IV. **Motor development**

  A. **Gross motor**

    1. A newborn can turn its head from side to side from a prone position unless the surface is very soft, which may lead to suffocation.

    2. At about 3 months, infant exhibits almost no head lag.

    3. **At about 5 months, infant rolls from front to back.**

    4. At 7 months, infant sits leaning forward.

    5. At 8 months, infant sits unsupported.

    6. At 9 months, infant pulls up to stand.

    7. At 10 months, infant cruises.

    8. At about 12 months, infant walks holding someone's hand.

  B. **Fine motor**

    1. At about 1 month, infant has strong grasp.

    2. At about 3 months, infant's grasp reflex fades and he or she can actively hold a rattle.

    3. At 5 months, infant can grasp voluntarily.

    4. At about 7 months, infant can make a hand-to-hand transfer.

    5. **At about 9 months, infant develops a pincer grasp.**

    6. At about 12 months, infant attempts to build a two-block tower.

  C. **Related safety concerns**

    1. Accidental injuries are a major cause of death during infancy; they include:

        a. Falling off beds and down stairs

        b. Aspiration of small objects

        c. Poisoning from overdose of medication or ingestion of toxic household substances

        d. Suffocation caused by inadvertently covered nose and mouth, pressure on the throat or chest, prolonged lack of air (possibly in a closed, parked car), or strangulation (from crib rails or household cords)

  e. Burns from hot liquids, foods, scalding bath water, excessive sun exposure, or electrical injury

  f. Motor vehicle accidents, most commonly linked to improper use, or nonuse, of infant car seat

 2. Nursing interventions for accident prevention

  a. Instruct parents to maintain a safe environment by placing breakable or sharp objects, hazardous cords, and harmful substances out of infant's reach.

  b. Alert parents to age-specific potential injury sources and accident prevention strategies.

  c. Encourage parents to avoid repetitive negative expressions ("No-no, don't touch") for the sake of safety and to stress the positive aspects of the infant's behavior, such as playing with suitable toys.

V. Psychosexual development

A. Overview (Freud)

 1. **The oral stage of development extends from birth to 18 months.**

 2. The infant sucks for enjoyment as well as nourishment and also gains gratification by swallowing, chewing, and biting.

B. Manifestations

 1. In this stage, the infant meets the world orally by crying, tasting, eating, and early vocalizing.

 2. Biting is interpreted as a way to get a hold on the environment and gain a greater sense of control; grasping and touching are used to explore variations in the environment.

VI. Illness and hospitalization

A. Reactions to illness

 1. There are no general findings regarding the response of preverbal children to illness or fear of bodily injury.

 2. Young infants respond to pain with generalized body responses including loud crying and some facial gestures.

 3. Older infants respond with a general body response and deliberate withdrawal of the stimulated area, loud crying, facial gestures and anger, and physical resistance.

B. Reactions to hospitalization

 1. Infants under age 3 months tolerate short-term hospitalization well if provided with a nurturing person to meet physical needs consistently.

 2. Between 4 and 6 months the infant begins to recognize mother and father as separate from self (known as "stranger anxiety");

therefore, the infant at this age may also experience separation anxiety when hospitalized.

C.   Nursing interventions

    1.   General guidelines

        a.   Spend time with parents within sight of infant so you are seen as a safe person.

        b.   **Allow parents to give as much care as possible.**

        c.   Follow home schedule as possible.

        d.   Provide sensorimotor stimulation.

    2.   Provide physical comfort and safety.

        a.   Keep infant warm and dry.

        b.   Meet hunger needs consistently: Follow home schedule; encourage breast-feeding, if possible; use type and amount of formula used at home; let parents feed infant when possible and give guidance on feeding position as needed; schedule treatments not to interfere with feeding.

        c.   Move safely: Keep crib side rails up; provide safe crib toys, bumper pads, and play areas.

    3.   Cognitive interventions

        a.   Provide a variety of stimulating toys (mobiles, music boxes, busy boxes, rattles).

        b.   Promote language development (make sounds, talk to the infant).

        c.   Encourage learning through sensorimotor experience (allow repetition of acts, variety of toys and textures for manipulation).

    4.   Psychosocial and emotional interventions

        a.   Maintain relationship with parents (encourage parent to give care).

        b.   **Maintain good relationship with parents of children in all age groups, encouraging them to give care, hold child, play with child, and room in with child as appropriate.**

        c.   Maintain consistent staffing.

        d.   Promote sense of security (handle gently, cuddle, talk, respond to cues).

Bibliography

Castiglia, P.T. & Harbin, R.B. (1993). *Child Health Care: Process and Practice.* Philadelphia: J.B. Lippincott.

Dixon, S.D. & Stein, M.T. (1992). *Encounters with Children: Pediatric Behavior and Development,* 2nd ed. St. Louis: Mosby–Year Book.

Erikson, E.G. (1986). *Childhood and Society.* New York: W.W. Norton.

Jackson, D.B. & Saunders, R.B. (1993). *Child Health Nursing: A Comprehensive Approach to the Care of Children and Their Families.* Philadelphia: J.B. Lippincott.

Wadsworth, B.J. (1989). *Piaget's Theory of Cognitive and Affective Development,* 4th ed. New York: Longman.

Wong, D.L. (1993). *Whaley and Wong's Essentials of Pediatric Nursing,* 4th ed. St. Louis: C.V. Mosby.

Wong, D.L. (1995). *Whaley and Wong's Nursing Care of Infants and Children,* 5th ed. St. Louis: C.V. Mosby.

STUDY QUESTIONS

1. Which of the following is true of weight gain in a 5-month-old infant?
   a. Weight doubles birth weight
   b. Weight triples birth weight
   c. Weight quadruples birth weight
   d. Weight remains stable

2. While performing physical assessment of an infant 12 months old, the nurse notes that the infant's anterior fontanel is still slightly open. What should the nurse do?
   a. Call the physician immediately
   b. Perform an intensive neurologic examination
   c. Perform an intensive developmental examination
   d. Nothing; this is normal for the age

3. What is the earliest age at which solids should be introduced to the diet?
   a. 1 month
   b. 2 months
   c. 3 months
   d. 4 months

4. A nurse can expect to note which of the following forms of language to appear by age 4 months?
   a. Cooing sounds
   b. Babbling sounds
   c. Imimitated sounds
   d. Combined syllables

5. The infant who experiences consistently delayed needs gratification will most likely develop a sense of:
   a. mistrust
   b. shame
   c. guilt
   d. inferiority

6. Which of the following is the most age-appropriate toy for a 5-month-old infant?
   a. A big red balloon
   b. A teddy bear with button eyes
   c. A push-pull wooden truck
   d. A colorful busy box

7. The mother of a 2-month-old infant is concerned that she may be spoiling her baby by picking her up when she cries. The nurse's best response to this concern would be:
   a. "Let her cry for a while before picking her up, so you don't spoil her."
   b. "Babies need to be held and cuddled; you won't spoil her by meeting these needs."
   c. "Crying at this age means the baby is hungry; give her a bottle."
   d. "If you leave her alone she will learn how to cry herself to sleep."

8. The primary nursing intervention to promote tolerance of hospitalization in a 1-month-old infant is:
   a. provide consistent caregivers
   b. provide sensorimotor stimulation
   c. follow home schedule as possible
   d. keep infant warm and dry

ANSWER KEY

1. **Correct response: a**
   Body weight doubles by age 5 months.
   b. Body weight triples by 1 year.
   c. Body weight quadruples by 4 years.
   d. Infants rapidly gain weight.
   Knowledge/Physiologic/Assessment

2. **Correct response: d**
   The anterior fontanel closes anywhere between 12 and 18 months of age.
   a, b, and c. These are all inappropriate because the lack of closure at this age is normal.
   Application/Physiologic/Intervention

3. **Correct response: d**
   Solids are not recommended before age 4 to 6 months because of the sucking reflex and the immaturity of the gastrointestinal tract.
   a, b, and c. All of these ages are inappropriate for introducing solid food for the same reason: the infant's sucking reflex and immature gastrointestinal system.
   Comprehension/Physiologic/Planning

4. **Correct response: b**
   Laughing and babbling sounds are apparent by age 4 months.
   a. Cooing occurs by 1 to 2 months.
   c. Imitated sounds are produced by 6 months.
   d. Combined syllables are uttered by 8 months.
   Knowledge/Psychosocial/Assessment

5. **Correct response: a**
   According to Erikson, infants need to have their needs met consistently and effectively to develop a sense of trust; those who do not will develop a sense of mistrust.
   b. A sense of shame is developed in toddlers when their autonomy needs are not met consistently.
   c. A sense of guilt is developed in preschoolers when their sense of initiative is thwarted.

   d. A sense of inferiority is developed in schoolagers when they do not develop a sense of industry.
   Comprehension/Psychosocial/Assessment

6. **Correct response: d**
   A busy box facilitates the fine motor development that occurs between 4 and 6 months.
   a. Balloons may be aspirated and are therefore unsafe for small children.
   b. Button eyes may detach and be aspirated, making this toy teddy bear unsafe for children younger than 3 years.
   c. A 5-month-old infant is too young to use a push-pull toy.
   Application/Health Promotion/Implementation

7. **Correct response: b**
   Infants need to have their security needs met; they are unable to make the connection between crying and attention until late infancy or early toddlerhood.
   a. Rationale is the same as for answer b.
   c. Infants cry for many reasons. Assuming that the child is always hungry will cause overfeeding problems.
   d. Rationale is the same as for answer b.
   Analysis/Psychosocial/Implementation

8. **Correct response: a**
   a. A consistent caregiver is the best way to meet the infant's security needs at this age.
   b. Provision of sensorimotor stimulation promotes cognitive growth, but it will not necessarily promote tolerance of the hospitalization.
   c. Following the home schedule and d, keeping the child warm and dry, will assist in maintaining security needs, but they are not the best ways to do so.
   Analysis/Health Promotion/Implementation

Toddler Growth and Development (Age 1 to 3 Years)

I. Physical growth and development

A. Growth parameters

1. General characteristics
   a. Size increases in steplike rather than linear patterns, reflecting the growth spurts and lags characteristic of toddlerhood.
   b. A toddler's characteristic protruding abdomen results from underdeveloped abdominal muscles.
   c. Bowleggedness typically persists through toddlerhood because the leg muscles must bear the weight of the relatively large trunk.

2. Height
   a. Average toddler grows about 3 inches (7.5 cm) per year.
   b. Average 2-year-old is about 34 inches (86.6 cm) tall.
   c. Height at 2 years is about half of expected adult height.

3. Weight
   a. Average toddler gains from 4 to 6 lb (1.8 to 2.7 kg) per year. Average 2-year-old weighs 27 lb (12.3 kg).
   b. Birth weight quadruples by 2.5 years.
4. Head circumference
   a. Within 1 to 2 years, head circumference (HC) equals chest circumference.
   b. The total increase in HC in the second year is 1 inch (2.5 cm); then the rate of increase slows to 0.5 inch per year until 5 years.

B.   Nutrition
1. **Growth rate slows dramatically, thereby decreasing the need for calories, protein, and fluid.**
2. Calorie requirement is 102 kcal/kg/d.
3. Protein requirement is 1.2 g/kg/d.
4. By 12 months, most toddlers are eating the same foods as the rest of the family.
5. At 18 months many toddlers experience physiologic anorexia and become picky eaters, experiencing food jags and eating large amounts one day and very little the next.
6. Toddlers are at risk for aspirating small food items such as peanuts.
7. Toddlers prefer to feed themselves and prefer small portions of appetizing foods. Frequent nutritious snacks can replace a meal.
8. Food should not be used as a reward or a punishment.
9. Milk should be limited to no more than 1 qt (about 1 L) daily to help ensure intake of iron-enriched foods. Hematocrit should be used to screen for anemia.

C.   Sleep patterns
1. Total sleep requirements decrease during the second year, averaging about 12 hours daily.
2. Most toddlers nap once a day until the end of the second or third year.
3. Sleep problems are common and may result from fears of separation.
4. **Bedtime rituals and transitional objects representing security, such as a blanket or stuffed toy, are helpful.**

D.   Dental health
1. Primary dentition (20 deciduous teeth) is completed by 2.5 years.
2. The first dental visit should be nontraumatic and should occur before the toddler is 2.5 years old.
3. Teeth should be cleaned with a soft toothbrush and water, then flossed. Toothpaste is not used as toddlers dislike its foaminess and, if fluoridated, it is dangerous if swallowed.

4. Fluoride supplementation is needed if the water is not fluoridated and the diet should be low in cariogenic foods, such as table sugar, which promote dental caries.

II. Cognitive development
A. Overview (Piaget)
   1. During toddlerhood, *the sensorimotor phase* (between ages 12 and 24 months) involves two substages:
      a. *Tertiary circular reactions* (age 12 to 18 months), involving trial-and-error experimentation and relentless exploration
      b. *Mental combinations* (age 18 to 24 months), during which the toddler begins to devise new means for accomplishing tasks through mental combinations
   2. In the *preconceptual substage of the preoperational phase,* which extends between age 2 and age 4, the child uses representational thought to recall the past, represent the present, and anticipate the future. During this phase, the child:
      a. Forms concepts that are not as complete or as logical as an adult's
      b. Makes simple classifications
      c. Associates one event with a simultaneous event (transductive reasoning)
      d. Exhibits egocentric thinking

B. Language
   1. At 15 months, the toddler uses expressive jargon.
   2. **At 2 years, the toddler says about 300 words, uses 2- to 3-word phrases, and also uses pronouns.**
   3. At 2.5 years, toddler gives first and last name and uses plurals.

III. Psychosocial development
A. Overview (Erikson)
   1. **Erikson terms the psychosocial crisis facing a child between ages 1 and 3 "autonomy versus shame and doubt."**
   2. The psychosocial theme is "to hold on; to let go."
   3. The toddler has developed a sense of trust and is ready to give up dependence to assert his or her budding sense of control, independence, and autonomy.
   4. The toddler begins to master social skills:
      a. Individuation (differentiation of self from others)
      b. Separation from parent(s)
      c. Control over bodily functions
      d. Communication with words
      e. Socially acceptable behavior
      f. Egocentric interactions with others
      (Note: Some of the interactive skills that the toddler is starting to develop may not be mastered until adolescence

when the child revisits uncomplicated tasks associated with early periods of development. Erikson refers to this as the "psychosocial moratorium.")

5. The toddler has learned that his or her parents are predictable and reliable; now the toddler begins to learn that his or her own behavior has a predictable, reliable effect on others.
6. The toddler learns to wait longer to gratify needs.
7. The toddler often uses "no," even when he or she means yes, to assert independence (negativistic behavior).
8. A sense of shame and doubt can develop if the toddler is kept dependent in areas where he or she is capable of using newly acquired skills or if he or she is made to feel inadequate when attempting new skills.
9. A toddler often continues to seek a familiar security object, such as a blanket, during times of uncertainty and stress.

B. Fears

1. Common fears of toddlers include:
    a. **Loss of parents (known as separation anxiety)**
    b. Stranger anxiety
    c. Loud noises (*e.g.*, vacuum cleaner)
    d. Going to sleep
    e. Large animals
2. Emotional support, comfort, and simple explanations may allay a toddler's fears.

C. Socialization

1. The toddler's interactions are dominated by ritualism, negativism, and independence.
2. **Separation anxiety peaks as toddlers differentiate themselves from significant others. Transitional objects are important, especially during periods of separation, such as a nap.**
3. **Tantrums may be used to assert independence and are best dealt with by "extinction" (ignoring them).**
4. **Negativism is also common. The best way to decrease the number of "nos" is to decrease the number of questions that can lead to a "no" response.**

D. Play and toys

1. **Toddlers engage in parallel play; they play alongside, not with, others.**
2. Imitation is one of the most common forms of play.
3. Locomotion skills can be enhanced with push-pull toys.
4. Toddlers' short attention span causes them to change toys frequently.

5. **Appropriate toys for toddlers should be safe (still no detachable or small parts) and should encourage imitation,
language development, and gross and fine motor skills, for
example:**
   a. Dolls, housekeeping toys
   b. Play phones, cloth books
   c. Appropriate rocking horses and ridable trucks, finger
      paints, play clay, large-piece wooden or plastic puzzles,
      large blocks

  E. **Discipline**
   1. Unrestricted freedom is a threat to a toddler's security despite
      limit testing.
   2. Discipline measures should be:
      a. Consistent
      b. Initiated after misbehavior
      c. Planned in advance
      d. Oriented to behavior, not the child
      e. Private and not shame-inducing
   3. Time-outs are effective measures and should be carried out in a
      safe, unstimulating area. Duration should be 1 minute per year
      of age, and an audible timer can be used.

IV. **Motor development**
  A. **Gross motor**
   1. Major gross motor skill: locomotion
   2. **At 15 months: walks without help**
   3. At 18 months: walks upstairs with one hand held
   4. At 24 months: walks up and down stairs one step at a time
   5. At 30 months: jumps with both feet

  B. **Fine motor**
   1. At 5 months: builds a 2-block tower and scribbles sponta-
      neously
   2. At 18 months: builds 3- to 4-block tower
   3. At 24 months: imitates vertical stroke
   4. At 30 months: builds 8-block tower, copies a cross

  C. **Related safety concerns**
   1. Toddlers are prone to the same injuries as infants, including:
      a. Falls
      b. Aspiration
      c. Poisoning
      d. Suffocation
      e. Burns
      f. Motor vehicle and other accidental injuries

2. Nursing interventions for accident prevention include:

    a. Falls: Instruct parents to keep crib rails up, place gates across stairways, secure screens on all open windows, and supervise the toddler at play.

    b. Aspiration and poisoning: Urge parents to place all toxic substances locked away from child's reach (child can now climb and open); secure safety caps on medications; and remove all small, easily aspirated objects from the child's environment. Urge parents to keep the phone number of the poison control center by the telephone at all times.

    c. Suffocation: Encourage the parents to teach the toddler water safety to help prevent accidental drowning in bathtubs and pools; instruct them to avoid storing plastic bags and balloons within the toddler's reach.

    d. Burns: Advise parents to avoid using tablecloths (a curious toddler may pull the cloth to see what is on the table, possibly spilling hot foods or liquids on himself or herself); to teach the toddler what "hot" means; to store matches and lighters in locked cabinets out of reach; and to secure safety plugs in all unused electrical outlets.

    e. Motor vehicle and other accidents: Instruct parents to continue properly using an appropriate-sized car seat at all times. Also advise parents to lock cabinets and drawers that contain hazardous items, such as knives, firearms, and ammunition. Encourage parents to teach the toddler how to cross a street safely, but not to play in it. Urge parents to supervise tricycle riding and outdoor play.

V. Psychosexual development

A. Overview (Freud)

1. In the *anal stage,* extending from age 8 months to 4 years, the erogenous zone consists of the anus and buttocks, and sexual activity centers on the expulsion and retention of body waste.

2. In this stage, the child's focus shifts from the oral to the anal area, with emphasis on bowel control as he or she gains neuromuscular control over the anal sphincter.

3. The toddler experiences both satisfaction and frustration as he or she gains control over withholding and expelling, containing and releasing.

4. The conflict between "holding on" and "letting go" gradually resolves as bowel training progresses; resolution occurs once control is firmly established.

B. Developing sexuality

1. Masturbation can result from body exploration.

2. Learned words may be associated with anatomy and elimination.

3. Sex differences become evident.

    C.   **Toilet training**
1. Toilet training is a major task of toddlerhood.
2. Training readiness is unusual before 18 (up to 24) months. Signs of the toddler's readiness include:
   a. Stays dry for 2 hours, regular bowel movements
   b. Can sit, walk, and squat
   c. Can verbalize the desire to void or defecate
   d. Exhibits willingness to please parents
   e. Wants to have soiled diapers changed immediately (Note: Toilet training should not be initiated during times of stress such as a new baby, a move, a divorce, or a vacation.)
3. Bowel training is accomplished before bladder; complete night bladder training usually does not occur until age 4 or 5.
4. The training "potty" should offer security; the toddler's feet should reach the floor (needed for defecation).

VI. Moral development
    A.   **Overview (Kohlberg)**
1. A toddler is typically at the first substage of the preconventional stage, which involves punishment and obedience orientation. The toddler bases judgments on avoiding punishment or obtaining a reward.
2. Discipline patterns affect a toddler's moral development:
   a. Physical punishment and withholding privileges tend to give the toddler a negative view of morals.
   b. Withholding love and affection as a form of punishment leads to feelings of guilt in the toddler.

    B.   **Appropriate discipline measures include providing simple explanations why certain behaviors are unacceptable, praising appropriate behavior, and using distraction to avoid unacceptable behaviors.**

VII. Hospitalization
    A.   **Overview: The concept of body image, especially body boundaries, is poorly defined in toddlers. Therefore intrusive procedures are extremely anxiety producing. Toddlers react to pain in much the way as infants do and they may be affected by previous experiences as well. They may also react with great upset even when pain is perceived. Most are affected by separation and view it as abandonment (18 months is the peak age for separation anxiety).**

    B.   **Reactions to hospitalization**
1. In response to stressful events, such as hospitalization, the toddler's primary defense mechanism is regression.
2. The toddler may also sense a loss of control related to physical

restriction, a loss of routine and rituals, dependency, and fear of bodily injury or pain.

3. **Hospitalization may promote separation anxiety, which has three distinct phases:**
   a. **Protest: normal response to hospitalization, verbal cries for the parents, verbal or physical attack on others, attempts to find parents, clinging to parents, and inconsolableness**
   b. **Despair: disinterest in environment and play, passivity, depression, loss of appetite**
   c. **Detachment (denial): superficial adjustment in which the toddler exhibits apparent interest but in reality remains detached, usually occurs after prolonged separation, rarely seen in hospitalized children.**

C. Nursing interventions
   1. General guidelines
      a. Allow protest, and allow rooming in.
      b. **Encourage the use of transitional objects or parental objects (things child associates with parents) that can be left with child.**
      c. Instruct parents never to sneak out of room or away from hospital while the child is asleep.
      d. Be honest about the time of parents' return.
      e. Find out and use the words child uses (for transitional object, toileting, and so forth). Continue home routines as much as possible.
   2. Physical comfort and safety
      a. Explore toddler's already developed muscle skills (assess prehospital abilities) then give manipulable toys; provide supervised activities; use playroom.
      b. **After assessing child's level of function, prompte self-care (in all age groups), for example self-feeding, toileting as at home, dressing (with assistance as needed), and hygiene (washing face and hands, brushing teeth).**
   3. Cognitive interventions
      a. Promote sensorimotor learning through imitation.
      b. Enhance language skills (assess vocabulary, avoid speaking for child, reinforce mastered words; use activities that use language).
      c. Provide simple explanation for procedures (use equipment).
   4. Psychosocial and emotional interventions
      a. Promote toddler's sense of autonomy by encouraging self-

       care, participation in bedtime rituals, some control (give "OK" choices).

  b. Support toddler as he or she learns to separate from parents (assist family with coping with separation, encourage visiting, use primary nurse, encourage pictures of parents).

  c. Promote social adaptation (reinforce socially acceptable behaviors; encourage parallel play).

  d. Maintain usual routines and rituals (assess usual routines, especially bedtime; identify preferences; maintain as many of the home rituals as possible).

Bibliography

Castiglia, P.T. & Harbin, R.B. (1993). *Child Health Care: Process and Practice.* Philadelphia: J.B. Lippincott.

Dixon, S.D. & Stein, M.T. (1992). *Encounters with Children: Pediatric Behavior and Development,* 2nd ed. St. Louis: Mosby–Year Book.

Engel, J. (1993). *Pocket Guide to Pediatric Assessment,* 2nd ed. St. Louis: C.V. Mosby.

Jackson, D.B. & Saunders, R.B. (1993). *Child Health Nursing: A Comprehensive Approach to the Care of Children and Their Families.* Philadelphia: J.B. Lippincott.

Kohlberg, L. (1984). *The Psychology of Moral Development.* New York: Harper & Row.

Marino, B.L. (1991). Studying infant and toddler play. *Journal of Pediatric Nursing, 6,* 16.

Wong, D.L. (1993). *Whaley and Wong's Essentials of Pediatric Nursing,* 4th ed. St. Louis: C.V. Mosby.

Wong, D.L. (1995). *Whaley and Wong's Nursing Care of Infants and Children,* 5th ed. St. Louis: C.V. Mosby.

STUDY QUESTIONS

1. The characteristic protruding abdomen seen in toddlers results from:
   a. increased food intake owing to age
   b. underdeveloped abdominal muscles
   c. bow-legged posture
   d. linear growth curve

2. If a toddler is kept dependent in areas where he or she is capable of using skills, the toddler will develop a sense of:
   a. mistrust
   b. shame
   c. guilt
   d. inferiority

3. Common fears in toddlerhood include all of the following except:
   a. mutilation
   b. strangers
   c. separation
   d. going to sleep

4. A 2-year-old's mother has just left the hospital to check on her other children. Which of the following would best help the 2-year-old who is now crying inconsolably?
   a. Taking a nap
   b. A peer play group
   c. A large cuddly dog
   d. A favorite blanket

5. Which of the following is an appropriate toy for an 18-month-old child?
   a. Multiple-piece puzzle
   b. Miniature cars
   c. Finger paints
   d. Comic book

6. A mother is concerned that her 1-year-old is not yet walking. The nurse's response is based on the knowledge that most children should be able to walk by what age?
   a. 12 months
   b. 15 months
   c. 18 months
   d. 24 months

7. When teaching about readiness for toilet training, which of the following signs should the nurse instruct mothers to watch for in the toddler?
   a. Demonstrates dryness for 4 hours
   b. Demonstrates ability to sit and walk
   c. Has a new sibling for stimulation
   d. Verbalizes desire to go to the bathroom

8. The mother of a 20-month-old boy asks the nurse why her son has temper tantrums. The nurse's best response would be:
   a. "It is the only way he can get attention from his mother."
   b. "He is probably spoiled and needs discipline."
   c. "He cannot express his feelings or frustrations verbally."
   d. "He is expressing his need for identity."

9. A 30-month-old girl always puts her teddy bear on the left side of her bed immediately after her mother reads a bedtime story. What is the purpose of this repeated behavior?
   a. To manipulate the adults in the child's environment
   b. To establish learning behaviors
   c. To provide a sense of security
   d. To establish a sense of identity

10. Which of the following most typifies a toddler's eating patterns?
    a. Food "jags"
    b. Preference to eat alone
    c. Consistent table manners
    d. Increased appetite

ANSWER KEY

1. *Correct response: b*

   Underdeveloped abdominal muscula-
   ture gives the toddler a protruding abdomen.

   b. Food intake decreases in toddlerhood.

   c. Toddlers are characteristically bow-
   legged.

   d. Toddler growth patterns are steplike, not linear.

   Comprehension/Health Promotion/
   Assessment

2. *Correct response: b*

   According to Erikson, toddlers experience a sense of shame when they are
   not allowed to develop appropriate independence and autonomy.

   a. Infants develop mistrust when their
   needs are not consistently gratified.

   c. Preschoolers develop guilt when
   their initiative needs are not met.

   d. Schoolagers develop a sense of inferiority when their industry needs are
   not met.

   Comprehension/Psychosocial/Planning

3. *Correct response: a*

   Mutilation is a common fear among
   preschoolers, not toddlers.

   b, c, and d. All are common fears of
   toddlers and all are related to the
   separation-individuation process.

   Knowledge/Psychosocial/Assessment

4. *Correct response: d*

   The mother's departure has triggered
   the protest stage of separation anxiety
   in this child. A favorite blanket or other
   transitional object (representation of
   parent) will ease separation fears.

   a. A nap may actually increase separation fears.

   b. A 2-year-old is too young to interact
   with peers, other than in parallel
   play.

   d. Toddlers are usually fearful of large
   dogs.

   Analysis/Psychosocial/Implementation

5. *Correct response: c*

   Young toddlers are still sensorimotor
   learners and they enjoy the experience
   of feeling different textures.

   a. Multiple-piece toys are too difficult
   to manipulate and may be hazardous
   if the pieces are small enough to be
   aspirated.

   b. Miniature cars have the potential to
   be aspirated.

   d. Comic books are on too high a level
   for toddlers. Although they may
   enjoy looking at some of the pictures, toddlers are more likely to rip
   a comic book apart.

   Analysis/Psychosocial/Safe-Care/
   Implementation

6. *Correct response: b*

   Normal neuromuscular development
   should allow most children to walk by
   age 15 months.

   a. Many children walk by age 1 year,
   but a child is not considered abnormal if he or she is not walking by
   this age.

   c and d. Most children walk by age 15
   months.

   Comprehension/Physiologic/Assessment

7. *Correct response: d*

   The child must be able to state the
   need to go to the bathroom to initiate
   toilet training.

   a. Child needs to be dry for only 2
   hours.

   b. Child must also be able to squat.

   c. A new sibling would probably hin-
   der toilet training.

   Analysis/Physiologic/Planning

8. *Correct response: c*

   Temper tantrums decrease when a child
   learns words to express himself or herself.

   a. Toddlers use many methods to get
   their parents' attention.

   b. It is inappropriate to tell a parent
   that the child is spoiled.

    d. Identity is not an issue for toddlers; separation and individuation is.
Application/Psychosocial/Implementation

9. *Correct response: c*
   Rituals provide a sense of security for toddlers so that they may achieve autonomy.
   a. Toddlers' cognitive development is not at a level that would allow them to manipulate the environment.
   b. There is no evidence that rituals support learning.
   d. Identity is not an issue for toddlers.
Application/Psychosocial/Evaluation

10. *Correct response: a*
    Toddlers' food jags express a preference for the ritualism of eating one type of food for several days at a time.
    b. Toddlers typically enjoy socialization and imitating others at meal time.
    c. Toddlers are too young to have table manners.
    d. Toddlers' appetites usually decrease owing to the decrease in growth rate.
Comprehension/Psychosocial/Planning

Preschool Growth
and Development
(Age 3 to 6 Years)

I. Physical growth and development
A. Growth parameters
   1. General characteristics
      a. A healthy preschooler is slender, graceful, and agile, and has good posture.
      b. Major development occurs in fine motor coordination as demonstrated by an improved ability to draw.
      c. Gross motor skills also improve; the preschooler can hop, skip, and run more smoothly. Athletic abilities such as skating and swimming can be developed.
   2. Height
      a. Growth averages 2.5 to 3 inches (6.25 to 7.5 cm) per year.
      b. Average 4-year-old is 40.5 inches (101.25 cm) tall.

    3. Weight
        a. Weight gain averages 5 lb (2.3 kg) per year.
        b. Average 4-year-old weighs 37 lb (16.8 kg).

B. Nutrition
    1. Requirements are similar to those of the toddler although the calorie requirement decreases to 90 Kcal/kg/d.
    2. Protein requirement remains 1.2 g/kg/d.
    3. Fluid requirement is 100 mL/kg/d, depending on the activity level of the child.
    4. The 4-year-old is a picky eater.
    5. Most 3- and 4-year-olds may still be restless or fussy during meals with the family.
    6. The 5-year-old is influenced by food habits of others. A 5-year-old tends to focus on the "social" aspects of eating, including table conversation, manners, willingness to try new foods, and help with meal preparation and clean up.

C. Sleep patterns
    1. The average preschooler sleeps 11 to 13 hours per day.
    2. Most preschoolers need an afternoon nap until age 5 when most begin kindergarten.
    3. Bedtime rituals persist.

    4. Sleep problems are common and include nightmares, night terrors, difficulty settling down after a busy day, extending bedtime rituals to delay sleep.
    5. Continuing reassuring bedtime rituals with relaxation time before bedtime should help child settle down.
    6. The daytime nap may be eliminated if it seems to interfere with nighttime sleep.
    7. For many preschoolers, a security object and a night-light continue to provide help with sleep.

D. Dental health
    1. All 20 deciduous teeth should be in by age 3.
    2. The preschooler's fine motor development enables him or her to use a toothbrush properly; the child should brush twice a day.
    3. Parents should supervise the child's brushing and perform flossing.
    4. The child should avoid cariogenic foods to help prevent dental caries.

II. Cognitive development
    A. Overview (Piaget)
    1. The stage of cognitive development known as preoperational thought (ages 2 to 7 years) has two phases: preconceptual and intuitive.

a. Preconceptual phase (ages 2 to 4):
  (1) Forms concepts that are not as complete or as logical as an adult's
  (2) Makes simple classifications
  (3) Associates one event with a simultaneous one (transductive reasoning)
  (4) Exhibits egocentric thinking
b. Intuitive phase (ages 4 to 7)
  (1) Becomes capable of classifying, quantifying, and relating objects but remains unaware of the principles behind these operations
  (2) Exhibits intuitive thought processes (aware that something is right but cannot say why)
  (3) Unable to see viewpoint of others
  (4) Uses many words appropriately but lacks real knowledge of their meaning
2. Preschoolers exhibit *magical thinking* and believe that their thoughts are all powerful. They may feel guilty and responsible for "bad" thoughts, which sometimes may coincide with a wished-for event (*e.g.*, wishing a sibling were dead and the sibling coincidentally becomes ill and is hospitalized).

B. Language
1. The average 3-year-old says 900 words, speaks three- to four-word sentences, and talks incessantly.
2. The average 4-year-old says 1500 words, tells exaggerated stories, sings simple songs.
3. **Age 4 is the peak age for "why" questions.**
4. The average 5-year-old says 2100 words, knows four or more colors, and can name the days of the week and the months.

III. Psychosocial development
A. Overview (Erikson)
1. **Between ages 3 and 6, a child faces a psychosocial crisis that Erikson terms initiative versus guilt.**
2. The child's significant other is the family.
3. At this age, the child has normally mastered a sense of autonomy and moves on to master a sense of initiative.
4. A preschooler is an energetic, enthusiastic, and intrusive learner with an active imagination.
5. Conscience (an inner voice that warns and threatens) begins to develop.
6. The child explores the physical world with all of his or her senses and powers.
7. **Development of a sense of guilt occurs when the child is**

made to feel that his or her imagination and activities are unacceptable; guilt, anxiety, and fear result when the child's thoughts and activities clash with parental expectations.

8. A preschooler begins to use simple reasoning and can tolerate longer periods of delayed gratification.

B. **Fears**

1. **A child commonly experiences more fears during the preschool period than at any other time.**

2. Common fears of preschoolers include:
   a. The dark
   b. Being left alone, especially at bedtime
   c. Animals, particularly large dogs
   d. Ghosts
   e. **Body mutilation, pain, and objects and people associated with painful experiences**

3. The preschooler is prone to parent-induced fears stemming from his or her parent's remarks and actions; parents are typically unaware that their behavior or words instill fear in the child.

4. Allowing preschoolers to have a night-light and encouraging them to play out fears with dolls or other toys may help them develop a sense of control over the fear.

5. Exposing the child to a feared object in a controlled setting may provide an opportunity for desensitization and reduction of fear.

C. **Socialization**

1. In the preschool years, a child's radius of significant others expands beyond the parents to include grandparents, siblings, and preschool teachers.

2. The child needs regular interaction with age mates to help develop social skills.

3. Preschool programs
   a. The primary purpose of preschool is to foster the child's social skills.
   b. Criteria to consider when selecting a preschool program include:
      (1) Accreditation, licensing, and standards followed
      (2) Daily schedule of activities, materials available
      (3) Teacher's qualifications
      (4) Environment: safety, noise level, teacher-child ratio, and sanitary practices
      (5) Recommendations of other parents
      (6) Observations of the children at play and work, and their interactions with teachers
      (7) Alternative plans offered when child is ill and parents work

D. Play and toys

1. **Typical preschoolers' play is associative (*i.e.*, interactive and cooperative with sharing).**
2. Preschoolers need contact with age mates.
3. Activities should promote growth and motor skills, such as jumping, running, and climbing.
4. **This is the typical age for imaginary playmates.**
5. Imitative, imaginative, and dramatic play are important.
6. TV and video games should be only a part of the child's play and parents should monitor content and amount of time spent in use. Parents can encourage toys and games that promote gross and fine motor development, including:

   a. **Tricycle, big wheels, gym sets, wading pools, and sandboxes to enhance gross motor skills**
   b. **Large blocks, puzzles, crayons, paints, simple crafts, and age-appropriate electronic games to enhance fine motor skills**
   c. **Dress-up clothes and dolls, housekeeping toys, play tents, puppets, and doctor and nurse kits to enhance imitative play and imagination**
7. **Curious and active preschoolers need adult supervision, especially near water, gym sets, and other potential hazards.**

F. Discipline

1. Authority figures must apply discipline fairly, firmly, and consistently.
2. The child needs simple explanations of why certain behavior is inappropriate.
3. In a situation involving conflict, a short time-out can help the child relieve intense feeling, regain control, and think about his or her behavior.

IV. Motor development

A. Gross motor

1. At age 3 a preschooler can ride a tricycle, go upstairs using alternate feet, stand on one foot for a few seconds, and broad jump.
2. At age 4, the child can skip, hop on one foot, catch a ball, and go downstairs using alternate feet.
3. At age 5, the child can skip on alternate feet, throw and catch a ball, jump rope, and balance on alternate feet with eyes closed.

B. Fine motor

1. At age 3 the child can build a 9- or 10-block tower, construct a 3-block bridge, copy a circle, and draw a cross.
2. **At age 4 the child can lace shoes, copy a square, trace a diamond, and add three parts to a stick figure.**

3. At age 5 the child can tie shoe laces, use scissors well, copy a diamond and a triangle, add 7 to 9 parts to a stick figure, and print a few letters and numbers and his or her first name.

C. **Related safety concerns**

1. Although preschoolers are somewhat less accident prone than toddlers, they are still at risk for the same type of injuries (*e.g.*, falls, aspiration, burns) and require many of the same type of safety precautions.

2. Parents and other caretakers should emphasize safety measures; preschoolers listen to adults and can understand and heed precautions.

3. Because preschoolers are keen observers and imitate adults, parents and other caretakers need to "practice what they preach" regarding safety.

4. When a child weighs 40 lb and is 40 inches tall, the child can use a safety belt instead of a car seat.

V. **Psychosexual development**

A. **Overview (Freud)**

1. According to Freud, the phallic stage, extends from about age 3 to age 7. During this time the child's pleasure centers on the genitalia and masturbation.

2. During the phallic stage, the child experiences what Freud termed the *Oedipal* conflict, marked by jealousy and rivalry toward the same-sex parent and love of the opposite-sex parent.

3. The Oedipal stage typically resolves in the late preschool period with a strong identification with the same-sex parent.

B. **Sexual development**

1. Many preschoolers masturbate for physiologic pleasure.

2. Preschoolers form strong attachments to parents of the opposite sex but identify with the parent of the same sex.

3. As sexual identity develops, modesty may become a concern as well as castration fears.

4. Because preschoolers are keen observers but poor interpreters, they may recognize but not understand sexual activity.

5. Before answering a child's questions about sex, clarify:
   a. What the child is really asking
   b. What the child already thinks about the specific subject

6. Answer questions about sex simply and honestly, providing only the information that the child requests; additional details can come later.

VI. **Moral development**

A. Overview (Kohlberg): A preschooler is in the *preconventional stage* of moral development, which extends to age 10. In this phase, conscience emerges, and the emphasis is on external control.

B. **Standards:** The child's moral standards are those of others, and he or she observes them either to avoid punishment or to reap rewards.

VII. Illness and hospitalization

A. **Overview:** Preschoolers differentiate poorly between self and the external world. They have a limited understanding of language and can see only one aspect of an object or situation at a time.

B. **Reactions to illness**

1. Preschoolers perceive unrelated concrete phenomena as causes of illness.

2. Magical thinking causes a preschooler to think of illness as a punishment. Moreover, the preschooler experiences psychosexual conflicts and fear of mutilation.

C. **Reactions to hospitalization**

1. The primary defense mechanism of preschoolers is regression. They will react to separation by regression and refusal to cooperate.

2. They sense a loss of control because they experience a loss of their own power.

3. Fear of bodily injury and pain lead to fear of mutilation and intrusive procedures.

4. Their limited knowledge of the body enhances typical preschooler fears; for example, castration fears (evoked by enemas, rectal thermometers, catheters), fear that damage to skin (*e.g.*, from intravenous [IV] line, blood work procedures) will cause the insides of their body to leak out.

5. They interpret hospitalization as punishment and parental separation as loss of love.

D. **Nursing interventions**

1. General guidelines

   a. **Use puppets and dolls to demonstrate procedures.**
   b. Use terms that are appropriate for the child's age and level of understanding (*e.g.*, say "fix" rather than "cut out").

   c. **Use adhesive bandages after giving injections.**
   d. Stay with child during procedures.

   e. **Avoid performing invasive procedures, if possible.**
   f. Give stars, badges, and other rewards.
   g. Play out the hospital experience (improvise doctor and nurse kits).

   h. **Reassure the preschooler that he or she is not responsible for illness.**
   i. Assess for secondary gains.

2. Physical comfort and safety
   a. Allow child to maintain control over body functions (allow normal patterns; reassure when accidents occur; praise success; provide motor stimulation).
   b. Promote self-care and allow child to wear his or her own clothes.
3. Cognitive interventions
   a. Protect from guilt (no one to blame, explain procedures).
   b. Protect from fears (therapeutic play; do not talk over the child's head).
   c. Promote language (encourage questions; allow child to tell stories, teach new words).
4. Psychosocial and emotional interventions
   a. Encourage independence (permit self-care, allow some decisions, praise competence; respect suggestions).
   b. Allow child to experience limits to feel secure (safety rules, define limits due to illness, follow home rules whenever possible).
   c. Allow rituals.
   d. Allow for separation without conflict (use primary nurse, encourage visiting, have parents do as much care as possible, encourage sibling and peer contact).
   e. Promote sexual identity (reassure child about genitalia, use child's hand to handle genitalia; avoid intrusive procedures).

Bibliography

Castiglia, P.T. & Harbin, R.B. (1993). *Child Health Care: Process and Practice*. Philadelphia: J.B. Lippincott.

Dixon, S.D. & Stein, M.T. (1992). *Encounters with Children: Pediatric Behavior and Development*, 2nd ed. St. Louis: Mosby–Year Book.

Engel, J. (1993). *Pocket Guide to Pediatric Assessment*, 2nd ed. St. Louis: C.V. Mosby.

Jackson, D.B. & Saunders, R.B. (1993). *Child Health Nursing: A Comprehensive Approach to the Care of Children and Their Families*. Philadelphia: J.B. Lippincott.

Piaget, J. (1966). *The Origins of Intelligence in Children*. New York: International Universities Press.

Robinson, P. (1993). *Freud and His Critics*. Berkeley: University of California Press.

Wong, D.L. (1993). *Whaley and Wong's Essentials of Pediatric Nursing*, 4th ed. St. Louis: C.V. Mosby.

Wong, D.L. (1995). *Whaley and Wong's Nursing Care of Infants and Children*, 5th ed. St. Louis: C.V. Mosby.

STUDY QUESTIONS

1. According to Piaget, a preconceptual preschool child should be able to:
   a. see another's point of view
   b. make simple classifications
   c. exhibit intuitive thought
   d. see relationships in reverse

2. A preschooler who is made to feel that his or her imagination and activities are unacceptable is likely to develop a sense of:
   a. mistrust
   b. shame
   c. guilt
   d. inferiority

3. A 4-year-old boy resists going to bed at night. Which of the following suggestions should the nurse offer the parents?
   a. "Allow him to fall asleep in your room, then move him to his own bed."
   b. "Tell him that you will lock his room if he gets out of bed one more time."
   c. "Encourage active play at bedtime to tire him out so he will fall asleep faster."
   d. "Read him a story and allow him to play quietly in his bed until he falls asleep."

4. Which of the following toys would best promote imaginative play in a 4-year-old?
   a. large blocks
   b. dress-up clothes
   c. wooden puzzle
   d. big wheels

5. Which of the following is an expected gross motor behavior in a 3-year-old?
   a. riding a tricycle
   b. hopping on one foot
   c. catching a ball
   d. skipping on alternate feet

6. Which of the following best describes preschool sexual identification?
   a. identification with same sex parent; attachment to opposite sex parent
   b. identification with opposite sex parent; attachment to same sex parent
   c. identification and attachment to same sex parent
   d. identification and attachment to opposite sex parent

7. Why do preschoolers view hospitalization as punishment?
   a. egocentrism
   b. past experience
   c. magical thinking
   d. Oedipal conflict

8. When can a child be safely restrained in a regular automobile seat belt?
   a. 35 lb or 3 years of age
   b. 30 lb or 30 inches tall
   c. 40 lb or 40 inches tall
   d. 60 lb or 6 years of age

9. A preschooler typically views parents as:
   a. a necessary evil
   b. persons who keep order
   c. omnipotent
   d. too rigid

10. The main reason for using adhesive bandages after giving injections to preschoolers is because:
    a. they use them to get attention from their parents
    b. they are afraid that they will leak from the "hole"
    c. bandages help to alleviate fear of strangers
    d. children collect bandages to show their peers

ANSWER KEY

1. **Correct response: b**
   The preconceptual child, age 2 to 4 years, is capable of making simple classifications.
   a. Seeing another's point of view occurs during concrete operations (ages 7 to 11 years).
   c. Intuitive thinking occurs during the intuitive phase, ages 4 to 7 years.
   d. Seeing relationships involving the reverse occurs in formal operations, ages 11 to 15 years.
   Comprehension/Psychosocial/NA

2. **Correct response: c**
   According to Erikson, preschoolers develop a sense of guilt when made to feel that their imagination and activities are wrong, thus disallowing the child to develop a sense of initiative.
   a. Mistrust develops when an infant's needs are consistently not met and the infant cannot develop a sense of trust.
   b. Shame develops when a toddler is not allowed to develop appropriate autonomy.
   d. Inferiority develops when a school-ager is not allowed to have a sense of industry.
   Comprehension/Psychosocial/NA

3. **Correct response: d**
   Quiet play and time with parents is a positive bedtime routine that provides security and readies the child for sleep.
   a. The child should sleep in his own bed.
   b. The child will see this as a threat; a locked door is frightening and potentially hazardous.
   c. Vigorous activity at bedtime stirs up the child and makes it more difficult to fall asleep.
   Comprehension/Psychosocial/Implementation

4. **Correct response: b**
   Dress-up clothes allow preschoolers to use their imaginations and engage in rich fantasy play.
   a. Building blocks encourage fine motor development.
   c. Wooden puzzles encourage fine motor development.
   d. Big wheels encourage gross motor development.
   Comprehension/Psychosocial/Implementation

5. **Correct response: a**
   A 3-year-old should have the gross motor ability to balance on and ride a tricycle.
   b. Hopping on one foot is accomplished by 4 years.
   c. Catching a ball is accomplished by 4 years.
   d. Skipping on alternate feet is accomplished by 5 years.
   Comprehension/Physiologic/Assessment

6. **Correct answer: a**
   Preschoolers identify with the parent of the same sex, but attach to the parent of the opposite sex (Oedipal conflict).
   b, c, and d. Alternate identifications and attachments are unusual in this age group.
   Knowledge/Psychosocial/Assessment

7. **Correct response: c**
   The fantasies of preschoolers can result in a sense of guilt; because they cannot discern cause and effect, they see hospitalization as punishment for some real or fantasized misdoing.
   a. Egocentrism accounts for the preschooler's inability to see another's point of view.
   b. Past experience can certainly affect the preschooler's reaction to hospitalization, but it is not the primary precipitant here.
   d. Oedipal conflicts do not directly affect hospitalization.
   Comprehension/Psychosocial/Planning

8. *Correct response: c*

   A child of this weight and height has sufficiently developed bone structure and muscle mass to use regular restraints.

   a. A child of this size is too small.

   b. A child of this size is too small.

   d. Use of a car seat can be discontinued much earlier than this.

   Application/Safe Care/Implementation

9. *Correct response: c*

   The preschooler typically believes that parents can do no wrong and enjoys their guidance.

   a. This is more typical of an adolescent.

   b. The preschooler has not yet developed this view of parents.

   d. Preschoolers are not bothered by rigidity; in fact, guidelines give them a sense of security.

   Analysis/Health Promotion/Evaluation

10. *Correct response: b*

    Preschoolers have poorly defined body boundary images; therefore they are afraid that their body parts will come out of the injection site.

    a. This may happen, but it is secondary.

    c. Fear of strangers is more apparent in toddlers.

    d. Schoolagers are more likely to collect things to show their peers.

    Analysis/Health Promotion/ Implementation

School-Age Growth and Development (Age 6 to 12 Years)

I. Physical growth and development
A. Growth parameters
   1. General characteristics
      a. During this period, girls usually grow faster than boys and commonly surpass them in height and weight.
      b. During preadolescence, extending from about age 10 to 13, a child commonly experiences rapid and uneven growth compared with age mates.
      c. The immune system becomes more efficient, allowing for more localization of infections and better antibody-antigen response. Therefore, school-age children develop immunity to a wide number of organisms. However, many develop several infections in the first and second year of

school because of increased exposure to other children with germs.

2. Height
   a. Average schoolager grows 2 inches (5 cm) per year.
   b. Average 6-year-old is 45 inches (112.5 cm) tall.
   c. Average 12-year-old is 59 inches (147.5 cm) tall.
3. Weight
   a. Average schoolager gains 4.5 to 6.5 lb (2 to 3 kg) per year.
   b. Average 6-year-old weighs 46 lb (21 kg).
   c. Average 12-year-old weighs 88 lb (40 kg).

B. Nutrition
1. A school-age child's daily caloric requirements diminish in relation to body size.
2. Caregivers should continue to stress the need for a balanced diet from the food pyramid; resources are being stored for the increased growth needs of adolescence.
3. The child is exposed to broader eating experiences in the school lunchroom; he or she may still be a "picky" eater but should be more willing to try new foods. Children may trade, sell, or throw away home-packed school lunches.
4. At home the child should eat what the family eats; the patterns that develop now stay with the child into adulthood.

C. Sleep patterns
1. Individual sleep requirements for schoolagers vary but typically range from 8 to 9.5 hours nightly. Because growth rate has slowed, schoolagers actually need less sleep now than they will during adolescence.
2. The child's bedtime can be later than during the preschool period but should be firmly established and adhered to on school nights.
3. Reading before bedtime may facilitate sleep and set up a positive bedtime pattern.
4. Children may be unaware of fatigue; if allowed to remain up, they will be tired the next day.

D. Dental health
1. Beginning around age 6, permanent teeth erupt and deciduous teeth are gradually lost.
2. Regular visits to the dentist are important, and fluoride supplements should be continued when the water supply is insufficiently fluoridated.
3. The child should brush teeth after meals with a soft nylon toothbrush; because of the child's better coordination, parental supervision and assistance usually are not necessary.
4. Flossing should be done by parents until the child reaches age 8 or 9.

5. Caries, malocclusion, and periodontal disease become evident in this age group.

II. Cognitive development

A. Overview (Piaget)

1. **Between ages 7 and 11, a child is in the stage of concrete operations, marked by inductive reasoning, logical operations, and reversible concrete thought.**

2. Specific characteristics of this stage include:
   a. Transition from egocentric to objective thinking (*i.e.*, seeing another's point of view, seeking validation, and asking questions)
   b. Focus on immediate physical reality with inability to transcend the here and now
   c. Difficulty dealing with remote, future, or hypothetical matters
   d. Development of various mental classifying and ordering activities
   e. Development of the principle of conservation (*i.e.*, of volume, weight, mass, and numbers)

3. Typical activities of a child at this stage may include:
   a. Collecting and sorting objects (*e.g.*, baseball cards, dolls, marbles)
   b. Ordering items according to size, shape, weight, and other criteria
   c. Considering options and variables when problem solving

B. Language

1. **Child has developed formal adult articulation patterns between ages 7 and 9.**

2. Child learns that words can be arranged in terms of structure.

3. The ability to read is one of the most significant skills learned.

III. Psychosocial development

A. Overview (Erikson)

1. **Erikson terms the psychosocial crisis faced by a child between ages 6 and 12 industry versus inferiority.**

2. During this period, the child's radius of significant others expands to include schoolmates and instructive adults.

3. A school-age child normally has mastered the first three developmental tasks, which are *trust, autonomy,* and *initiative,* and now focuses on mastering industry.

4. A child's sense of *industry* grows out of a desire for real achievement.

5. The school-age child engages in tasks and activities that he or she can carry through to completion.

6. The child learns rules, how to compete with others, and how to cooperate to achieve goals.
7. Social relationships with others become increasingly important sources of support.
☼ 8. **In the school-age group, the child can develop a sense of inferiority stemming from unrealistic expectations or a sense of failing to meet standards set for him or her by others. When the child feels inadequate, his or her self-esteem sags.**

B. Fears
1. During the school-age years, many fears of earlier childhood resolve or decrease.
2. Common fears may include:
   a. Failure at school
   b. Bullies
   c. Intimidating teachers
3. Parents and other caregivers can help reduce a child's fears by communicating empathy and concern without being overprotective.

C. Socialization
1. The school-age years are a period of dynamic change and maturation as the child becomes increasingly involved in more complex activities, decision making, and goal-directed activities.
2. As a school-age child learns more about his or her body, social development centers on the body and its capabilities.
☼ 3. **Peer relationships gain new importance.**
4. Group activities, including team sports, typically consume much time and energy.

D. Play and toys
1. Play becomes more competitive and complex during the school-age period.
2. Characteristic activities include team sports, secret clubs, "gang" activities, scouting or other organizations, complex puzzles, collections, quiet board games, reading, and hero worship.
3. Rules and rituals are important aspects of play and games.
☼ 4. **Toys, games, and activities that encourage growth and development include:**
   a. **Increasingly complex board and card games**
   b. **Books, crafts**
   c. **Music, art**
   d. **Athletic activities (*e.g.*, swimming)**
   e. **Team activities**
   f. **Video games**

E. **Discipline**
   1. School-age children begin to internalize their own controls and need less outside direction.
   2. School-age children, however, do need a parent or other caretaker to answer questions and provide guidance for decisions and responsibilities.
   3. Regular household responsibilities help schoolagers feel that they are an important part of their family and increase their sense of accomplishment.
   4. A weekly allowance, set in accordance with a schoolager's needs and duties, assists in teaching skills, values, and a sense of responsibility.
   5. When disciplining schoolagers, parents and other caretakers should set reasonable concrete limits (and provide plausible explanations) and keep rules to a minimum.
   6. Children should be included in problem solving as the best approach to limit setting.

IV. **Motor development**
   A. **Gross motor skills acquired during the school years include:**
      1. Bicycling
      2. Roller skating, rollerblading, skateboarding
      3. Progressively improved running and jumping
      4. Swimming
   B. **Fine motor skills include:**
      1. Printing in early years; script in later years (by age 8)
      2. Greater dexterity for crafts and video games
      3. Computer competence (manual skills)
   C. **Related safety concerns**
      1. School-age children learn to accept more responsibility for personal health care and injury prevention.
      2. School-age children who learn safe swimming and diving practices, fire safety, use of seat belts and bicycle helmets, and other safety practices are at reduced risk for injury.
      3. The children's developing cognitive skills complement their own judgment and assist in helping them avoid many types of injuries.
      4. School-age children are still prone to accidents, however, mainly owing to increasing motor abilities and independence (*e.g.*, a bicycle can take a child farther from home independently).
      5. Major sources of injuries include bicycles, skateboards, and team sports. Learning proper techniques, using safe equipment, and, in the case of organized sports, good coaching and well-matched teams (playing with children of similar size) can reduce the risk of injury.

6.   Parents should continue to provide guidance for new situations and threats to safety.

7.   School-age children should receive education about the use and abuse of alcohol, tobacco, and other drugs.

V.   Psychosexual development

A.   Overview (Freud)

☀ **1.   The latency period, extending from about age 5 to 12 years, represents a stage of relative sexual indifference before puberty and adolescence.**

2.   During this period, development of self-esteem is closely linked with a developing sense of industry to produce a concept of one's value and worth.

B.   Sexual development

1.   Preadolescence begins near the end of schoolage at which time discrepancies in growth and maturation between the genders becomes apparent.

2.   A school-age child has acquired much of his or her knowledge of, and many of his or her attitudes toward, sex at a very early age.

3.   During the school-age years, the child refines this knowledge and these attitudes.

4.   Questions about sex require honest answers based on the child's level of understanding.

VI.   Moral development

According to Kohlberg, children arrive at the conventional level of the *role conformity stage,* generally, between ages 10 and 13. They have an increased desire to please others. They also observe and to some extent externalize the standards of others and want to be considered "good" by those persons whose opinions matter to them.

VII.   Hospitalization

A.   Overview

1.   Stressors include immobilization, fear of mutilation and death, and modesty concerns.

2.   School-age children have difficulty with forced dependency.

3.   They may be unable to express themselves verbally and their self-consciousness may interfere with care.

B.   Reactions to illness

1.   School-age children perceive illness as being caused by external forces.

2.   They are aware of the significance of different illnesses.

C.   Reactions to hospitalization

1.   School-age children's primary defense mechanism is reaction formation.

2. Schoolagers may react to separation by demonstrating loneliness, boredom, isolation, and depression. They may also show aggression, irritability, and inability to relate to siblings and peers.
3. The sensed loss of control is related to enforced dependency and altered family roles.
4. Fear of bodily injury and pain results from fear of illness, disability, and death.

C. Nursing interventions
 1. General guidelines
     a. Encourage verbalization.
     b. Encourage self-care.
     c. **Encourage peer interactions.**
     d. **Inform schoolagers that it is "OK" to cry.**
     e. Give factual information; use models to demonstrate concepts or procedures.
     f. Provide diversions.
 2. Physical comfort and safety
     a. Allow schoolager control over body functions.
     b. Assist in developing fine motor skills (encourage construction toys, such as Lego sets; drawing; computer games; drawing body parts; "taking notes" during patient education).
     c. Allow schoolagers to participate in treatment.
 3. Cognitive interventions
     a. Assist in developing rational thinking (scientific explanations, rationales, rules) and provide for decision making.
     b. Assist child with mastering concepts of conservation, constancy and reversibility, classification and categorization (*e.g.*, allow child to chart intake and output and vital signs; tell nurse when procedures are due; create a scrapbook; use concepts, such as cards and board games, in teaching and games; and do school work.
     c. Provide time and encourage verbalization (talk time).
 4. Psychosocial/emotional interventions
     a. Provide the opportunity to channel drives (encourage peer interaction, group education, and limit setting; avoid coed rooms).
     b. Promote achievement of industry (praise cooperative play; assign tasks that can be accomplished; involve child in care).

Bibliography

Castiglia, P.T. & Harbin, R.B. (1993). *Child Health Care: Process and Practice*. Philadelphia: J.B. Lippincott.

60

Curry, D.M. & Duby, J.C. (l994). Developmental surveillance by pediatric nurses. *Pediatric Nursing, 20,* 40.

Dixon, S.D. and Stein, M.T. (1992). *Encounters with Children: Pediatric Behavior and Development,* 2nd ed. St. Louis: Mosby–Year Book.

Engel, J. (1993). *Pocket Guide to Pediatric Assessment,* 2nd ed. St. Louis: C.V. Mosby.

Jackson, D.B. & Saunders, R.B. (1993). *Child Health Nursing: A Comprehensive Approach to the Care of Children and Their Families.* Philadelphia: J.B. Lippincott.

Schuster, S. & Ashburn, A. (1992). *The Process of Human Development: A Holistic Life-Span Approach,* 3rd ed. Philadelphia: J.B. Lippincott.

Wong, D.L. (1993). *Whaley and Wong's Essentials of Pediatric Nursing,* 4th ed. St. Louis: C.V. Mosby.

Wong, D.L. (1995). *Whaley and Wong's Nursing Care of Infants and Children,* 5th ed. St. Louis: C.V. Mosby.

STUDY QUESTIONS

1. One of the reasons for maintaining a consistent bedtime schedule for schoolagers is:
   a. They require more sleep now than in adolescence.
   b. They are prone to nightmares and night terrors.
   c. They may be unaware of their own fatigue.
   d. They all need 10 hours of sleep per night.

2. All of the following are characteristics of school-age cognition, except:
   a. Collecting baseball cards and marbles
   b. Ordering dolls according to size
   c. Considering simple problem-solving options
   d. Developing plans for the future

3. When do the deciduous teeth usually begin to fall out?
   a. Age 5
   b. Age 6
   c. Age 7
   d. Age 8

4. Unrealistic expectations or a sense of failing to meet standards would cause a schoolager to develop a sense of:
   a. Shame
   b. Guilt
   c. Inferiority
   d. Role confusion

5. A hospitalized schoolager states: "I'm not afraid of this place, I'm not afraid of anything." This is most likely an example of:

   a. Regression
   b. Repression
   c. Reaction formation
   d. Rationalization

6. Which of the following best describes typical annual growth during the school-age period?
   a. The child grows an average of 2 inches (5 cm) per year.
   b. The child gains an average of 3 lb (1.4 kg) per year.
   c. Few differences are noted between age mates.
   d. Increased number of fat pads give them a chubby appearance.

7. Which of the following statements associated with a schoolager's eating patterns is true?
   a. The child should develop impeccable table manners.
   b. The child's preferences should reflect family culture.
   c. A rigid mealtime environment is recommended.
   d. High-energy activity requires high-energy snacks.

8. Which of the following statements about causes of accidents during the school years is inaccurate?
   a. Schoolagers are more active and adventurous.
   b. Schoolagers are more susceptible to home hazards.
   c. Schoolagers are unable to understand potential dangers.
   d. Schoolagers are less subject to parental control.

For additional questions, see
Lippincott's Self-Study Series Software
Available at your bookstore

ANSWER KEY

1. *Correct response: c*
   Schoolagers are often unaware of their own fatigue and, if allowed to remain up, they will be tired the next day.
   a. Schoolagers require less sleep than adolescents because their growth rate is slower.
   b. Preschoolers are prone to nightmares and night terrors.
   d. The typical range of sleep hours for this age is 8 to 9.5 hours.
   Comprehension/Health Promotion/ Implementation

2. *Correct response: d.*
   The ability to consider the future requires formal thought operations, which are not developed until adolescence.
   a, b, and c. All are examples of the concrete operational thinking of the schoolager.
   Comprehension/Health Promotion/ Assessment

3. *Correct response: b*
   The deciduous, or primary, teeth typically begin to fall out by age 6.
   a. Age 5 is too young.
   c and d. Age 7 or 8 is too old.
   Knowledge/Health Promotion/ Assessment

4. *Correct response: c*
   According to Erikson, feelings of inadequacy and a failure to develop a sense of industry result in a sense of inferiority in the schoolager.
   a. Failure to develop a sense of autonomy results in a sense of shame in the toddler.
   b. Failure to develop a sense of initiative results in a sense of guilt in the preschooler.
   d. Failure to develop a sense of identity results in a sense of role confusion in the adolescent.
   Comprehension/Psychosocial/Assessment

5. *Correct response: c*
   Reaction formation is the typical defensive response of the schoolager when hospitalized. In reaction formation, expression of unacceptable thoughts or behaviors is prevented (or overridden) by the exaggerated expression of opposite thoughts or types of behaviors.
   a. Regression (seen in toddlers and preschoolers) is the retreating to an earlier level of development.
   b. Repression is the involuntary blocking of unpleasant feelings and experiences from one's awareness.
   d. Rationalization is the attempt to make excuses to justify unacceptable feelings or behaviors.
   Analysis/Psychosocial/Assessment

6. *Correct response: a*
   School-age children usually grow about 2 inches per year.
   b. Schoolagers normally gain about 5 lb per year.
   c. Schoolagers grow at different rates.
   d. Fat pads normally do not increase until adolescence.
   Analysis/Physiologic/Evaluation

7. *Correct response: b*
   The overriding value of nutrition and eating is determined by the family's cultural values.
   a. Table manners are important, but peer pressure and society will help mold them in later life.
   c. Mealtime should be relaxed with conversation that includes the children and their interests.
   d. School-age children need nutritious snacks, not empty calories.
   Application/Physiologic/Planning

8. *Correct response: c*
   The schoolager's cognitive level is sufficiently developed to enable good understanding of and adherence to rules.

a. With greater freedom, children become more adventurous and daring.
b. Home hazards are different for this age; firearms, alcohol, and medications become tempting.
d. The child is away from home more and therefore needs safety education to protect self from harm.

Comprehension/Safe Care/Evaluation

Adolescent Growth and Development (Age 12 to 18 Years)

I. Physical growth and development
A. General characteristics
1. Adolescence encompasses puberty, the period when primary and secondary sex characteristics begin to develop and mature.
2. In girls, puberty begins between ages 8 and 14 and usually is completed within 3 years; in boys, puberty begins between the ages of 9 and 16 and is completed by age 18 or 19.
3. During adolescence, hormonal influence causes important developmental changes:
   a. Body mass reaches adult size.
   b. Sebaceous glands become active.

      c.   Eccrine sweat glands become fully functional.

      d.   Apocrine sweat glands develop with hair growth in the axillae, breast areolae, and genital and anal regions.

      e.   Body hair assumes characteristic distribution patterns and texture changes.

      f.   During puberty, girls experience increases in height, weight, breast development, and pelvic girth with expansion of uterine tissue. Menarche (onset of menstrual periods) typically occurs about 2.5 years after the onset of puberty.

      g.   During puberty, boys experience increases in height, weight, muscle mass, and penis and testicle size; facial and body hair grows, and the voice deepens. The onset of spontaneous nocturnal emissions of seminal fluid is an overt sign of puberty and is analogous to menarche in girls.

B.   **Growth parameters**

    1.   Height

      a.   About 20% to 25% of adult height is achieved in adolescence.

      b.   Girls grow 2 to 8 inches (5 to 20 cm). Growth ceases at about age 16 or 17.

      c.   Boys grow 4 to 12 inches (10 to 30 cm). Growth ceases between ages 18 and 20.

    2.   Weight

      a.   About 30% to 50% of adult weight is gained during adolescence.

      b.   On average, girls gain between 15 and 55 lb (6.8 to 25 kg).

      c.   On average, boys gain 15 to 65 lb (6.8 to 29.5 kg).

C.   **Sex characteristics (Tanner's stages):**

    1.   Female breast development

      a.   Stage 1: prepubertal

      b.   Stage 2: breast buds

      c.   Stage 3: further enlargement of the breasts and areolae with no separation of contours

      d.   Stage 4: projection of areola and papilla to form a secondary mound

      e.   Stage 5: adult configuration

    2.   Male genitalia development

      a.   Stage 1: prepubertal

      b.   Stage 2: initial enlargement of scrotum and testes with ruggation and reddening of the scrotum

      c.   Stage 3: lengthening of the penis; testes and scrotum further enlarge

      d.   Stage 4: increase in length and width of the penis and the development of the glans; scrotum darker

      e.   Stage 5: adult

3. Pubic hair (male and female)
   a. Stage 1: prepubertal
   b. Stage 2: sparse, long, straight downy hair
   c. Stage 3: darker, coarser, curly; sparse over entire pubis
   d. Stage 4: dark, curly, and abundant, but just in pubic area
   e. Stage 5: adult pattern

D. Nutrition
1. An adolescent's daily intake should be balanced among the foods groups (Fig. 6-1); average daily caloric intake requirements vary with gender and age as follows:
   a. Girls, ages 11 to 14: 48 kcal/kg/d
   b. Girls, ages 15 to 18: 38 kcal/kg/d
   c. Boys, ages 11 to 14: 60 kcal/kg/d
   d. Boys, ages 15 to 18: 42 kcal/kg/d
2. Adolescents typically eat whenever they have a break in their activities; readily available nutritious snacks provide good insurance for a balanced diet.

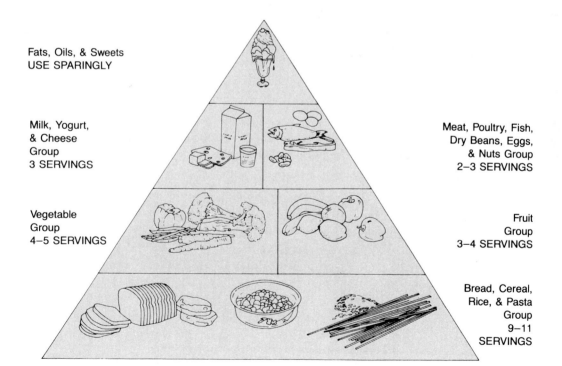

Fats, Oils, & Sweets
USE SPARINGLY

Milk, Yogurt,
& Cheese
Group
3 SERVINGS

Meat, Poultry, Fish,
Dry Beans, Eggs,
& Nuts Group
2–3 SERVINGS

Vegetable
Group
4–5 SERVINGS

Fruit
Group
3–4 SERVINGS

Bread, Cereal,
Rice, & Pasta
Group
9–11
SERVINGS

Smaller number of servings for Teen Girls—Larger number of servings for Teen Boys

FIGURE 6-1.
Food guide pyramid adapted for adolescents. (From United States Department of Agriculture)

       3.   Milk (calcium) and protein are needed in sufficient quantity to promote bone and muscle growth.

       4.   Maintaining adequate quality and quantity of daily intake may be difficult because of such factors as busy schedule, influence of peers, and easy availability of fast foods and fatty, empty-calorie foods.

       5.   Family eating patterns established during the school years continue to influence an adolescent's food selection.

       6.   Female adolescents are very prone to negative dieting behaviors.

       7.   Common dietary deficiencies include iron, folate, and zinc.

E. Sleep patterns

       1.   During adolescence, rapid growth, overexertion in activities, and a tendency to stay up late commonly interfere with sleep and rest requirements.

       2.   In an attempt to "catch up" on missed sleep, many adolescents sleep late at every opportunity.

F. Dental health

       1.   Regular and preventive dental check-ups should continue during adolescence.

       2.   Many adolescents must wear orthodontic appliances, which may be a source of embarrassment.

       3.   Adolescents must pay special attention to careful brushing and care of teeth.

II. Cognitive development

A. Overview (Piaget)

       1.   In the stage known as formal operations, which commonly occurs from ages 11 to 15, the adolescent develops abstract reasoning.

       2.   This period consists of three substages:

          a.   Substage 1: The adolescent sees relationships involving the inverse of the reciprocal.

          b.   Substage 2: The adolescent develops the ability to order triads of propositions or relationships.

          c.   Substage 3: The adolescent develops the capacity for true formal thought.

B. Formal thought

       1.   In true formal thought, the adolescent thinks beyond the present and forms theories about everything, delighting especially in considerations of "that which is not."

       2.   Relationships are hypothesized as causal and are analyzed for effects that they bring.

       3.   Random cognitive behavior is replaced by a systematic approach to problems.

III. Psychosocial development

A. Overview (Erikson)

1. Erikson terms the psychosocial crisis faced by adolescents between ages 13 and 18 **identity versus role diffusion**.
2. For adolescents, the radius of significant others is the peer group.
3. To adolescents, development of who they are and where they are going becomes a central focus.
4. Adolescents continue to redefine their self-concepts and the roles that they can play with certainty.
5. As rapid physical changes occur, adolescents must reintegrate previous trust in their body, themselves, and how they appear to others.
6. Adolescents who cannot develop a sense of who they are and what they can become may experience role diffusion and an inability to solve core conflicts.

B. Fears

1. Common fears of adolescents include:
   a. Relationships with persons of the opposite sex
   b. Homosexual tendencies
   c. Ability to assume adult roles
2. Listening to an adolescent's concerns and encouraging open communication help the adolescent develop increased confidence in his or her ability to cope with fearful situations.

C. Socialization

1. To free themselves from family domination, adolescents must define an identity separate from parental authority.
2. This period of rebellion and uncertainty, which constitutes the final separation and individuation process of childhood, can resemble the toddler period in certain respects.
3. Requisites for this emancipation from home include acceptance by peers, a few close friends, and secure love from a supportive family.
4. Relationships with parents change as the adolescent achieves competence and authority.
5. Peers and peer relationships become all important providers of advice and support.
6. Being found attractive by members of the opposite sex is important to an adolescent's self-esteem.
7. Group parties and teams typically occupy much of an adolescent's social time.
8. Heterosexual relationships typically begin with groups of teens, followed by group dating, paired dating in groups, and then a couple on a double-date or alone.

9. The degree of sexual intimacy that an adolescent experiences depends in large part on peer-group codes and the adolescent's expectations and value system.
10. Movies and music provide enjoyable diversions for most adolescents.
11. Older adolescents of both genders commonly are interested in the independence and status represented by driving an automobile.
12. Common early jobs for adolescents include baby sitting and lawn mowing.
13. Starting at age 16, an adolescent can obtain a more formal job for earning money and learning responsibility.
14. The adolescent typically spends money on dates, clothes, and other items important to him or her.

D. Activities and toys that are appropriate for adolescents include:
   1. **Sports, camping, fishing gear**
   2. **Videos, video games, computer games; radios and compact disk players**
   3. **Personal telephones**
   4. **Models and collectibles**

E. Discipline
   1. Firm but reasonable limit setting is still necessary and appreciated by most adolescents.
   2. A supportive, yet noninterfering, family is essential.
   3. An adolescent's privileges and responsibilities should be balanced in accordance with his or her maturity.

IV. Motor development

A. Gross motor development has reached adult levels.
B. Fine motor development continues to be refined.
C. Related safety concerns
   1. When teaching adolescents about safety, keep in mind that adolescents commonly feel that they are invulnerable. They are more likely to take risks and often do not consider safety before action.
   2. Adolescents contribute substantially to motor vehicle accidents through:
      a. Inexperience and poor judgment
      b. Reckless driving or speeding
      c. Driving under the influence of alcohol or other drugs
      d. Failure to use seat belts
      e. Unsafe driving practices in response to peer pressure
   3. Similarly, adolescents also are prone to accidents from unsafe use of bicycles, skateboards, motorcycles, boats, all-terrain vehicles, and snowmobiles.

      4. Accidental injury can result from improper use of firearms; safety instruction on proper use and storage of firearms and other weapons, such as nonpowder arms (*e.g.*, BB guns), should be provided.

      5. Adolescents are particularly prone to swimming and diving accidents as well; swimming and diving safety should be taught.

      6. Safety teaching should also reinforce the need for proper respect for gasoline, electricity, and fire.

      7. Adolescents need instruction on avoiding sports injuries (*e.g.*, avoiding overexertion and using proper equipment and techniques).

      8. Use of sunscreen during sun exposure should be encouraged.

      9. Smoking and use of alcohol and other drugs should be discouraged.

     10. Problem-solving techniques should be taught to decrease use of physical violence as a coping mechanism.

V. Psychosexual development

  A. Overview (Freud)

      1. In the genital stage, which extends from about age 12 to 20, adolescents focus on the genitals as an erogenous zone and engage in masturbation and in sexual relations with others.

      2. During this period of renewed sexual drive, adolescents experience conflict between their own needs for sexual satisfaction and society's expectations for control of sexual expression.

      3. Core concerns of adolescents include body image development and acceptance by the opposite sex.

  B. Sexual development

      1. Relationships with the opposite sex are important.

      2. Adolescents engage in sexual activity for pleasure, to satisfy drives and curiosity, as a means of conquest or power, to express and receive affection, and in response to peer pressure.

      3. Education about sexual function, begun during the school years, should expand to cover the physical, hormonal, and emotional changes of puberty.

      4. An adolescent needs accurate, complete information on sexuality and cultural and moral values; information must include:

         a. How pregnancy occurs

         b. Methods of preventing pregnancy, stressing that male and female partners both are responsible for contraception

         c. Transmission of and protection against sexually transmitted diseases (STDs), especially acquired immunodeficiency syndrome (AIDS)

VI. **Moral development: According to Kohlberg, the postconventional level of morality occurs at about age 13 and is marked by the development of an individual conscience and a defined set of moral values. For the first time, the adolescent can acknowledge a conflict between two socially accepted standards and try to decide between them. Control of conduct is now internal, both in standards observed and in reasoning about right or wrong.**

VII. **Hospitalization**

A. Overview: Hospitalized adolescents' concerns focus on:

1. Alterations in body image
2. Separation from peers
3. Illness as punishment (12 to 14 years of age)
4. Restricted independence (because of confinement)

B. **Reactions to hospitalization**

1. Primary defense mechanisms include denial and displacement (shifting focus from undesired object or feeling to a more acceptable object or feeling).
2. Loss of control is related to loss of identity and enforced dependence, possibly causing adolescents to react by rejection, uncooperativeness, self-assertion, anger, or frustration. They may withdraw, even from peers.
3. Adolescents' fears of mutilation and sexual changes may be evidenced by their numerous questions, rejecting others, questioning adequacy of care, psychosomatic complaints, and sexual reactions. Separation, especially from the peer group, may result in further withdrawal, loneliness, and boredom.

C. **Nursing interventions**

1. General guidelines
   a. Relate to adolescents on their level.
   b. Be genuine.
   c. Allow them to wear their own clothes.
   d. Allow them to decorate room.
   e. Provide a telephone whenever possible.
   f. **Respect an adolescent's privacy.**
   g. Set limits.
   h. Do not flirt with adolescents.
   i. Do not assign an adolescent to a hospital room with a small child.

2. Physical comfort and safety
   a. Provide nutritional information; utilize the skills of the dietitian; offer nutritious snacks.
   b. Provide counseling about issues related to puberty and health (personal hygiene, breast self-examination, testicu-

  lar self-examination, contraception, AIDS, and other STDs).

  c. Promote exercise and mobility (schedule activities, acknowledge need for physical expression of frustration).

3. Cognitive interventions

  a. Provide scientific explanations.

  b. **Encourage adolescents to participate in health management (include them as well as their parents in planning and instruction).**

  c. Support them in achieving academic and career goals (help them complete school work, involve their teachers, reinforce realistic goals).

4. Psychosocial/emotional interventions

  a. Assist adolescents to develop healthy attitudes about body image and sexuality by allowing them to verbalize fears and concerns, providing privacy, permitting them to have their own belongings, assisting with and promoting grooming.

  b. Promote independence (compliment strengths; promote self-care; provide flexible limits; assist with goal setting, and support decision making).

  c. Promote peer contact (allow visits and calls; sponsor group activities).

  d. Promote family support (encourage visiting, allow family to discuss issues, support family unit, assist with finding community resources).

Bibliography

Castiglia, P.T. & Harbin, R.B. (1993). *Child Health Care: Process and Practice.* Philadelphia: J.B. Lippincott.

Department of Health and Human Services. (1991). *Healthy People 2000.* Washington, DC: Public Health Service.

Dixon, S.D. & Stein, M.T. (1992). *Encounters with Children: Pediatric Behavior and Development,* 2nd ed. St. Louis: Mosby–Year Book.

Engel, J. (1993). *Pocket Guide to Pediatric Assessment,* 2nd ed. St. Louis: C.V. Mosby.

Jackson, D.B. & Saunders, R.B. (1993). *Child Health Nursing: A Comprehensive Approach to the Care of Children and Their Families.* Philadelphia: J.B. Lippincott.

North American Nursing Diagnosis Association. (1994). *Nursing Diagnoses: Definitions and Classification 1995–1996.* Philadelphia: NANDA.

Wong, D.L. (1993). *Whaley and Wong's Essentials of Pediatric Nursing,* 4th ed. St. Louis: C.V. Mosby.

Wong, D.L. (1995). *Whaley and Wong's Nursing Care of Infants and Children,* 5th ed. St. Louis: C.V. Mosby.

STUDY QUESTIONS

1. Which of the following best describes puberty in females?
   a. It begins between ages 8 and 14 and ends within 3 years.
   b. It begins between ages 9 and 16 and ends by age 18 or 19.
   c. It begins between ages 8 and 14 and ends by age 18 or 19.
   d. It begins between ages 9 and 16 and ends within 3 years.

2. Projection of the areola and papilla to form a secondary mound on the breast occurs during which stage (Tanner's) of sexual development?
   a. 2
   b. 3
   c. 4
   d. 5

3. The inability of an adolescent to develop a sense of who he or she is and what he or she can become results in a sense of:
   a. Shame
   b. Guilt
   c. Inferiority
   d. Role diffusion

4. Typical adolescent rebellion against parents is done at the:
   a. Final separation-individuation phase
   b. Start of aggressive behavior
   c. Start of peer relationships
   d. Final phase of relationships

5. What is the primary cause of accidental injuries in the adolescent age group?
   a. Falls
   b. Motor vehicle accidents
   c. Firearms
   d. Diving accidents

6. After learning that he will need surgery to repair his knee, an adolescent throws a cup at the nurse. This is an example of:
   a. Displacement
   b. Reaction formation
   c. Projection
   d. Denial

7. According to Erikson, why may an adolescent have difficulty mastering appropriate psychosocial tasks?
   a. The basic focus is on mastery of sexual relationships.
   b. Only a limited interaction occurs between culture and individual development.
   c. Modern culture tends to make identity crisis the most challenging to resolve.
   d. The adolescent commonly lacks positive role models.

8. What is menarche?
   a. A female's first menstruation
   b. The first year of menstruation
   c. The entire menstrual cycle
   d. The onset of uterine maturation

9. A 14-year-old boy has acne and, according to his parents, dominates the bathroom by using the mirror all the time. Which of the following remarks by the nurse would be least helpful in talking to the boy and his parents?
   a. "This is probably the only concern he has about his body, so don't worry about it."
   b. "Teenagers are anxious about how they are perceived by their peers and spend a lot of time grooming."
   c. "A teen may develop a poor self-image when experiencing acne; do you feel this way sometimes?"
   d. "You appear to be keeping your face well-washed, would you feel comfortable discussing your cleansing method?"

10. A 15-year-old girl became sexually active with her boyfriend 6 months ago. She is worried that her parents will "kill her" if they find out. Based on this information, what is the most appropriate nursing diagnosis?
    a. Altered growth and development related to sexual activity
    b. Impaired social interaction related to parental limitations
    c. Altered sexuality patterns related to parental expectations
    d. Fear related to expectations of boyfriend

ANSWER KEY

1. **Correct response: a**
   In females, puberty generally begins between ages 8 and 14 and generally ends within 3 years.
   b. In males, puberty generally begins between ages 9 and 15 and ends by age 18 or 19.
   c. It begins between age 8 and 14 but ends within 3 years.
   d. It ends within 3 years but begins between age 8 and 14.
   Comprehension/Physiologic/Planning

2. **Correct response: c**
   The papilla and areola project during stage 4.
   b. Stage 2 is breast buds.
   c. Stage 3 demonstrates no separation of contours.
   d. Stage 5 is the adult configuration.
   Comprehension/Physiologic/Assessment

3. **Correct response: d**
   According to Erikson, role diffusion develops when the adolescent does not develop a sense of identity and a sense of where he or she fits in.
   a. Toddlers develop a sense of shame when they do not achieve autonomy.
   b. Preschoolers develop a sense of guilt when they do not develop a sense of initiative.
   c. School-age children develop a sense of inferiority when they do not develop a sense of industry.
   Comprehension/Psychosocial/Assessment

4. **Correct response: a**
   This process, which occurs during the last phase of separation-individuation, assists the adolescent in developing a sense of identity.
   b. Typical adolescent rebellion is not a sign of an aggressive personality.
   c. Peer relationships start in the school-age years.
   d. There is no final relationship phase.
   Analysis/Psychosocial/Planning

5. **Correct response: b**
   Inexperience, poor judgment, use of drugs and alcohol, and peer pressure make motor vehicle accidents number one.
   a. Falls are more common in younger children.
   c. Although increasing, injuries caused by firearms are not yet the leading cause of accidental injury in adolescents.
   d. Diving accidents are a common cause of injuries, but not the leading cause.
   Knowledge/Safe Care/Planning

6. **Correct response: a**
   Displacement is a common defense mechanism in the hospitalized adolescent. Displacement is the transferring of emotional reactions from one object or person to another; it is the "kick-the-dog" defense mechanism.
   b. Reaction formation involves the person acting in a way that is opposite of the way the person feels.
   c. Projection is the projection of one's feelings on another.
   d. Denial involves ignoring unacceptable realities.
   Comprehensive/Psychosocial/Evaluation

7. **Correct response: c**
   An adolescent must resolve many choices and demands to master the task of identity.
   a. Mastery of sexual relationships is part of the young adult task of intimacy.
   b. Adolescents have several interactions with culture.
   d. Peers, teachers, parents, and extended family all serve as role models.
   Analysis/Psychosocial/Evaluation

8. **Correct response: a**
   Menarche refers to the onset of the first menstruation.

b and c. Menarche refers to the first cycle only.

d. Uterine growth and broadening of the pelvic girdle occurs before menarche.

Knowledge/Physiologic/Assessment

9. *Correct response: a*

   This response shuts off further investigation and is likely to make the adolescent and his parents feel defensive.

   b. Time spent in front of the mirror is important to the development of self-image.

   c. This response will encourage the adolescent to share his feelings.

d. This response can help to identify any patient-teaching needs for the adolescent regarding cleansing.

Application/Physiologic/Implementation

10. *Correct response: c*

    The adolescent is expressing concern about the conflict between parental expectations and her own desires.

    a and b. This is a normal experimental pattern for many adolescents, but this adolescent verbalizes parental expectations against this behavior.

    d. The adolescent is not expressing any conflict with her boyfriend.

Application/Safe Care/Analysis

Common Pediatric

Problems

C. Pathophysiology and management
D. Clinical assessment findings
E. Diagnostic assessment findings
F. Nursing diagnoses

G. Planning and implementation
H. Evaluation
Bibliography
Study questions

I. Fluid and electrolyte balance and imbalance

A. Body water percentages

1. Body water is expressed as a percentage of body weight; this percentage varies with age:
   a. In infants, total body water constitutes 80% of body weight.
   b. By age 3 years, total body water constitutes about 65% of body weight.
   c. By age 15 years, total body water constitutes 60% of body weight.
2. Age-specific fluid requirements include:
   a. Newborn: 80 to 100 mL/kg/d
   b. Infant: 120 to 130 mL/kg/d
   c. Age 2 years: 115 to 125 mL/kg/d
   d. Age 6 years: 90 to 100 mL/kg/d
   e. Age 15 years: 70 to 85 mL/kg/d
   f. Age 18 years: 40 to 50 mL/kg/d
3. Fluid and electrolyte disturbances (*e.g.*, caused by diarrhea, vomiting, and fever) occur more frequently and develop more rapidly in infants and young children than in older children and adults.
4. **Infants and very young children are more vulnerable to alterations in fluid and electrolyte balance because their bodies have:**
   a. A higher proportion of water content and a greater surface area
   b. A greater proportion of fluid in the extracellular spaces
   c. A higher metabolic rate that increases the rate at which body water must be replenished (also called water turnover)
   d. An immature homeostatic regulation (buffer) system
   e. Greater insensible water loss
   f. An inability to shiver or sweat to control temperature

TABLE 7-1.
Acid-Base Disturbances

DISTURBANCE	INITIAL METABOLIC CHANGE	EFFECT ON BLOOD pH	COMPENSATORY REACTION
Respiratory acidosis	Increased PCO_2	Decreased	Increased HCO_3
Metabolic acidosis	Decreased HCO_3	Decreased	Decreased PCO_2
Respiratory alkalosis	Decreased PCO_2	Increased	Decreased HCO_3
Metabolic alkalosis	Decreased H^+; increased HCO_3	Increased	Increased PCO_2

B. Acid-base disturbances

    1. Acid-base imbalances are common complications of diarrhea, vomiting, and febrile conditions in infants and young children as well as possible complications of respiratory, endocrine, renal, and metabolic disorders.

    2. Acid-base disturbances include acidosis, resulting from an accumulation of acid or a loss of base, and alkalosis, resulting from an accumulation of base or a loss of acid (Tables 7-1 and 7-2).

        a. Respiratory acidosis results from diminished or inadequate pulmonary ventilation, leading to an elevated PCO_2 level and a decreased plasma pH.

        b. Metabolic *acidosis* results from a gain of nonvolatile acids

TABLE 7-2.
Problems that Result in Acid-Base Disturbances

SYSTEM AFFECTED	ACIDOSIS	ALKALOSIS
Respiratory	Factors that depress respiratory center: head injury, narcotic drugs, CNS infections	Primary CNS stimulation from emotions, CNS infections, salicylate ingestion, mechanical respiration
	Lung disorders: cystic fibrosis, obstructive pulmonary disease, pneumonia, atelectasis.	Reflex CNS stimulation from fever, CHF, anemia
	Factors that affect chest wall action: chest wall trauma, muscular dystrophy	Lung disease: irritant inhalation, pulmonary edema
Endocrine/ Metabolic	Acid gain from salicylate ingestion, diabetic ketoacidosis, starvation, infection	Acid loss from vomiting, diuretic therapy
	Bicarbonate loss from diarrhea, renal tubular acidosis	Bicarbonate gain from (uncommon) bicarbonate ingestion

CNS = central nervous system; CHF = congestive heart failure.

or the loss of base and leads to decreased plasma pH and decreased plasma HCO_3 concentration.

    c.   *Respiratory alkalosis* results from an increase in the rate and depth of pulmonary ventilation leading to a decreased PCO_2 level and an elevated plasma pH.

    d.   *Metabolic alkalosis,* produced by a gain in base or a loss of acid, results in elevated urine pH, elevated plasma pH, and elevated plasma HCO_3 concentrations.

  3. Compensatory mechanisms reflect the body's attempts to correct an acid-base imbalance through changes in the component of the acid-base equation not primarily affected.

  4. To sustain a child with an acid-base imbalance until the primary disorder resolves, interventions may include:

    a.   Providing adequate hydration

    b.   Replacing electrolytes

    c.   Correcting the acid-base imbalance

II. Diarrhea

A. **Description: the frequent passage of loose, abnormally watery stools. Diarrhea may be mild, moderate, or severe; acute or chronic; inflammatory or noninflammatory.**

B. **Etiology and incidence**

  1. Diarrhea is one of the most common problems in childhood. The disorder is a manifestation of abnormal water and electrolyte transport.

  2. Predisposing factors include young age, malnutrition, chronic disease, use of antibiotics, contaminated water, poor sanitation or hygiene, improper food preparation and storage, and travel to underdeveloped areas.

  3. Chronic diarrhea usually is associated with malabsorption disorders, anatomic defects, allergic reactions, and inflammatory response.

  4. Rotavirus is the most common cause of acute nonbacterial diarrhea (gastroenteritis).

  5. Bacterial causes include *Escherichia coli,* and *Salmonella* and *Shigella* organisms. Diarrhea from *Clostridium difficile* may follow antibiotic therapy.

  6. Additional causes of acute diarrhea include other infections (upper respiratory infections, urinary tract infections), overfeeding, antibiotics, ingested toxins, irritable bowel syndrome, enterocolitis, and lactose intolerance.

C. **Pathophysiology and management**

  1. Invading pathogens cause diarrhea in several ways. For example, in infectious diarrhea the disease-causing organisms produce enterotoxins that invade and destroy intestinal epithelial cells, thereby promoting fluid and electrolyte secretion.

D. Clinical assessment findings
1. History reveals exposure to infection, contaminated foods, or other causative agents; allergy; or travel.
2. Severity of diarrhea
   a. *Mild:* few loose stools without other symptoms
   b. *Moderate:* several loose or watery stools; possibly elevated temperature, vomiting, and irritability; usually no signs of dehydration; weight loss or failure to gain weight
   c. *Severe:* numerous stools, signs of moderate to severe dehydration (see Section III), drawn appearance, weak cry, irritability, purposeless movements, inappropriate responses, and, possibly lethargic, moribund, or comatose appearance

E. Diagnostic assessment findings
1. Extensive testing is unnecessary for uncomplicated diarrhea without dehydration.
2. Stool specimens may reveal:
   a. Polymorphonuclear leukocytes, differentiating bacterial infections from viral infections
   b. Culture positive for offending organisms
   c. Ova and parasites
   d. *C. difficile* toxin
3. Stool pH value under 6 and presence of reducing substances suggesting carbohydrate malabsorption.
4. For other test findings indicative of dehydration, see Section III, E.).

F. Nursing diagnoses
1. Diarrhea
2. Hyperthermia
3. Fluid volume deficit
4. Altered nutrition: less than body requirements
5. Impaired skin integrity

G. Planning and implementation
1. Assist in correcting fluid and electrolyte imbalance and, when prescribed, treating the underlying cause of the diarrhea.
2. Because mild to moderate diarrhea usually is managed at home, teach parents about providing oral rehydrating solutions (ORS), followed by reintroducing normal nutrients. Providing nonhuman milk is controversial because of concerns related to possible lactose intolerance. Older children may be treated with ORS followed by a regular diet.
3. Because severe diarrhea warrants hospitalization, nursing care usually involves management of parenteral fluid replacement (see Section III).

4. Administer antimicrobial therapy if indicated and prescribed.
5. Assess frequency, duration, consistency, appearance, and odor of stools; assess hydration status.
6. Assess any connection between loose stools and diet.
7. Monitor intake and output (I&O); weigh diapers for accuracy; also monitor urine specific gravity.
8. Record daily body weights, weighing child in minimal amount of clothing at same time every day—usually in early morning before feeding—and on the same balanced scale. This is the best way to determine hydration status.
9. Obtain stool specimens and test stools for reducing substances as prescribed.
10. Assess skin integrity around perineal area.
11. Assess and monitor hydration status.
12. Keep child on NPO (nothing by mouth) status as prescribed, monitor intravenous (IV) lines and fluids, add to diet as prescribed from ORS and clear fluids to banana, rice, apple, toast (BRAT) regimen to light diet without milk or milk products for about 1 week.
13. Maintain enteric precautions.
14. Provide adequate skin care (expose diaper area to air, keep clean, avoid commercial wipes that may contain irritating chemicals, apply ointments as prescribed).
14. Avoid using rectal thermometers.

H. Evaluation

1. Child has normal fluid and electrolyte balance as noted by well-hydrated appearance, taking of prescribed nourishment, satisfactory weight gain, and normal serum electrolyte values (Table 7-3).
2. Child's perineal area remains intact.
3. Infection does not spread to other people.

TABLE 7-3.
Normal Serum Electrolyte Ranges in Children

AGE GROUP	SODIUM (mEq/L)	POTASSIUM (mEq/L)	CHLORIDE (mEq/L)	CO_2 (mEq/L)	BUN (mg/dL)	CREATININE (mg/dL)
Newborn	136–146	3.0–6.0	97–110	13–22	3–12	0.3–1.0
Infant	139–146	3.5–5.0	98–106	20–28	5–18	0.2–0.4
Child	138–145	3.5–5.0	98–106	20–28	5–18	0.3–0.7
Adolescent	136–146	3.5–5.0	98–106	23–30	7–18	0.5–1.0

III. Dehydration
A. **Description: excessive loss of water from the body tissues.**
B. **Etiology and incidence**
   1. Common disturbance in infants and children whenever total fluid output exceeds intake
   2. Can result from several problems that cause insensible water loss from the skin and respiratory tract and that cause increased renal and gastrointestinal excretion
   3. Possible causes include:
      a. Excessive vomiting and diarrhea
      b. Insufficient fluid intake
      c. Diabetic ketoacidosis
      d. Severe burns
      e. Prolonged high fever
      f. Hyperventilation
C. **Pathophysiology and management**
   1. Depending on the cause and nature of the fluid loss, a child will lose both water and electrolytes. Dehydration is classified as isotonic, hypertonic, or hypotonic.
   2. Isotonic dehydration
      a. Electrolyte and water deficits occur in approximately balanced proportions.
      b. **Isotonic dehydration is the most common type of dehydration (accounting for about 70% of the dehydration cases linked to diarrhea in infants).**
      c. The major loss involves extracellular components and circulating blood volume, making the child susceptible to hypovolemic shock.
      d. Serum sodium (Na^+) level decreases or remains within normal range; chloride (Cl^-) level decreases; and potassium (K^+) level stays normal or decreases.
      e. Deficits should be corrected over 24 hours.
   3. Hypertonic dehydration
      a. Water loss exceeds electrolyte loss.
      b. Hypertonic dehydration accounts for about 20% of dehydration cases related to severe diarrhea in infants.
      c. It results in fluid shifts from the intracellular to the extracellular compartment, which can lead to neurologic disturbances such as seizures.
      d. Serum sodium (Na^+) level increases; serum potassium (K^+) level varies; chloride (Cl^-) level increases.
   4. Hypotonic dehydration
      a. Electrolyte deficit exceeds water deficit.
      b. Hypotonic dehydration may be caused by excessive per-

spiration, severe diarrhea, or administration of oral or IV fluids without electrolytes added; in infants, it accounts for 10% of dehydration cases resulting from severe diarrhea.

   c. In hypotonic dehydration, water shifts from the extracellular to the intracellular compartments in an attempt to establish osmotic equilibrium, which further increases extracellular fluid loss and commonly results in hypovolemic shock.

   d. Serum sodium (Na^+) level decreases; chloride (Cl^-) decreases and potassium (K^+) level varies.

   e. Volume and Na^+ should be replaced within 24 to 36 hours.

6. The degree of dehydration can be estimated by comparing the child's current weight with his or her weight before the illness.

7. As with diarrhea, dehydration can be classified by severity:

   a. **Mild: loss of up to 5% of pre-illness weight.**

   b. **Moderate: loss of 5% to 10% of pre-illness weight.**

   c. **Severe: loss of more than 10% of preillness weight.**

D. Clinical assessment findings (Table 7-4)

1. Weight loss
2. Dry mucous membranes
3. Decrease or absence of tear production
4. Poor skin turgor, increased capillary refill time
5. Sunken eyes
6. Depressed fontanels
7. Decreased urine output

TABLE 7-4.
Clinical Findings According to Degree of Dehydration

	DEGREE OF DEHYDRATION		
SIGN	MILD	MODERATE	SEVERE
Fluid Loss	Under 5%	5% to 9%	10% or more
Skin Color	Pale	Gray	Mottled
Skin Turgor	Decreased	Poor	Very poor
Mucous Membranes	Dry	Very dry	Parched
Urine Output	Decreased	Oliguria	Marked oliguria
Blood Pressure	Normal	Normal or lowered	Lowered
Pulse Rate	Normal or increased	Increased	Rapid and thready

(Adapted from Wong, D.L. [1995]. Whaley and Wong's Nursing Care of Infants and Children, 5th ed. St. Louis: C.V. Mosby, p. 1210.)

8. Tachycardia
9. Tachypnea
10. Decreased blood pressure
11. Excessive thirst

E. Diagnostic assessment findings

1. Concentrated urine with high specific gravity (>1.030) and high osmolarity
2. Elevated hematocrit
3. Elevated blood urea nitrogen (BUN) level
4. Decreased urine sodium concentration
5. Altered serum electrolyte (Na^+, K^+, Cl^-) values
6. Low serum pH value if the child is acidotic

F. Nursing diagnoses

1. Fluid volume deficit
2. Hyperthermia
3. Risk for infection
4. Knowledge deficit
5. Altered nutrition: less than body requirements

G. Planning and implementation

1. Nursing management aims at correcting fluid and electrolyte imbalance and treating underlying cause as prescribed.
2. Maintain IV lines and fluids. Administer parenteral fluids as prescribed. The selected solution is usually a saline solution containing 5% dextrose. The selection is based on the probable type and cause of dehydration. Sodium bicarbonate and K^+ may be added when appropriate.
3. **Do not add potassium to the IV solution until the child voids.**
4. Obtain an accurate initial weight, and monitor weight changes indicating fluid gains and losses.
5. Evaluate the child's health history, physical assessment findings, and laboratory test results to help identify the underlying cause of the dehydration.
6. Administer ORS and other fluids, as prescribed, to correct fluid balance.
7. Offer oral fluids in small quantities (*e.g.*, 1 to 2 oz every hour); withhold a full diet until the child is well hydrated and the underlying problem is under control.
8. If the child cannot ingest sufficient fluid orally, start an IV line and administer an appropriate replacement solution, as prescribed.
9. Monitor IV replacement therapy and check the IV site frequently.

10. Teach parents about positioning, moving, and caring for a child with an IV line.

11. Evaluate the child's hydration status by observing for signs and symptoms of dehydration.

12. Monitor and record accurate I&O and note urine specific gravity value.

13. Maintain skin integrity by providing hygienic skin care, using aseptic technique when inserting IV catheters and monitoring the IV infusion for signs of infiltration.

14. Prevent spreading infection by maintaining good hygiene, washing hands as required, and instituting necessary isolation techniques appropriate to the cause of the dehydration.

15. Gradually reintroduce the child to a regular diet, as prescribed, and monitor the child's response.

16. Provide support to the family and explain all tests and procedures.

17. Provide family education, covering:
   a. Diet and oral fluid instructions
   b. Causes of dehydration
   c. Signs and symptoms of dehydration to watch for and report
   d. Hand washing and hygiene instructions as indicated
   e. Follow-up appointments

   H. **Evaluation**

1. The child displays signs of normal hydration and tolerates a regular diet.

2. The family verbalizes an understanding of managing the child's home diet and fluid intake, causes of dehydration, signs and symptoms of dehydration, the importance of hand washing and good hygiene, and of scheduling follow-up appointments.

IV. Upper respiratory tract infections

   A. Definition: Upper respiratory tract infections include *nasopharyngitis, pharyngitis,* and *tonsillitis.* Also called the common cold, nasopharyngitis is a viral infection of the nose and throat. *Pharyngitis,* an inflammation of the pharynx, and *tonsillitis,* an inflammation of the tonsils, are also upper respiratory tract infections.

   B. Etiology and incidence

1. Of the upper respiratory tract inflammations, nasopharyngitis is the most common illness in infancy and childhood. Uncommon under age 1 year, pharyngitis peaks between ages 4 and 7. It usually is caused by viral, or group A beta hemolytic streptococcus, which has the potential to lead to complications such as rheumatic fever or acute glomerulonephritis.

C. **Pathophysiology and management**
1. In young children, the tonsils commonly are enlarged, becoming smaller with age. Upper respiratory tract infections usually are caused by a viral or bacterial pathogen, with the disease course following the events of the inflammatory process.
2. Nonbacterial tonsillitis is a mild disorder characterized by gradual onset, low-grade fever, mild headache, sore throat, hoarseness, and a cough.
3. Bacterial tonsillitis is a more dramatic disorder marked by rapid onset of high fever, headache, generalized muscle aches, and vomiting.

D. **Clinical assessment findings**
1. Difficulty eating and swallowing
2. Frequent sore throats and ear infections
3. History of allergic disorders

E. **Diagnostic assessment findings**
1. Throat culture may be positive for streptococcal organisms

F. **Nursing diagnoses**
1. Risk for fluid volume deficit
2. Risk for injury
3. Knowledge deficit
4. Pain
5. Ineffective breathing pattern
6. Impaired swallowing

G. **Planning and implementation**
1. Nursing management of upper respiratory tract viral infections is symptomatic (focused on relieving symptoms).
   a. In nasopharyngitis, keep nasal passages clear, especially in infants younger than 4 months, who are obligatory nose breathers, by using normal saline nose drops and a nasal aspirator.
   b. Provide liquids and soft foods.
   c. Use a cool mist vaporizer to keep mucous membranes moist.
2. If child has streptococcal infection, give antibiotics as prescribed. An antibiotic (usually penicillin, but erythromycin if child is allergic to penicillin) is prescribed, typically for about 10 days to prevent the complication of rheumatic fever.
3. Pre- and postoperative nursing care is required if surgery is performed (*e.g.*, to remove the tonsils). Tonsillectomy or adenoidectomy, or both, may be indicated in chronic enlargement that interferes with swallowing or breathing, or in recurrent streptococcal infections, peritonsillar abscess, or retropharyngeal abscess.

4. Preoperative nursing care for tonsillectomy and adenoidectomy includes:
   a. Prepare child for hospitalization and surgery according to developmental level.
   b. Explain that the child will have a sore throat after surgery but will be able to talk and swallow.
   c. Explain postoperative care measures (*e.g.*, proper positioning, ingesting cool liquids, using an ice collar).
5. Postoperative nursing care
   a. Observe for and report unusual bleeding.
   b. Intervene for bleeding as appropriate.
   c. Monitor vital signs.
   d. Assess child's color.
   e. Help prevent bleeding by discouraging the child from coughing and clearing throat.
   f. Position the child on the side or the abdomen to facilitate drainage from the throat.
6. Provide appropriate teaching. Instruct the child and parents to:
   a. Observe activity restrictions, including when the child can return to school.
   b. Avoid persons with known infections.
   c. Provide a soft diet with adequate fluid intake.
   d. Avoid acidic or other irritating foods.
   e. **Monitor the child for bleeding, especially immediately postoperatively and 5 to 10 days postoperatively when tissues sloughing occurs.**

   H. Evaluation
   1. Vital signs remain within normal limits for the child's age.
   2. The child does not exhibit restlessness or frequent swallowing.
   3. No signs of bleeding are evident.
   4. The child demonstrates adequate oral fluid intake.
   5. The child experiences minimal to no pain.

V. Fever
  A. Definition: abnormally elevated body temperature.
  B. Etiology and incidence
   1. Common causes of fever in infants include upper and lower respiratory tract infections, pharyngitis, otitis media, and generalized and enteric viral infections.
   2. More serious causes of fever include urinary tract infections, pneumonia, bacteremia, meningitis, osteomyelitis, septic arthritis, cancer, immunologic disorders, poisoning or drug overdose, immunization reactions, and dehydration.
  C. Pathophysiology and management
   1. Fever most commonly results from disruption of the hypothalamic set point caused by infection, allergy, endotoxins, or tumor.

        2. Disrupted thermoregulation leads to increased heat production and decreased heat loss.

        3. Associated clinical findings provide clues regarding the seriousness of the fever (*e.g.*, an active, alert child with a fever of 104°F [40.0°C] generally is of less concern than a listless, lethargic infant with a temperature of 102.2°F [39.0°C]).

  D. **Clinical assessment findings**

        1. Temperature 102°F to 105°F (38.9°C to 40.6°C) measured by the axillary route.

        2. Skin flushing, diaphoresis, chills

        3. Restlessness or lethargy

  E. **Diagnostic assessment findings**

        1. Tests and results vary depending on underlying cause of fever

  F. **Nursing diagnoses**

        1. Risk for altered body temperature

        2. Risk for injury

  G. **Planning and implementation**

        1. Monitor temperature.

        2. Administer antipyretics as prescribed.

          a. **As prescribed, administer acetaminophen instead of aspirin because of the association between aspirin and Reye's syndrome.**

          b. Administer ibuprofen, if prescribed. Ibuprofen also is approved for reducing fever in children as young as 6 months.

        3. Give tepid sponge baths, as needed.

        4. Teach parents how to take child's temperature and implement fever control measures.

  H. **Evaluation**

        1. Temperature decreases by no more than 1°F each hour.

        2. The infant or child rests comfortably.

VI. **Febrile seizures**

  A. **Definition: a seizure associated with a febrile illness**

  B. **Etiology and incidence**

        1. Affects 3% to 5% of children; usually occurs after 6 months and before 3 years; unusual after 5 years

        2. Boys affected more than girls; increased susceptibility in families

        3. Cause unknown; usually associated with upper respiratory tract infections, urinary tract infections, and roseola

  C. **Pathophysiology and management**

        1. Most often a grand mal seizure manifested by an active tonic-clonic pattern, usually lasting less than 1 minute associated with an acute, benign febrile illness

2. Usually results from the rapid rise in temperature, with the initial fever
3. Considered benign if underlying neurologic and physical problems are ruled out; the electroencephalograph (EEG) is usually normal; there is a family history of febrile convulsions

D. Clinical assessment findings

1. Most seizure activity ceases by the time the child is brought in for medical attention.
2. Most seizures consist of tonic and clonic manifestations.

E. Diagnostic assessment findings

1. Diagnostic evaluation is performed to rule out other disease processes; for example, a lumbar puncture may be done to rule out meningitis and an EEG to rule out a seizure disorder.
2. Computed tomography (CT) and magnetic resonance imaging (MRI) may be performed as well.

F. Nursing diagnoses

1. Hyperthermia
2. Risk for injury

G. Planning and implementation

1. Reassure parents.
2. Observe for signs and symptoms of illness.
3. Provide safe environment.
4. Assist with procedures and prepare family for same.
5. Use temperature control implementations.
6. Educate parents on temperature control and how to protect child during seizure.
7. When appropriate, use anticonvulsant therapy as prescribed, keeping in mind that prophylactic therapy does not reduce the risk of future seizures. Anticonvulsant therapy may be prescribed for children who meet certain criteria: a focal or prolonged seizure; neurologic abnormalities; afebrile seizures in a first-degree relative; age under 1 year; multiple seizures in less than 24 hours.

H. Evaluation

1. Child remains injury free.
2. Child has no further seizures.
3. Child's temperature becomes regulated.

VII. Enuresis

A. Definition: repeated involuntary (usually nocturnal) urination in a child who should have bladder control (usually by age 4 or 5 years).

B. Etiology and incidence

1. Incidence is approximately 5% to 17% in otherwise normal children between ages 3 and 15.

      2. Boys are affected more than girls.

      3. Enuresis may have a familial component; typically, a child with enuresis has siblings or a parent who experienced the problem.

C. Pathophysiology and management

      1. Enuresis is primarily a problem of delayed or incomplete neuromuscular maturation of the bladder. The condition is benign and self-limiting.

D. Clinical assessment findings

      1. Nocturnal bed wetting

      2. Possibly urinary urgency, dysuria, restlessness, and frequency

E. Diagnostic assessment findings

      1. A physical and psychosocial evaluation is performed to rule out pathology such as urinary tract infections, sickle cell anemia, neurologic deficits, diabetes, and psychogenic problems.

F. Nursing diagnoses

      1. Altered urinary elimination

      2. Low, situational self-esteem

      3. Anxiety

G. Planning and implementation

      1. Assist with therapeutic treatment plan, which may include:

          a. Bladder retention training, motivational therapy, or behavior modification

          b. Drug therapy such as imipramine (Tofranil), which has an anticholinergic effect on the bladder or desmopressin (DDAVP) nasal spray which reduces nighttime output

      2. Provide emotional support.

      3. Encourage parents and other caretakers to accept the child's problem and to avoid placing blame or adopting attitudes that may foster feelings of worthlessness and hopelessness in the child.

H. Evaluation

      1. Episodes of enuresis become less frequent.

      2. Enuresis ceases.

VIII. Lead poisoning (plumbism)

A. Definition: a common pediatric problem that results from ingesting or inhaling lead-containing substances.

B. Etiology and incidence

      1. Highest incidence in late infancy and toddlerhood

      2. Sources include lead in paint chips, powder from paint, gasoline, soil or dust contamination, unglazed ceramic containers, lead crystal, water from lead pipes, batteries, folk remedies, fishing weights, refinishing furniture, art supplies, cosmetics, and even certain industries. Lead poisoning is one of the most common health problems in the United States.

C. **Pathophysiology and management**

1. Lead, which is very slowly excreted through the kidney, gastrointestinal (GI) tract, and slightly through sweat, is stored chiefly in the bone. When the rate of absorption surpasses the rate of excretion, lead is deposited into soft tissues of the body and bone and attaches itself to red blood cells (RBCs). In the RBCs, it interferes with the production of heme and the formation of hemoglobin, which results in a microcytic, hypochromic anemia.

2. Lead affects the kidneys by altering the permeability of the proximal tubules, resulting in increased urinary elimination of glucose and protein.

3. Lead deposits also increase vascular permeability resulting in fluid shifts that lead to encephalopathy and increased intracranial pressure (ICP).

D. **Systemic clinical assessment findings**

1. Hematologic: signs of anemia
2. Renal: glycosuria, proteinuria, ketonuria, hyperphosphaturia
3. Gastrointestinal: (may have pica) acute crampy abdominal pain, vomiting, constipation, anorexia
4. Musculoskeletal: short stature, lead lines in bones on x-ray films
5. Neurologic (central nervous system)

   a. **Mild lead poisoning causes such behavioral changes as irritability, hyperactivity, aggressive behavior, lethargy, learning problems, developmental delays, short attention span, clumsiness, and deficits in sensory perception.**

   b. **Severe, chronic lead poisoning causes such problems as seizures, mental retardation, encephalopathy, increased ICP, paralysis, sensory loss, coma, and death.**

E. **Diagnostic assessment findings**

1. A serum lead level exceeding 10 mcg/dL is considered positive for lead poisoning.

2. Traditionally, elevated erythrocyte protoporphyrin (EP) levels were considered positive for lead poisoning, but the Centers for Disease Control (CDC) currently suggests not using EP levels because they do not always detect elevated lead levels in children.

F. **Nursing diagnoses**

1. Risk for activity intolerance
2. Altered nutrition: less than body requirements
3. Risk for injury

G. Planning and implementations

1. Prepare child and family for interventions, which vary according to lead level scores (per Centers for Disease Control, 1991):
   a. 9 and under: rescreen
   b. 10 to 14: rescreen
   c. 15 to 19: rescreen; look for sources and educate parents
   d. 20 to 44: conduct medical examination; identify and eliminate sources of lead
   e. 45 to 69: begin treatment and environmental clearance in 48 hours
   f. 70 and over: begin treatment and environmental clearance immediately

2. Prepare child and family for chelation therapy, and administer as prescribed. Chelators include: d-penicillamine, CaNa2EDTA, BAL (dimercaprol), succimer.

3. Encourage fluids to enhance lead excretion.

4. Monitor I&O to evaluate kidney function.

5. Perform prescribed serial urine testing during chelation to monitor kidney status and the rate and volume of lead excretion. Draw blood for analysis of serum lead and EP levels. Additional routine analyses of serum BUN and creatine levels and urine protein concentration detect are done to detect possible drug toxicity.

7. Monitor for encephalopathy resulting from medications.

8. Provide parent teaching regarding lead-poisoning risks.

9. Make home referral for lead removal.

10. Review nursing implications for various chelators:
    a. d-penicillamine: assess for penicillin allergy
    b. Edathamil calcium disodium (CaNa2EDTA)
       (1) Use CaNa2EDTA, *not* Na2EDTA, which induces fatal hypocalcemia.
       (2) Carefully monitor renal functioning; appearance of sediment in urine may signal renal failure.
       (3) Give medication by IV route, if medication must be given intramuscularly (IM) (*e.g.*, if client has encephalopathy), administer with procaine. Draw up edathamil calcium disodium first, then procaine, then air bubble, then inject; air bubble pushes last bit of EDTA into muscle and prevents tracking into dermal layers.
    c. Dimercaprol (BAL)
       (1) Do not give to children allergic to peanuts (medication contains peanut oil).
       (2) Because medication forms toxic compound with

iron, start iron therapy at least 24 hours after BAL administration finishes; give deep IM.

    d.   Succimer: Experience using this agent in children with lead levels exceeding 70 is limited.

H. **Evaluation**

1. Lead sources are removed.
2. Lead is removed from the body and further accumulation is stopped.
3. The child does not have injuries from seizure activity.
4. The child functions developmentally at optimal level.

Bibliography

Carpenito, L.J. (1995). *Nursing Diagnosis: Application to Clinical Practice*, 6th ed. Philadelphia: J.B. Lippincott.

Castiglia, P.T. & Harbin, R.B. (1993). *Child Health Care: Process and Practice*. Philadelphia: J.B. Lippincott.

Centers for Disease Control. (1991). *Preventing Lead Poisoning in Young Children*. Atlanta: U.S. Department of Health and Human Services.

Engel, J. (1993). *Pocket Guide to Pediatric Assessment*, 2nd ed. St. Louis: C.V. Mosby.

Jackson, D.B. & Saunders, R.B. (1993). *Child Health Nursing: A Comprehensive Approach to the Care of Children and Their Families*. Philadelphia: J.B. Lippincott.

North American Nursing Diagnosis Association. (1994). *NANDA Diagnoses: Definitions and Classification 1995–1996*. Philadelphia: NANDA.

Pillitteri, A. (1995). *Maternal and Child Health Nursing: Care of the Childbearing and Childrearing Family*, 2nd ed. Philadelphia: J.B. Lippincott.

Wong, D.L. (1993). *Whaley and Wong's Essentials of Pediatric Nursing*, 4th ed. St. Louis: C.V. Mosby.

Wong, D.L. (1995). *Whaley & Wong's Nursing Care of Infants and Children*, 5th ed. St. Louis: C.V. Mosby.

STUDY QUESTIONS

1. Which of the following is true about fluid and electrolyte balance and imbalance in infants?
   a. Infants can concentrate urine at an adult level.
   b. Water turnover in infants is two to three times slower than in adults.
   c. Infants have more intracellular water than adults.
   d. Infants have greater body surface areas than adults.

2. Which of the following is produced by an aspirin overdose or vomiting?
   a. Metabolic alkalosis
   b. Respiratory alkalosis
   c. Metabolic acidosis
   d. Respiratory acidosis

3. What organism is responsible for most of the cases of acute viral gastroenteritis?
   a. Respiratory syncytial virus (RSV)
   b. Shigella
   c. Rotavirus
   d. Salmonella

4. A physician orders KCl to be added to a child's IV infusion. Which of the following is an appropriate nursing intervention?
   a. Add sodium bicarbonate to the IV.
   b. Hold the KCl until the child voids.
   c. Give the KCl by IV push (bolus).
   d. Never add KCl to a child's IV.

5. When planning care for an 8-month-old child with dehydration, which of the following would be a priority intervention for monitoring hydration status?
   a. Measuring intake and output (I&O)
   b. Monitoring daily weight
   c. Checking electrolyte status
   d. Checking skin turgor

6. Which of the following clinical assessments would most likely be demonstrated in severe dehydration?
   a. Pale skin turgor
   b. Normal skin turgor
   c. Marked oliguria
   d. Normal blood pressure

7. When caring for a 7-year-old with nasopharyngitis, which of the following would be the most appropriate nursing diagnosis?
   a. Impaired gas exchange
   b. Ineffective airway clearance
   c. Altered tissue perfusion
   d. Impaired swallowing

8. Aspirin is contraindicated for children with viral syndromes because of the possibility of:
   a. Reye's syndrome
   b. Reflux syndrome
   c. Raynaud's syndrome
   d. Reiter's syndrome

9. What diagnostic procedure is performed to rule out seizure disorder in a child with a febrile convulsion?
   a. Brain scan
   b. Electroencephalogram (EEG)
   c. Serum chemistry
   d. Lead level analysis

10. What is the most likely cause of primary enuresis?
    a. Urinary tract infection
    b. Psychogenic stress
    c. Vesicoureteral reflux
    d. Delayed bladder maturation

11. Assessment of early lead poisoning includes all of the following signs except:
    a. Anorexia
    b. Irritability
    c. Seizures
    d. Anemia

ANSWER KEY

1. *Correct response: d*
   Infants have greater body surface areas than adults, which makes them more predisposed to fluid and electrolyte imbalance.
   a. Infants cannot concentrate urine at the adult level.
   b. Water turnover in infants is two to three times higher than adults.
   c. Infants have more extracellular fluid.
   Comprehension/Physiologic/Planning

2. *Correct response: a*
   Aspirin overdose (a gain in base) and vomiting (a loss of acid) can both lead to metabolic alkalosis.
   b. Respiratory alkalosis occurs from a decreased PCO_2 level and increased respiratory rate.
   c. Metabolic acidosis results from a gain in acid or a loss of base.
   d. Respiratory acidosis results from decreased ventilation that increases PCO_2.
   Analysis/Physiologic/Assessment

3. *Correct response: c*
   Most cases of viral gastroenteritis are caused by rotavirus.
   a. RSV causes bronchiolitis and other respiratory problems.
   b and d. Both are bacterial but do cause acute gastroenteritis.
   Knowledge/Physiologic/NA

4. *Correct response: b*
   KCl should be held until the nurse can verify kidney functioning by monitoring the child's voiding.
   a. There is no order to add this.
   c. Never give KCL by IV push as it can induce a cardiac arrhythmia and death or, at the least, severe burning.
   d. KCl is commonly needed to restore electrolyte balance in children.
   Application/Safe Care/Implementation

5. *Correct response: b*
   Daily weight is the most accurate way to measure a child's fluid loss or gain as insensible water loss in children cannot be measured.
   a. Measuring I&O is necessary, but doing so cannot measure insensible loss.
   c and d. Both are necessary, but they are not the priority measure.
   Application/Physiologic/Evaluation

6. *Correct response: c*
   Marked oliguria is a sign of severe dehydration, loss of more than 10% of body weight.
   a. Mild dehydration, loss of less than 5%.
   b. Moderate dehydration, 5% to 10% loss.
   d. Mild dehydration.
   Application/Physiologic/Assessment

7. *Correct response: d*
   Nasopharyngitis is another name for the common cold; therefore the child will most likely have a sore throat that will impair swallowing.
   a, b, and c. All are unlikely due to the benign nature of the disorder.
   Comprehension/Physiologic/Analysis (Dx)

8. *Correct response: a*
   In children with viral illnesses, the use of aspirin is linked with the development of Reye's syndrome, an acute encephalitis with fatty infiltrates of the internal organs.
   b. There is no association with any type of reflux syndrome.
   c. This is a disorder of extremity ischemia.
   d. This is an arthritic disorder of adult males.
   Comprehension/Physiologic/Planning

9. *Correct response: b*
An electroencephalogram (EEG) is used to determine if a child has a seizure disorder.
  a. A brain scan may be used to rule out a lesion.
  c. Serum chemistry findings may rule out electrolyte imbalance.
  d. Lead level determination will rule out lead poisoning.
Comprehension/Physiologic/Assessment

10. *Correct response: d*
The most likely cause of primary enuresis is delayed or incomplete maturation of the bladder.
  a. A urinary tract infection may cause either primary or secondary enuresis, but it is not the leading cause of primary enuresis.

  b. Psychogenic stress may cause either primary or secondary enuresis, but it is not the leading cause of primary enuresis.
  c. Vesicoureteral reflux may cause either primary or secondary enuresis, but it is not the leading cause of primary enuresis.
Comprehension/Physiologic/NA

11. *Correct response: c*
Seizures usually are associated with encephalopathy, a late sign of lead poisoning, in which lead levels have already exceeded 70.
  a, b, and d. All are early signs of lead poisoning.
Analysis/Physiologic/Assessment

Common Psychosocial Problems

I.   Death and dying
   ### A.   Developmental reactions
   1.   Infancy to 2 years: The question whether children of this age grieve or mourn evokes controversy.
   2.   Ages 2 to 7 years: Children this age typically believe that they have caused a death. They also believe that death is reversible.

99

A strong possibility exists that they are aware of the seriousness of their illnesses.

    a. **Between ages 3 and 5:**
- (1) **Death is denied.**
- (2) **Death is equated with sleep and separation.**
- (3) **Death is reversible.**
- (4) **Life is attributed to the dead (*e.g.*, the dead can eat).**

    b. **Between ages 5 and 6:**
- (1) **Death is temporary.**
- (2) **Death has degrees (*e.g.*, "not real dead").**
- (3) **Life and death are interchangeable.**

3. Ages 7 to 11: aware that death is irreversible; can give specific examples of death; when fatally ill, can express death themes and fear of body intrusion

    a. **Between ages 7 and 9:**
- (1) **Death is personified (*e.g.*, "Boogie man").**
- (2) **Death can be avoided by being good.**

    b. **Between ages 9 and 11:**
- (1) **Death is universal.**
- (2) **Death may be defied by daredevil behavior and jokes.**

4. Adolescence
    a. Adolescents normally respond with appropriate grief and reactions. Typical adolescent reactions to death indicate an almost adult understanding and a search for meaning in death.
    b. Adolescent are unable to prioritize their losses; therefore, the loss of a friend may be as debilitating as the loss of a mother.
    c. Death may seem remote and adolescents typically test the boundaries between life and death.

B. **Clinical assessment findings**
When evaluating a child's psychosocial health in relation to death and dying, assessment findings usually focus on:
1. Developmental level of child
2. Cultural and spiritual issues
3. Socioeconomic implications
4. Support network and family themes
5. Grief symptoms
6. Unfinished business between parents and child

C. **Nursing diagnoses**
1. Anxiety
2. Fear
3. Powerlessness
4. Ineffective individual coping

        5.   Anticipatory grieving
        6.   Dysfunctional grieving

D.   **Planning and implementation**
1. Assist the family and child to understand the process of death and dying and to maintain a healthy grieving process.
2. Discuss child's experiences with death and dying.
3. Determine comforting and security measures or objects.
4. Decrease anxiety.
5. Utilize child's and family's customs and rituals whenever possible; refer to clergy if needed.
6. Allow child and family to express feelings.
7. Determine need for financial assistance.
8. Mobilize support systems.
9. Assist family in completing unfinished business; refer to specialist if needed.

E.   **Evaluation**
1. Child and family avail themselves of support.
2. Child and family express feelings freely.
3. Child experiences minimal or no physical discomfort.

II. Nonorganic failure to thrive (NFTT)

A.   **Description: weight remains below the fifth percentile of weight for children of same age.**

      1. **Failure to gain weight results from psychosocial causes, such as deficient parent–child relationship (most common cause).**

B.   **Etiology and incidence**
1. NFTT is seen most often in infants.
2. Problem may result from parental deprivation. If so, growth and development should improve with nurturing.
3. Other causes include parents' inadequate nutritional information, deficient parental care, and disturbance in parent–child attachment.

C.   **Clinical assessment findings**
1. Growth below 5%; developmental retardation; apathy
2. Poor hygiene, withdrawn behavior, feeding problems
3. No fear of strangers, eye contact avoidance, stiff or flaccid posture, minimal smiling

D.   **Nursing diagnoses**
1. Anxiety
2. Compromised, ineffective family coping
3. Altered family processes
4. Altered growth and development
5. Ineffective infant feeding pattern
6. Risk for injury
7. Knowledge deficit

        8. Altered nutrition: less than body requirements
        9. Altered parenting
       10. Altered role performance

  D. **Planning and implementation**
        1. Monitor feeding patterns.
        2. Observe parent–child interaction and temperament; observe parents' general behaviors.
        3. Structure feeding.
        4. Provide appropriate developmental stimulation, parental instruction, and referrals.

  E. **Evaluation**
        1. Child will gain appropriate weight and reach appropriate developmental status.
        2. Parents will exhibit appropriate parenting behaviors.

III. Child abuse

  A. **Description: acts of commission or omission by caregivers that prevent a child from actualizing his or her potential growth and development.**

  B. **Etiology and incidence**
        1. In 1992, about 2.7 million children were reported abused or neglected in the United States.
        2. Predisposing influences
            a. *Parental factors* involve severe punishment as children, poor impulse control, free expression of violence, social isolation, poor social-emotional support system, low self-esteem, substance abuse
            b. *Child factors* involve temperament ("misfit"); illness, disability, and developmental delay; typically no other siblings; illegitimacy; hyperkinesis; resemblance to someone the parent does not like; bonding failure; problem pregnancy, delivery or prematurity
            c. *Environmental factors* (all socioeconomic groups) involve chronic stress (divorce, poverty) and frequent relocation

  C. **Clinical assessment findings**
        1. Physical abuse (intentional infliction of injury to child)
            a. Physical indicators include cutaneous injuries (different stages of bruises in odd locations, possibly shaped like object responsible for bruise); burns (cigarette marks, "glove-stocking marks"); fractures (*e.g.*, femoral spiral fracture in infant); head injuries (especially in a young child); eye injuries (*e.g.*, conjunctival hemorrhages seen in "shaken baby syndrome"); mouth injuries; poisonings; drownings; repetitive accidents.
            b. Behavioral indicators include wariness of adults; frightened

of parents; suffers pain without crying; afraid to go home; superficial relationships; overly friendly; reports injury by parents; exhibits attention-seeking behaviors.

2. **Munchausen's syndrome by proxy (illness that is fabricated or induced by one person onto another, usually mother to child)**
   a. Munchausen's syndrome by proxy is difficult to confirm.
   b. Indicators include unexplained, prolonged, or extremely rare illnesses; discrepancies between history and clinical findings; illness that is unresponsive to treatment; symptoms that occur only when the parent is present; parent overly interested in health care team members; parent overly attentive to the child; and family members with similar symptoms.

3. Emotional abuse (deliberate attempt to destroy child's self-esteem or competence)
   a. Physical indicators include failure to thrive; developmental lags; feeding problems; enuresis; sleep problems.
   b. Behavioral indicators include habit disorders (rocking, biting, hair pulling); withdrawal; unusual fearfulness; conduct problems; behavioral extremes (very passive or very aggressive); age-inappropriate behaviors; attempted suicide.

4. Neglect (deprivation of necessities)
   a. Physical indicators include failure to thrive (FTT), malnutrition, constant hunger, poor hygiene, inappropriate clothing, bald patches on infant, lack of adequate supervision, abandonment, and poor health care.
   b. Behavioral indicators include dull, inactive infant; begging or stealing food; school attendance problems (arrives early, leaves late); drug and alcohol (D & A) abuse; delinquency; reports having no caretaker.

4. Sexual abuse (contacts or interactions between a child and an adult when the child is used for sexual stimulation of an adult)
   a. **In many cases, there are no overt signs of sexual abuse.**
   b. Possible physical indicators include difficulty walking or sitting; torn, stained, bloody underclothes; gross evidence of trauma (genital, oral, anal); pain; itching; sexually transmitted diseases (STDs); discharge; pregnancy; weight loss; eating disorders; vague somatic complaints.
   c. Behavioral indicators
      (1) Under age 5: regression, feeding or toileting disturbances, temper tantrums, requests for frequent panty changes, seductive behavior
      (2) Ages 5 to 10: school problems, night terrors, sleep

problems, anxieties, withdrawal, refusal of physical activity, inappropriate behaviors

    (3) Adolescence: school problems, running away, delinquency, promiscuity, drug and alcohol abuse, eating disorders, depression, and other significant psychological problems, such as suicide attempts

D. Nursing diagnoses
1. Post-trauma response
2. Unilateral neglect
3. Altered role performance
4. Risk for injury
5. Powerlessness

E. Planning and implementation

1. **See that the child is free from further harm and report the incident to the proper authorities.**
2. Demonstrate acceptance of child during physical assessment.
3. Carefully assess the child's emotional status and behavior.
4. Provide the child with positive attention and age-appropriate play and activities.
5. Document assessment findings carefully and objectively.
6. Collaborate with the multidisciplinary team concerning immediate and long-term therapies to prevent further abuse.
7. Work with caregivers on changing factors that led to the abuse.

F. Evaluation
1. The child experiences no further harm.
2. The child's physical injuries heal.
3. The child's emotional injuries are healing with therapy through an appropriate health care professional.
4. Appropriate interventions aimed at effecting behavioral changes in caregivers are progressing.

IV. School phobia
A. Description: an abnormal, persistent fear of attending school.
B. Etiology and incidence
1. Typically related to a dreaded school situation (*e.g.*, a bully), fear of leaving home, or separation anxiety

C. Clinical assessment findings
1. Common physiologic manifestations include nausea, vomiting, headache, and stomachache.
2. Physical symptoms tend to resolve when child is allowed to stay home from school.

D. Nursing diagnoses
1. Fear
2. Ineffective individual coping

       3. Altered growth and development

       4. Impaired social interaction

  E. **Planning and implementation**

       1. Collaborate with the child's parents, teacher, and school counselor to determine the cause of the problem and identify possible solutions.

       2. Discuss the problem and possible causes and solutions with the child.

       3. Implement plans to return the child to school. The child should attend school even during resolution of the problem; keeping the child out of school only reinforces feelings of worthlessness, dependency, and inability to cope.

  F. **Evaluation**

       1. The child attends school regularly.

       2. The child freely discusses any problems with parents, teacher, or school counselor.

       3. The child experiences no physiologic symptoms.

V. **Adolescent pregnancy**

  A. **Description: pregnancy before age 19, usually unplanned and out of wedlock.**

       1. Traditionally, but no longer, considered hazardous to the fetus, but still viewed as socially, economically, psychologically, and educationally handicapping to the mother

       2. Mortality declining, but morbidity high

  B. **Etiology and incidence**

       1. Various theories explain the causes of adolescent pregnancy, among them, earlier sexual activity and ignorance of reliable contraceptive methods.

       2. In the United States, about 1 million females under age 20 (or 1 in 10 female adolescents) become pregnant each year.

  C. **Complications**

       1. **Complications of teenage pregnancy include preeclampsia, iron-deficiency anemia, prolonged labor, and an increased incidence of premature births.**

       2. A pregnant adolescent commonly faces many crises:

          a. Early crises include recognizing the pregnancy and informing her partner and her parents.

          b. Prenatal crises include deciding whether to carry the fetus to term or seek an abortion; providing financial, medical, and nutritional needs; and dealing with interpersonal relationships at home and at school.

          c. Intrapartal crises revolve around environmental control and depersonalization issues.

          d. Common postpartal crises include deciding whether to keep the infant or put it up for adoption, coping with body image changes, and dealing with bonding and parenting issues.

D. **Clinical assessment findings**
1. Because an adolescent commonly denies pregnancy, early recognition by a parent or health care provider may be crucial to timely initiation of prenatal care.
2. Initial signs include cessation of menstrual periods and breast enlargement.

E. **Nursing diagnoses**
1. Knowledge deficit
2. Altered sexuality patterns
3. Risk for altered parenting

F. **Planning and implementation**
1. In collaboration with the pregnant adolescent and her support persons, implement a plan of care that includes prenatal health care; proper nutritional intake; exercise; avoidance of alcohol, nonprescribed drugs, cigarettes, and illicit drugs; emotional support; plans for delivery; plans for infant care; and anticipatory guidance about birth control and future sexual conduct.
2. Assess for complications of pregnancy.

G. **Evaluation**
1. The adolescent understands and follows the plan of care.
2. The adolescent who decides to carry the fetus to term delivers a healthy infant.
3. The adolescent is comfortable with the decision she has made.

VI. **Suicide**

A. **Description: estructive, self-inflicted actions that result in actual or attempted self-harm or death; the intentional ending of one's life.**

B. **Etiology and incidence**
1. **Suicide is the third leading cause of death in adolescents.**
2. The common stresses of adolescence, compounded by limited problem-solving abilities, sometimes lead to harmful, life-threatening behaviors. Adolescents who are depressed, psychotic, or substance abusers are at highest risk.
3. Common contributing factors include family dysfunction and low self-esteem. An adolescent who attempts or successfully completes suicide typically has a family history of suicide or suicidal behavior.

C. **Clinical assessment findings**
1. Depression usually precedes suicide; signs of depression may be overt or subtle.
2. **Danger signs include lethargy, malaise, inability to sleep or early morning awakening, loss of appetite or overeating, ex-**

cessive crying, giving away cherished possessions, preoccu-
pation with death or death themes (*e.g.*, music, art, or
movies with death themes), and statement of intention to
commit suicide.

D. **Nursing diagnoses**

1. Altered thought process
2. Social isolation
3. Chronic low self-esteem
4. Ineffective individual coping
5. Hopelessness
6. Spiritual distress

E. **Planning and implementation**

1. Provide information for teachers, parents, and adolescents about
   risk factors, counseling available to adolescents, and stress-re-
   duction and problem-solving strategies.
2. Provide crisis intervention for an adolescent who gestures or attempts suicide and plan for family follow-up care. Ensure that
   the adolescent understands that he or she must cease or not implement this destructive behavior.
3. Arrange for counseling and hospitalization if necessary; refer the
   adolescent and the family to a professional therapist who will
   work with them through the crisis.
4. After a successful suicide, counsel the adolescent's family and
   friends to help them understand and work through their grief.

G. **Evaluation**

1. An adolescent who has made suicide attempts or gestures displays improved self-esteem, positive behaviors, and more effective coping and problem-solving strategies.
2. Family and friends of an adolescent who successfully committed
   suicide work through their grief and resolve the loss over time.

VII. **Attention deficit/hyperactivity disorder (ADHD)**

A. **Description: ADHD is the latest terminology used to refer to a
persistent pattern of inattention or hyperactivity with impulsivity. The pattern is pronounced and more frequent than in other
children at comparable development levels.**

1. The disorder is classified in three subtypes:
   a. Combined type (most common type): The individual has
      six or more symptoms of inattention and six or more
      symptoms of hypersensitivity and impulsivity.
   b. Predominantly inattentive type: The individual has six or
      more symptoms of inattention but fewer than six of hyper-
      activity with impulsivity.
   c. Predominantly hyperactive/impulsive type: The individual
      has six or more symptoms of hyperactivity and impulsivity
      but fewer than six of inattention.

3. For most children, the disorder is relatively stable through early adolescence and, in most, symptoms subside between late adolescence and early adulthood. A few individuals experience the full range of ADHD symptoms into middle adulthood.

B. **Etiology and incidence**

1. The etiology is uncertain and may be related to any illness or trauma affecting the brain at any stage of development. Multiple causes are probably involved. Some experts think the disorder is physiologic because many persons with ADHD respond to medications classified as central nervous system (CNS) stimulants.

2. The disorder is more prominent in boys than girls, with ratios reported from 4:1 to 7:1.

C. **Clinical assessment findings**

1. The behaviors observed are not unusual aspects of child behavior; the difference is in the quality of motor activity and developmentally inappropriate inattention, impulsivity, and hyperactivity the child displays.

2. Manifestations vary in number and severity.

3. Most behaviors are observed at an early age, but learning disabilities may not become apparent until the child is in school.

4. The diagnosis of ADHD is based on the following specific criteria proposed by the American Psychiatric Association in the *Diagnostic and Statistical Manual of Mental Disorders (DSM IV)*:

   a. Either (1) or (2)

      (1) Six or more symptoms of inattention that have persisted for at least 6 months to a degree that is maladaptive and inconsistent with developmental level. The child fails to give close attention to details or makes careless mistakes; often has difficulty sustaining attention in tasks or play; often does not seem to listen when spoken to; often does not follow through on instructions; often has difficulty organizing; often avoids or dislikes tasks that require sustained mental effort; often loses things necessary for tasks; is often easily distracted; is often forgetful of daily activities.

      (2) Six or more symptoms of hyperactivity/impulsivity that have persisted for at least 6 months to a degree that is maladaptive and inconsistent with developmental level–(hyperactivity) often fidgets or squirms; often leaves seat in classroom; often runs or climbs excessively or during inappropriate times; often has difficulty playing quietly; is often "on the go"; often talks excessively; (impulsivity) often blurts out answers before questions are complete; often has difficulty waiting turn; often interrupts or intrudes on others.

       b. Some symptoms causing impairment were present before age 7 years.

       c. Some impairment is present in two or more settings (home, school).

       d. There must be clear evidence of social, academic, or occupational functioning.

       e. Symptoms do not occur during episodes of pervasive developmental disorder, schizophrenia or other psychotic disorder, and are not better accounted for by any other mental disorder.

D. Nursing diagnoses

    1. Impaired adjustment

    2. Anxiety

    3. Risk for ineffective individual coping

    4. Risk for ineffective family coping

    5. Potential for altered family processes

    6. Altered growth and development

    7. Risk for altered parenting

    8. Risk of impaired social interaction

    9. Risk for injury

E. Planning and implementation

    1. Actively participate in all aspects of managing child with ADHD.

    2. Serve as a liaison between other health care professionals and educators.

    3. Allow parents to vent their feelings.

    4. Assist parents in understanding the importance and longevity of treatment.

    5. Evaluate effectiveness of medication by questioning parents, child and teachers, and by direct observation.

    6. Teach the parents and the child about the nature of the disorder; provide reading material and refer to support groups.

    7. Teach parents about treatment plan and medications:

       a. Advise them that management usually involves a multiple approach including medication, such as methylphenidate (Ritalin), dextroamphetamine (Dexedrine), magnesium pemoline (Cylert), and tricyclic antidepressants; family counseling and education; behavioral and psychotherapy; proper classroom placement; and environmental manipulation.

       b. Explain that some medications (*e.g.*, pemoline) require 2 to 3 weeks to achieve the desired effects; others begin at low dosages, which are increased until the desired effect is achieved.

       c. Inform parents about possible medication side effects such as anorexia, blurred vision, and sleeplessness.

       d. If the child takes methylphenidate (Ritalin):

(1) Suggest small frequent meals and finger-food snacks to help compensate for anorexia induced by medication.

(2) Reduce sleeplessness by administering medication earlier in the day.

(3) Carefully monitor growth because methylphenidate may also retard growth. As appropriate, the health care team may recommend medication "holidays and vacations" on weekends and during the summer or other nonschool periods.

e. If the child takes tricyclic antidepressants, point out the importance of regular dental care because these medications cause increased dental caries. Meticulous dental care is needed.

f. To prevent accidents, warn parents to keep these drugs out of children's reach.

8. Assist families in learning environmental manipulation: using organizational charts; decreasing distractions; and modeling positive behaviors. Encourage consistency both at home and at school.

9. Encourage appropriate placement in classrooms equipped for special training.

10. Encourage counseling for children and families who demonstrate anxiety or depression.

F. Evaluation

1. The child will function to his or her fullest capacity at both home and at school.

2. The family demonstrates the ability to manage the child's behavior.

Bibliography

American Psychiatric Association (1994). *Diagnostic and Statistical Manual of Mental Disorders*, 4th ed. Washington, DC: APA.

Castiglia, P.T. & Harbin, R.B. (1993). *Child Health Care: Process and Practice*. Philadelphia: J.B. Lippincott.

Derstewitz, R.A. (1993). *Ambulatory Pediatric Care*. Philadelphia: J.B. Lippincott.

Engel, J. (1993). *Pocket Guide to Pediatric Assessment*, 2nd ed. St. Louis: C.V. Mosby.

Garfinkel, B., Carlson, G., & Weller, E. (1990). *Psychiatric Disorders in Children and Adolescents*. Philadelphia: W.B. Saunders.

Jackson, D.B. & Saunders, R.B. (1993). *Child Health Nursing: A Comprehensive Approach to the Care of Children and Their Families*. Philadelphia: J.B. Lippincott.

Rankin, S.H. & Stallings, K.D. (1990). *Patient Education: Issues, Principles, and Practices*, 2nd ed. Philadelphia: J.B. Lippincott.

Wong, D.L. (1993). *Whaley and Wong's Essentials of Pediatric Nursing*, 4th ed. St. Louis: C.V. Mosby.

Wong, D.L. (1995). *Whaley & Wong's Nursing Care of Infants and Children*, 5th ed. St. Louis: C.V. Mosby.

STUDY QUESTIONS

1. A 6-year-old boy's pet gerbil just died. Which of the following is he most likely to say?
   a. "He's not real dead."
   b. "The boogieman got him."
   c. "What can he eat now?"
   d. "I'll be good so I won't die."

2. All of the following are appropriate nursing diagnoses for nonorganic failure to thrive (NFTT) except:
   a. Altered growth and development
   b. Altered breathing pattern
   c. Altered parenting
   d. Risk for injury

3. The nurse notes that a 3-year-old is engaging in explicit sexual behavior during doll play. The nurse should suspect that:
   a. The child is exhibiting normal preschool curiosity.
   b. The child is acting out personal experiences.
   c. The child does not know how to play with dolls.
   d. The child is probably developmentally delayed.

4. When assessing a family for potential child abuse risks, the nurse would observe for all of the following, except:
   a. Chronic stress
   b. Low socioeconomic status
   c. Developmental delays
   d. Problem pregnancies

5. A mother administers laxatives to her infant to deliberately induce diarrhea. This is an example of:
   a. Nonorganic failure to thrive
   b. Munchausen's by proxy
   c. Emotional child abuse
   d. Medical child neglect

6. Appropriate nursing interventions for a child with school phobia include all of the following except:
   a. Keeping child home until phobia subsides
   b. Collaborating with teachers and counselors
   c. Allowing child to verbalize the problem
   d. Discussing possible solutions with child and parents

7. Which of the following must be monitored carefully in the child with ADHD who is receiving methylphenidate (Ritalin)?
   a. Dental health
   b. Mouth dryness
   c. Height and weight
   d. Excessive appetite

For additional questions, see
Lippincott's Self-Study Series Software
Available at your bookstore

ANSWER KEY

1. **Correct response: a**
   A 6-year-old views death in "degrees," so the child could consider that the pet is "not real dead."
   b. Personification of death occurs in ages 7 to 9 years.
   c. Attributing life qualities to the dead occurs during ages 3 to 5.
   d. The thinking that being good will avoid death occurs in children between ages 7 and 9.
   Analysis/Psychosocial/Planning

2. **Correct response: b**
   There is no organic cause for NFTT; therefore, the diagnosis of Altered breathing pattern is unlikely.
   a, c, and d. All are appropriate nursing diagnoses for NFTT because it is usually caused by parental deprivation (altered parenting), leads to abnormal development (altered growth and development), and deficits may lead to injury (risk for injury).
   Application/Psychosocial/Analysis(Dx)

3. **Correct response: b**
   Preschoolers should be developmentally incapable of demonstrating explicit sexual behavior. If a child does so, the child has been exposed to such behavior, and sexual abuse should be suspected.
   a. This is not characteristic of preschool development.
   c. This is irrelevant.
   d. This is not symptomatic of developmental delay.
   Analysis/Psychosocial/Assessment

4. **Correct response: b**
   Child abuse occurs in all socioeconomic groups.
   a, c, and d. All of these are risk factors for child abuse and, therefore, should be assessed.
   Analysis/Psychosocial/Assessment

5. **Correct response: b**
   Munchausen's by proxy is a syndrome by which one person (the mother of father) deliberately fabricates or causes illness in another (the child) in order to call attention to themselves.
   a. NOFTT is a syndrome in which a child's growth falls below the fifth percentile for nonorganic reasons, such as parental deprivation.
   c. Emotional child abuse occurs when an adult deliberately attempts to destroy the self-esteem of a child.
   d. Medical neglect occurs when the responsible adult fails to procure needed medical care for his or her child.
   Analysis/Psychosocial/Assessment

6. **Correct response: a**
   Keeping the child home reinforces feelings of worthlessness and dependency.
   b. Allowing the child to verbalize helps the child to ventilate feelings and may help to uncover causes and solutions.
   c. Collaboration may lead to uncovering the cause of the phobia and to the development of solutions.
   d. The child should participate in developing possible solutions.
   Application/Psychosocial/Implementation

7. **Correct response: c**
   Methylphenidate (Ritalin) can suppress growth; therefore, growth must be carefully monitored.
   a and b. Dental caries and mouth dryness are associated with tricyclic antidepressants.
   d. Ritalin is more likely to suppress appetite, not increase it.
   Knowledge/Physiologic/Assessment

Immunity and

Infectious Diseases

9

I. Immune system overview

A. Purpose of immune system

1. The immune system acts to neutralize, eliminate, or destroy microorganisms that penetrate or invade the body's internal environment before the invaders (organisms and substances) can multiply or overwhelm the body's defense mechanisms.

2. The immune system must work against invaders (antigens) so as not to harm the host.

    a. Increased immune function (too much immune activity) may damage healthy tissue.

    b. Decreased immune system function (too little activity) increases the risk of infection.

B. Structures and functions

1. The white blood cells (WBCs) (*i.e.*, the leukocytes) are the workhorses of the immune system. The various kinds of WBCs protect the body from invaders by:

    a. Recognizing and distinguishing indigenous cells ("self") from foreign, invading organisms ("nonself")

    b. Activating phagocytic cells (monocytes and macrophages) to engulf and destroy the invaders and unhealthy cells

    c. Mobilizing complement (immune system substances that trigger a disintegration process known as cytolysis)

    d. Producing antibodies against foreign invaders

2. The WBCs are composed of various kinds of cells: granulocytes, such as neutrophils, eosinophils, and basophils, and agranulocytes, such as monocytes (or macrophages) and lymphocytes. The lymphocytes, which differentiate into B lymphocytes (B cells) and T lymphocytes (T cells), play major roles in humoral and cell-mediated immunity, respectively.

3. The immune system is responsible for three kinds of responses: inflammation (or inflammatory response), humoral (or antibody) immunity, and cell-mediated (or cellular) immunity.

C. Inflammatory response (nonspecific response to invasion)

1. Offers immediate but short-term protection.

2. Generates symptoms (redness, heat, swelling, pain).

3. Occurs as a response to infection (*e.g.*, otitis media) or tissue injury (*e.g.*, sprain, incision, blister).

4. Mobilizes leukocytes (neutrophils, macrophages, eosinophils, basophils) in a search-and-destroy-type action known as phagocytosis, whereby the phagocytic cells are exposed, attracted to, and adhered to the invader. Then they ingest and destroy the invader.

D. Humoral (antibody) immunity

1. B lymphocytes become sensitized to specific proteins or antigens ("invaders") and produce antibodies directly against specific proteins as follows:

      a.   Antigen exposure: Circulating immune cells encounter invaders (antigens).

      b.   Antigen recognition: Circulating macrophages and CD4+ marker cells (a kind of T cell) recognize antigens.

      c.   Lymphocyte sensitization: Lymphocytes differentiate into two types of cells, *plasma cells* that immediately produce antibody (immunoglobulin) against specific antigen (Table 9-1), and *memory cells* that remain dormant and sensitized, responding later when the same antigen invades again.

      d.   Antibody release: Plasma cells release antibody.

      e.   Antibody binds with antigen (not lethal).

      f.   Antibody-binding reactions (lethal) occur. Possible reactions are known as agglutination, lysis, complement fixation, precipitation, and neutralization. All are aimed at destroying or incapacitating the antigen.

      g.   The immune system sustains memory (immunity).

    2.   Antibody activity mobilizes complement, a group of proteins (C1 through C9) that cause a cascade of enzymatic actions that kill the identified antigens.

E.   Cell-mediated (cellular) immunity

    1.   A variety of leukocyte actions. Leukocytes must recognize self and invaders and respond by exerting direct cytotoxic action or by assisting cytotoxic action of other cells.

    2.   There are 50 different known T cells active in cell-mediated immunity. Among them:

      a.   Helper T cells (CD4+): These cells act as phagocytes, stim-

TABLE 9-1.
Characteristics of Immunoglobulin

TYPE	CHARACTERISTIC
IgA	Prevents antigens from entering internal environment Inhibits viruses and bacteria from entering skin or mucosa Circulating levels normally low
IgG	Primarily responsible for most acquired immunity Neutralizes toxins Freely crosses placenta (natural passive immunity) Most abundant
IgM	Responds to bacteria Forms anti-A and anti-B antibodies in blood May initiate autoimmune response
IgE	Associated with basophil and mast cells Responsible for immediate hypersensitivity responses Plays role in parasitic infections
IgD	Function unclear

ulate other WBCs, such as B cells; secrete lymphokines (*e.g.*, interleukin-2, interferon); stimulate macrophages for inflammatory responses.

    b.   Cytotoxic cells: These cells form antibody-like substances and direct the lysis and death of invaders.

    c.   Suppressor cells ($CD8^+$): These cells prevent overreaction or hypersensitivity; directly oppose $CD4^+$ cells. The ratio of $CD4^+$ to $CD8^+$ cells is 2:1. A decrease in $CD4^+$ cells signifies immunosuppression; a decrease in $CD8^+$ cells signifies hypersensitivity reactions.

    d.   Killer T cells secrete lymphokines to destroy and remove toxins.

F. Immune system development

    1.   The newborn receives significant amounts of IgG from the mother, which confers immunity for about 3 months against antigens to which the mother was exposed. During the first 2 months of life, the infant begins to synthesize IgG and reaches about 40% of adult levels by 1 year.

    2.   Significant amounts of IgM are produced at birth, and adult levels are achieved by about 9 months. IgA, IgD, and IgE are produced more gradually. Maximal levels are reached in early childhood.

    3.   Cell-mediated immunity is poorly developed before age 6 years.

II. Immunizations

    A. Types of immunity

        1.   Naturally acquired active: Immune system makes antibodies after exposure to disease.

        2.   Naturally acquired passive: Antibodies are received passively but naturally (via placenta and colostrum).

        3.   Artificially acquired active: Ingested or injected medically engineered substances stimulate immune response against specific disease.

        4.   Artificially acquired passive: Injected antibodies provide immunity without stimulating immune response.

    B. Types of vaccines

        1.   Live attenuated

            a.   Pathogen is treated with chemicals or heat to reduce the virulence of the organism.

            b.   Examples include measles, mumps, rubella (MMR) vaccine and Sabin polio vaccine.

        2.   Inactivated

            a.   Toxoid (*e.g.*, tetanus, diphtheria) is treated with formalin or heat, which yields a nontoxic but still antigenic agent.

            b.   Killed or diffusible virus (*e.g.*, pertussis, Hib, HB) uses killed organisms or parts of organisms to produce immunity.

C. **Routine immunizations (Table 9-2)**

    1. Diphtheria

        a. Commonly administered with tetanus (in children <7 years old as DT, >7 years as dT) or with tetanus and pertussis (7 years and under as DPT)

        b. Contraindications: immediate anaphylaxis or encephalopathy within 7 days; not contraindicated in pregnancy, but should wait until second trimester.

        c. Side effects: relatively none.

    2. Pertussis

        a. Whole cell (used for primary series); acellular (used for boosters)

        b. Contraindications: previous severe reactions; neurologic problems such as uncontrolled or poorly managed seizure disorders

        c. Side effects

            (1) Local: redness, tenderness and swelling at site

            (2) Mild: fever (under 105°F), crying, irritability

            (3) Severe: high-pitched cry, fever (over 105°F), convulsions, hypotonia; encephalopathy with brain damage and death

            (4) Fewer side effects associated with acellular vaccine

    3. Tetanus

        a. Toxoid used as routine immunization (tetanus immunoglobulin is passive and tetanus antitoxin is rarely used)

TABLE 9-2.
Recommended Childhood Immunization Schedule

RECOMMENDED AGE	IMMUNIZATION	ROUTE
Birth–2 months	HB (1st)	IM
2–4 months	HB (2nd)	IM
2 months	DTP, Hib, OPV	IM, IM, PO
4 months	DTP, Hib, OPV	IM, IM, PO
6 months	DTP, Hib	IM, IM
6–18 months	HB (3rd), OPV	IM, PO
12–15 months	Hib, MMR	IM, SQ
12–18 months	DTP or DTaP (at 15 mo)	IM, IM
4–6 years	DTP or DTaP, MMR, OPV	IM, SQ, PO
11–12 years	MMR (if not received at 4–6 years)	SQ
11–16 years	Td	IM

(From Centers for Disease Control and Prevention. Recommended Childhood Immunization Schedule—United States January 1995. Approved by the Advisory Committee on Immunization Practices (ACIP), the American Academy of Pediatrics (AAP), and the American Academy of Family Physicians (AAFP).)

      b.   Contraindications: previous anaphylaxis or severe reaction

      c.   Side effects: pain at injection site, anaphylaxis (rare)

4.   Polio (both vaccine forms trivalent)

      a.   Oral polio vaccine (OPV) (*e.g.*, Sabin, oral polio)

          (1) Vaccine is attenuated and is the one usually used because it is more effective.

          (2) Contraindications include congenital immunodeficiency diseases; acquired immunodeficiency diseases; altered immune response (steroids, leukemia, chemotherapy) or family members with any of these; and pregnancy.

          (3) Side effects are few if any. OPV may shed in stools and be transmitted to others.

      b.   Trivalent inactivated polio vaccine (TIPV) (*e.g.*, Salk) injected

          (1) Vaccine is inactivated and usually is used when OPV is contraindicated.

          (2) Contraindications include anaphylactic reaction to streptomycin.

5.   Measles: Vaccine should be administered after 12 months of age after effectiveness of maternal antibodies subsides.

6.   Mumps: same as measles

7.   Rubella: same as measles

8.   MMR (measles, mumps and rubella)

      a.   Contraindications include immunosuppression, except human immunodeficiency virus (HIV) disease; pregnancy; allergy to eggs and neomycin.

      b.   Side effects include transient rash, pruritus, low-grade fever; arthralgia and transient arthritis from rubella, especially in adults. Measles vaccine can cause false-negative tine test (TB test) results.

9.   *Haemophilus influenzae* type B (Hib)

      a.   Second-generation, Hib conjugate, is primarily used. Vaccine comes in two types, which are not interchangeable:

          (1) HibTITER (Praxis Biologics) four-dose schedule of three primary injections plus booster at 15 months

          (2) PedvaxHIB (Merck Sharpe & Dohme) three-dose schedule of two primary injections plus booster at 12 months

      b.   No contraindications

      c.   Side effects: relatively none; possibly discomfort and low-grade fever.

10.   Hepatitis B (HB)

      a.   Recommended for universal immunization.

      b.   Two available vaccines include Recombivax HB (Merck Sharpe & Dohme) and Engerix-B (SmithKline Beecham).

       c.   Three doses recommended at 0- ,1- , and 6-month intervals.

       d.   Side effects include redness and tenderness at site (rare).

  11. Tetramune: combination diphtheria, tetanus, pertussis (DTP) and Hib

  12. Varivax (varicella)

       a.   Recommended at 12 months (later if not immunized and if did not have varicella; children over 13 years require two doses, 4 to 8 weeks apart)

       b.   Live vaccine

       c.   Contraindications: history of hypersensitivity to components; history of anaphylactoid reaction to neomycin; immunosuppression, including AIDS; active untreated tuberculosis; any active febrile illness; pregnancy

D. **Immunization schedule: Most children should have most of their scheduled immunizations by the time they enter elementary school (see Table 9-2 for the recommended order of immunizations).**

E. General contraindications

  1. Do not provide immunization during severe febrile illness.

  2. Avoid giving live virus to clients with impaired immune system (the exception is MMR for children with HIV disease).

  3. Postpone live virus immunization for 3 months in children who have just received passive immunity through blood transfusions, immunoglobulin, or maternal antibodies.

  4. Avoid live virus immunization in pregnancy and in women likely to become pregnant within 3 months.

  5. Do not give vaccine if client is allergic to vaccine or its components.

F. Nonmandatory immunizations

  1. Influenza virus vaccine

       a.   Provides protection against strains of influenza

       b.   Recommended for children over 6 months old who have chronic illnesses or HIV disease or who are receiving long-term aspirin therapy (risk for Reye's syndrome)

       c.   Should be administered in the fall and repeated yearly; two doses 4 weeks apart for children under 12 years; one dose for those over 12.

       d.   Contraindicated in children allergic to eggs

       e.   May be given with other childhood immunizations

  2. Pneumococcal vaccine

       a.   Provides protection against several strains of *Streptococcus pneumoniae*

       b.   Recommended for children age 2 and older who have sickle cell anemia, asplenia, HIV, and Hodgkin's lymphoma by subcutaneous (SQ) or intramuscular (IM) route; revaccination not recommended.

c.   Should be deferred in pregnancy
3.   Meningococcal vaccine
a.   Provides protection against *Neisseria meningitides*
b.   Recommended for children age 2 and older with terminal complement deficiencies and anatomic or functional asplenia
c.   Duration of protection unknown; safety during pregnancy not established

G.   Immunoglobulin

1.   Human serum fraction containing gamma globulin antibodies (IgG) that provide passive immunity in a variety of infections are useful in children with immunodeficiency syndromes and idiopathic thrombocytopenia purpura (ITP). Specific immunoglobulin are also available:
a.   TIG (tetanus immunoglobulin)
b.   HIG (hepatitis immunoglobulin)
c.   ZIG (zoster immunoglobulin, chicken pox)
2.   Specific immunoglobulin is used when client is exposed.
3.   Contraindications to use include hypersensitivity; safety in pregnancy has not been established.
4.   Side effects include pain, tenderness, muscle stiffness at site, and possible systemic reactions such as lightheadedness, headache, chest pain, nausea, urticaria, arthralgia.

III.   Sepsis

A.   Description: generalized bacterial infection occurring in the first month of life with high mortality.

B.   Etiology and incidence

1.   It is believed that all neonatal infections are opportunistic and that any bacteria is capable of causing sepsis.

2.   **Group B streptococcus is the most common cause of sepsis, followed by *Escherichia coli*, Group A streptococcus, and *Streptococcus viridans*.**

C.   Pathophysiology and management

1.   Immune defense mechanisms in neonates are immature, posing the potential for rapid invasion, spread, and multiplication of infecting organisms. The newborn is unable to localize infections.

D.   Clinical assessment findings

1.   Initial signs and symptoms include poor sucking and feeding, weak cry, lethargy, and irritability followed by pallor, cyanosis, or mottling; decreased pain response; hypotension; abnormal heartbeat (tachycardia); irregular respirations; jaundice; dehydration; temperature instability (may be hypothermic or hyperthermic); gastrointestinal disturbances; seizures; hypotonia; tremors; full fontanel; cardiac arrest.

        3. The most common presentation for late onset sepsis (up to age 4 months) is meningitis.

   E. **Diagnostic assessment findings**
        1. Blood culture may disclose offending organism.
        2. Urine culture and cerebrospinal fluid (CSF) analysis (by lumbar puncture) also are performed to detect organisms.
        3. Elevated WBC count with increased immature neutrophils suggests infection as do increased erythrocyte sedimentation rate (ESR) and C-reactive protein (CRP) levels.

   F. **Nursing diagnoses**
        1. Hypothermia or hyperthermia
        2. Risk for infection
        3. Risk for injury
        4. Altered tissue perfusion
        5. Ineffective breathing pattern

   G. **Planning and implementation**
        1. Provide care similar to that given to a high-risk newborn; set the following outcomes or goals:
            a. Maintain a patent airway.
            b. Provide a neutral thermal environment.
            c. Protect the infant from increased infection. As prescribed, administer antibiotic therapy for 7 to 10 days if culture results are positive and discontinue therapy as prescribed if culture results are negative (usually in 3 days).
            d. Provide adequate nutrition.
        2. **Anticipate sepsis. Immediate recognition of the onset of sepsis is crucial.**
        3. Administer medications as prescribed.
        4. Monitor the infant for signs of impending shock.

   H. **Evaluation**
        1. Infection has been detected early and vigorous treatment initiated.
        2. The chances for survival with little or no neurologic deficits have increased.

IV. **Meningitis**
   A. **Description: an infection of the meninges usually caused by bacterial invasion and less commonly by viruses. Prognosis depends on age, organism, and child's response to therapy.**
   B. **Etiology and incidence**
        1. Most cases occur between ages 1 month and 5 years, with infants under 12 months being the most susceptible to bacterial meningitis.

2. *Haemophilus influenzae, Neisseria meningitides,* and *Diplococcus pneumoniae* are the most common organisms after the neonatal period.
3. *Escherichia coli* and group B streptococcus are the most common organisms in the neonate.
4. Bacterial meningitis is fatal if not treated immediately.
5. Viral meningitis (caused by Coxsackie, echovirus, or mumps) is a self-limiting disease lasting 7 to 10 days.

C. Pathophysiology and management
1. In bacterial meningitis, the bacteria enter the meninges through the blood stream and spread through the CSF; the infection may also result directly through trauma or neurosurgery.
2. The pathogen acts as a toxin, creating a meningeal inflammatory response and a resultant release of purulent exudate; the infection spreads quickly through the exudate. Exudate can cover the choroid plexus and obstruct the arachnoid villi, causing hydrocephalus.
3. Vascular congestion and inflammation leads to cerebral edema, which may produce increased intracranial pressure (ICP); necrosis of brain cells can cause permanent damage and death.

D. Clinical assessment findings
1. **Children under 2 years old do not display the characteristic signs of meningitis. Instead, they may exhibit poor feeding, irritability and lethargy, high-pitched cry, bulging fontanel, fever or low temperature, and a resistance to being held; later in the disease opisthotonos (hyperextension of the neck and spine) may be apparent.**
2. **Older children may start with respiratory or gastrointestinal problems, then nuchal rigidity (stiff neck), headache, and tripod posturing. Kernig's sign (pain and resistance to knee extension when the child is in the supine position with knees and hips flexed) and Brudzinski's sign (flexion of the knees and hips when the neck is flexed with the child in the supine position). A petechial rash may also appear.**

E. Diagnostic assessment findings
1. CSF analysis (by lumbar puncture) establishes both the diagnosis (CSF may be cloudy, WBC count is elevated, protein level is elevated and glucose level is decreased) and the causative agent. Note: Lumbar puncture is not performed if the child has increased intracranial pressure (ICP). This is a measure to prevent brain herniation.
2. Complete blood count (CBC) reveals increased WBC count.
3. Blood culture may also identify causative agent.

F. **Nursing diagnoses**
1. Hypothermia or hyperthermia
2. Risk for infection (further infection)
3. Risk for injury
4. Altered tissue perfusion
5. Ineffective breathing pattern

G. **Planning and implementation**
1. Perform careful assessments to note clinical characteristics in their early stages.
2. Monitor temperature and vital signs frequently.
3. Monitor intake and output (I&O) and fluid and electrolyte balance; children with diminished consciousness should receive nothing by mouth, others are allowed liquids and diet progression as tolerated. Monitor I&O strictly. Fluid intake may be limited to two thirds of normal maintenance to prevent cerebral edema.
4. Check for neurologic signs and monitor level of consciousness. Measure head circumference to monitor for subdural effusions and obstructive hydrocephalus that may develop as complications.
5. Administer antibiotics, as prescribed (type depends on organism), and maintain intravenous (IV) line. In addition, provide supportive interventions including fever reduction, fluid and electrolyte balancing; monitor for hydrocephalus, increased ICP, and secondary infections. Steroids may be prescribed to relieve cerebral edema.
6. Implement isolation with respiratory precautions for 24 to 48 hours after antibiotic administration begins.
7. Keep room as quiet as possible to decrease environmental stimuli.

H. **Evaluation**
1. Early recognition and initiation of vigorous treatment has been instituted.
2. The chances for survival with few or no neurologic deficits have increased.

V. HIV and AIDS

A. **Description: Human immunodeficiency virus (HIV) leads to a broad spectrum of diseases and varied clinical courses. Acquired immunodeficiency syndrome (AIDS) is the most serious end of the spectrum.**

B. **Etiology and incidence**
1. **The predominant modes of HIV transmission are:**
   a. **Sexual contact (both homosexual and heterosexual)**
   b. **Percutaneous or mucous membrane exposure to contaminated needles or other sharp instruments**

   c. **Mother-to-infant transmission before or around the time of birth**
   d. **Although transfusion of blood, blood components, or clotting factor concentrates is now a rare mode of transmission, 11% to 13% of HIV-infected children were infected by transfusions (especially hemophiliacs receiving clotting factor) before 1985.**

2. AIDS in children and adolescents accounts for approximately 2% of all reported AIDS cases in the United States, and the numbers are increasing.

3. Most infected children are born to families in which one or both parents are infected. The remainder include children who received contaminated blood and blood products; adolescents with adult risk factors (sexual transmission and IV drug abuse), and children who have been sexually abused.

4. **The risk of infection for an infant whose mother is HIV-positive is 13% to 39%.**

5. The incubation period of symptomatic HIV infection varies and ranges from months to years. In infants infected perinatally, the median age for onset of symptoms is 3 years.

6. **The number of adolescents who are HIV positive is rapidly increasing.**

C. **Pathophysiology and management**

1. AIDS is caused by HIV, a retrovirus that produces lymphopenia and an inversion of the normal ratio of helper to suppressor lymphocytes. Immunosuppression is the result of this decrease in the number of $CD4^+$ T cells, as well as functional defects.

2. Abnormal B-cell function is apparent early in HIV infection in children. Because helper T cells control B-cell function, young children with HIV are deficient in both cell-mediated and humoral immunity.

3. Immunoglobulins are nonfunctional, rendering the child defenseless against recurrent bacterial infections. Additionally, HIV-infected children are unable to form antibodies after immunizations.

4. Currently there is no cure, so management is primarily supportive, with treatment given for opportunistic infections. The goals of therapy include slowing the growth of HIV, preventing and treating opportunistic infections, ensuring nutritional support, and relieving symptoms.

5. Medication regimens may use zidovudine (Azidothymidine, AZT [Retrovir]), dideoxycytidine (ddC), and didanosine (DDI) to slow the HIV infection and disease progression. Co-trimoxazole (Sulfamethoxazole-trimethoprim, Bactrim-Septra) and pen-

tamidine (NebuPent, Pentam 300) are used to treat *Pneumo-cystis carinii* pneumonia. Gamma globulin administration is helpful to compensate for B-cell deficiency.

6. Children are immunized as scheduled but receive inactivated polio vaccine (TIPV rather than OPV) and the pneumococcal and influenza vaccines. Children exposed to varicella (chicken pox) should receive ZIG (zoster immunoglobulin).

D. Clinical assessment findings

1. **Failure to thrive and multiple nutritional deficiencies**
2. **Lymphadenopathy, hepatosplenomegaly, recurrent bacterial infections and pulmonary diseases occur in two thirds of HIV-infected children.**
3. Other assessment findings include pulmonary diseases such as *P. carinii* pneumonia (PCP), lymphocytic interstitial pneumonitis (LIP), and pulmonary lymphoid hyperplasia (PLH).
4. Chronic diarrhea may be primary or secondary to opportunistic GI infections.
5. Neurologic problems may be assessed in 75% to 90% of children with HIV infection and include developmental delays, loss of developmental milestones and reflexes, lack of coordination, memory loss, ataxia, irritability, visual disturbances, and decreased brain growth evidenced by microcephaly.

E. Diagnostic assessment findings

1. Accurate testing in infants is complicated by maternal IgG, which may contribute to false-positive findings.
2. **Because infants may have maternal antibodies for up to 15 months, false-positive enzyme-linked immunosorbent assay (ELISA) test results are possible. Therefore other diagnostic measures are used, including HIV culture, detection of HIV-DNA sequences using the polymerase chain reaction (PCR), and identifying specific HIV antigen; for children over 18 months, traditional ELISA and Western blot assay tests are used.**
3. Findings on early peripheral smears may be normal; later, lymphopenia is noted. Additional findings include decreased $CD4^+$ and increased $CD8^+$ cells with a decreased ratio of normal $CD4^+$ to $CD8^+$ cells.

F. Nursing diagnoses

1. Risk for infection
2. Impaired social interaction
3. Altered sexuality
4. Pain
5. Altered nutrition: less than body requirements
6. Altered family processes

       7.   Anticipatory grieving

       8.   Altered growth and development

G. Planning and implementation

1. Institute the prescribed treatment plan.
2. Keep child away from infected persons and use good hand washing and medical asepsis. Use pulmonary hygiene (chest physiotherapy, deep breathing, and so forth) to prevent secretions from pooling and increasing susceptibility to infection.
3. Promote nutrition by offering foods that child likes as well as nutritious supplements. Child should only eat peeled or cooked fruits and vegetables to avoid infectious organisms. The child may also need enteral feeding or hyperalimentation, requiring the nurse to monitor these therapies.
4. Administer antibiotics and other medications as prescribed, and provide mouth care for conditions related to candidal organisms.
5. Assist child in maintaining self-esteem; also enhance growth and development by encouraging child to perform at his or her optimal level.
6. Allow child and family to verbalize their feelings and concerns. Be supportive and assist them in developing coping strategies.
7. Provide information and instruction to facilitate and sustain home care. Appropriately inform the child and family about the disease and its transmission; promote normalization of the child's lifestyle and protect the child from infections. If the client is a sexually active adolescent or a drug user, discuss ways to protect sexual partners or fellow drug users.
8. Discuss modes of transmission:
   a. Explain that no cases have been reported to be transmitted by casual contact.
   b. Identify precautions:
      (1) Avoid mixing the ill child's secretions with those of family members (*e.g.*, be sure to use separate linens, separate toothbrush, separate razor, separate eating utensils).
      (2) Observe blood and excretion precautions (use gloves to change dressings; clean up spilled body fluids with a 1:10 bleach solution; keep trash in a closed container; flush feces, urine, and other body fluids down the toilet; use proper container for needles).
      (3) Teach adolescents about safe sex.
9. Assist family in obtaining proper immunizations for the child.
10. Refer child and family to appropriate community agencies for support.
11. Assist child and family with the grieving process.

H. Evaluation
1. The child remains free of infection.
2. The child experiences growth and development that is as normal as possible.
3. The child and family cope effectively and have adequate support systems.
4. The family verbalizes adequate knowledge about caring for the child at home.

VI. Communicable diseases with rashes
    A. Measles (rubeola)
1. Infectious agent: virus
2. Mode of transmission: usually direct contact with droplets
3. Incubation period: 10 to 20 days
4. Period of communicability: from 4 days before to 5 days after rash appears
5. Clinical manifestations
    a. Prodromal stage: fever and malaise, followed by coryza, cough and conjunctivitis, and photophobia in 24 hours; Koplik's spots
    b. Rash: appears 3 to 4 days after onset of prodromal stage, begins as erythematous (reddened) maculopapular rash on face and gradually spreads downward; more severe in earlier sites, less in later sites; rash turns brownish after 3 to 4 days and fine desquamation occurs over severe areas.
6. Complications: otitis media, pneumonia, laryngotracheitis, encephalitis
7. Nursing implications: Show parents how to provide supportive management; use dimly lit room or sunglasses for photophobia.
8. Prevention: vaccine

    B. German measles (rubella)
1. Infectious agent: rubella virus
2. Mode of transmission: direct and indirect contact
3. Incubation period: 14 to 21 days
4. Period of communicability: 7 days before to about 5 days after rash
5. Clinical manifestations
    a. Prodromal stage: absent in children
    b. Rash: starts on face and rapidly spreads downward; discrete, pinkish red maculopapular rash; disappears in same order as it appeared
    c. General symptoms: possibly low-grade fever, headache, malaise, and lymphadenopathy
6. Complications: possible teratogenic effects on a fetus
7. Nursing implications: Provide supportive care.
8. Prevention: vaccine

C. Chicken pox (varicella)
   1. Infectious agent: varicella zoster
   2. Modes of transmission: direct contact and contaminated objects
   3. Incubation period: 2 to 3 weeks
   4. Period of communicability: from 1 to 2 days before rash develops until all lesions are crusted
   5. Clinical manifestations
      a. Prodromal stage: low-grade fever, malaise, anorexia
      b. Rash: maculas, papules, vesicles, pustules, and crusts; centripetal, spreading to face and proximal extremities, sparse on distal extremities; may affect mucous membranes; pruritus severe
      c. General symptoms: fever, lymphadenopathy, irritability from pruritus
   6. Complications: secondary infections, encephalitis, pneumonia, hemorrhagic varicella (in high-risk children)
   7. Nursing implications: Maintain strict isolation in hospital setting; isolate children at home until all vesicles dry; give skin care; administer antipyretics, but do not use aspirin; provide cool or Aveeno baths, loose clothing, fluids, and antihistamines, if prescribed. Also, if prescribed, administer acyclovir (for high-risk child) as well as zoster immune globulin (ZIG).
   8. Prevention: vaccine available for high-risk children and being considered for the general population. Provide ZIG for high-risk (immunosuppressed) children.

VII. Communicable diseases without rashes
   A. Diphtheria
      1. Infectious agent: *Corynebacterium diptheriae*
      2. Mode of transmission: direct contact, air, personal articles
      3. Incubation period: 1 to 6 days
      4. Period of communicability: 2 to 4 weeks without treatment; 1 to 2 days after start of treatment
      5. Clinical manifestations (depend on site of membrane):
         a. Nasal: resembles common cold; drainage becomes serosanguineous then mucopurulent; foul odor
         b. Tonsillar-pharyngeal: malaise; anorexia; sore throat; low-grade fever; pulse higher than expected for fever; lymphadenitis (bull-neck); when severe, toxemia, septic shock, and death.
         c. Laryngeal: fever, hoarseness, cough, potential airway obstruction
      6. Complications: myocarditis, neuritis
      7. Nursing implications: Maintain strict isolation; maintain airway and observe for signs of obstruction; promote hydration; administer antibiotics as prescribed; and maintain bed rest.

Institute orders for antitoxin, antibiotics, bed rest; tracheostomy may be needed for obstruction.

   8.   Prevention: vaccine, maintained by boosters

B.   Whooping cough (pertussis)

   1.   Infectious agent: *Bordetella pertussis*
   2.   Modes of transmission: direct contact, air, personal objects
   3.   Incubation period: 6 to 20 days (average 7)
   4.   Period of communicability: from catarrhal stage through the fourth week
   5.   Clinical manifestations
      a.   Catarrhal stage: symptoms of upper respiratory tract infection continuing for 1 to 2 weeks when hacking cough becomes more severe
      b.   Paroxysmal stage (generally 4 to 6 weeks): characteristic paroxysmal "whooping" cough (usually at night), accompanied by flushed or cyanotic cheeks, bulging eyes, protruding tongue; cough continuing until dislodgment of thick mucous plug; vomiting typical after attack
      c.   Convalescent stage: cough gradually decreasing, vomiting stopping, strength generally returning
   6.   Complications
      a.   Pneumonia, atelectasis, otitis media, convulsions, hemorrhage, weight loss, dehydration
      b.   **Respiratory arrest caused by mucous plug or apnea in young infants**
   7.   Nursing implications: Institute isolation and respiratory precautions and bed rest when febrile; provide reassurance during coughing; provide quiet environment to decrease paroxysmal spells; encourage fluids; provide humidity; observe for signs of obstruction; administer erythromycin if prescribed.
   8.   Prevention: vaccine

C.   Poliomyelitis

   1.   Infectious agent: three types of enteroviruses
   2.   Mode of transmission: direct contact; fecal-oral route
   3.   Incubation period: 14 to 21 days
   4.   Period of communicability: not known; virus is in throat for 1 week after onset and in feces intermittently for 3 to 4 weeks
   5.   Clinical manifestations (three forms)
      a.   Abortive or apparent: brief fever, malaise, anorexia, nausea, vomiting, constipation, headache, abdominal pain
      b.   Nonparalytic: same as abortive or apparent but more severe pain; progresses to nuchal and spinal rigidity with changes in reflexes
      c.   Paralytic: same as nonparalytic plus muscular weakness

> progressing to paralysis, including paralysis of bowel and
> bladder muscles and paresis of respiratory muscles

6. Complications: permanent paralysis, respiratory arrest, hypertension, kidney stones, pulmonary edema, and pulmonary emboli
7. Nursing implications: Promote anxiety relief; participate in physiotherapy techniques; maintain body alignment; observe for respiratory paralysis; treatment is supportive with airway maintenance and bowel and bladder programs when needed.
8. Prevention: vaccine

D. Mumps (parotitis)

1. Agent: paramyxovirus
2. Mode of transmission: direct contact or droplet
3. Incubation period: 14 to 21 days
4. Period of communicability: immediately before to immediately after swelling appears
5. Clinical manifestations:
   a. Prodromal stage: fever, headache, anorexia followed by earache aggravated by chewing
   b. Acute stage: by third day, glandular (parotid) swelling reaching maximal size in 1 to 3 days, accompanied by pain and tenderness
6. Complications: meningoencephalitis, orchitis, epididymitis, arthritis, sterility in males (rare)
7. Nursing implications: Institute isolation and respiratory precautions and bed rest; administer analgesics and fluids; provide warmth and support for orchitis; administer IV fluids if prescribed and if child refuses to drink.

Bibliography

Betz, C.L., Hunsberger, M.M., & Wright, S. (1994). *Family Centered Nursing Care of Children,* 2nd ed. Philadelphia: W.B. Saunders.

Castiglia, P.T. & Harbin, R.B. (1993). *Child Health Care: Process and Practice.* Philadelphia: J.B. Lippincott.

Committee on Infectious Diseases, American Academy of Pediatrics. (1994). *1994 Red Book: Report of the Committee on Infectious Diseases,* 23rd ed. Elk Grove, IL: American Academy of Pediatrics.

Jackson, D.B. & Saunders, R.B. (1993). *Child Health Nursing: A Comprehensive Approach to the Care of Children and Their Families.* Philadelphia: J.B. Lippincott.

Poon, C.Y. (1992). Childhood immunization, Part 1. *Journal of Pediatric Health Care,* 6(6), 370–376.

Poon, C.Y. (1992). Childhood immunization, Part 2. *Journal of Pediatric Health Care,* 7(3), 127–133.

Wong, D.L. (1993). *Whaley and Wong's Essentials of Pediatric Nursing,* 4th Ed. St. Louis: C.V. Mosby.

Wong, D.L. (1995). *Whaley and Wong's Nursing Care of Infants and Children,* 5th ed. St. Louis: C.V. Mosby.

STUDY QUESTIONS

1. Which of the following immune responses is a nonspecific response to invasion?
   a. Inflammatory response
   b. Antibody response
   c. Humoral response
   d. Cell-mediated response

2. When an infant is given a DTP injection, what type of immunity does he or she receive?
   a. Natural, active
   b. Natural, passive
   c. Artificial, active
   d. Artificial, passive

3. A nurse is administering immunizations at a Well Baby Clinic. Which of the following 4-year-olds would receive OPV?
   a. A child with AIDS
   b. A child with an upper respiratory tract infection
   c. The sibling of a leukemic child
   d. A child on long-term steroid therapy

4. After administering DTP to a child, the nurse provides home care instructions for the child's mother. These should include:
   a. Monitoring the child for a rash in 7 to 10 days
   b. Decreasing milk intake to prevent diarrhea
   c. Giving acetaminophen for fever and discomfort
   d. Warning that the virus may be shed in the child's stool

5. According to the routine immunization schedule, what immunizations should a 15-month-old child receive?
   a. DTP, OPV
   b. Hib, MMR
   c. HB, MMR
   d. Hib, HB

6. Which of the following organisms is the most common cause of neonatal sepsis?

   a. *E. coli*
   b. *Streptococcus viridans*
   c. Group B streptococcus
   d. *Haemophilus influenzae*

7. Common early manifestations of meningitis in a 2-month-old infant include:
   a. Opisthotonos
   b. Nuchal rigidity
   c. Kerning's sign
   d. Hypothermia

8. The risk of transmission of HIV from an HIV-positive mother to her unborn child is:
   a. No risk
   b. Less than 13%%
   c. 13% to 39%
   d. Greater than 39%

9. Which of the following is not an appropriate nursing intervention for a child with HIV?
   a. Offering large amounts of fresh fruits and vegetables
   b. Encouraging child to perform at optimal level
   c. Teaching family about disease transmission
   d. Using good hand washing before handling child

10. A child's parents seek attention for the child's generalized confluent red-pink maculopapular rash; the child appears ill and exhibits conjunctivitis and photophobia. These are common manifestations of:
    a. Rubella
    b. Roseola
    c. Rubeola
    d. Varicella

11. A thick whitish-gray pseudomembrane and a "bull-neck" are characteristic of:
    a. Pertussis
    b. Diphtheria
    c. Mumps
    d. Tetanus

ANSWER KEY

1. *Correct response: a*
   The inflammatory response is a nonspecific response to injury or infection.
   b and c. Humoral and antibody are the same response; B lymphocytes synthesize antibodies to specific proteins.
   d. Cell-mediated responses are varied but specific leukocyte actions.
   Knowledge/Physiologic/NA

2. *Correct response: c*
   Ingested or injected vaccines are medically altered substances that cause the body to make antibodies.
   a. Antibodies are developed naturally (through nature) (*e.g.*, when an infectious disease develops in an individual).
   b. Antibodies are directly received naturally (*e.g.*, through the placenta).
   d. Antibodies are artificially delivered to the body as in the administration of tetanus immunoglobulin.
   Analysis/Physiologic/Planning

3. *Correct response: b*
   Immunizations are not contraindicated in children with mild episodic illnesses.
   a and d. The live polio vaccine is contraindicated in children who are immunosuppressed as they may develop the disease.
   c. Live polio vaccine is shed into the stools and, therefore, may contaminate an immunosuppressed sibling.
   Application/Safe Care/Planning

4. *Correct response: c*
   Acetaminophen assists in decreasing the fever that may accompany the pertussis vaccine and the pain that may accompany the tetanus vaccine.
   a. A rash may be seen 7 to 10 days after the MMR.
   b. Diarrhea is not a side effect of DTP.
   d. The live polio vaccine may shed into the stools.
   Application/Safe Care/Implementation

5. *Correct response: b*
   Hib (HibTITER) and MMR are scheduled to be given at this age.
   a. DTP and OPV booster is scheduled at 18 months.
   c and d. HB is given at 0, 2, and 6 months or at 2, 4, and 6 months.
   Application/Health Promotion/Planning

6. *Correct response: c*
   Group B beta-hemolytic streptococcus is the most common cause of bacterial meningitis and sepsis in the neonate.
   a. *E. coli* is also a common cause in the neonate, but not the most common.
   b. *Streptococcus viridans* is not a common cause of sepsis.
   d. *Haemophilus influenzae* can cause sepsis and meningitis, but is less common in the neonate and now is less frequent in the older child as a result of the Hib vaccine.
   Comprehension/Physiologic/NA

7. *Correct response: d*
   Hypothermia and hyperthermia are early signs of meningitis in the small infant.
   a. Opisthotonos is a late and ominous sign.
   b and c. Nuchal rigidity and Kerning's sign are seen in older children and adults with meningitis; infants do not localize infections.
   Knowledge/Physiologic/Assessment

8. *Correct response: c*
   The risk of neonatal HIV transmission from an HIV-positive mother to her infant is 13% to 39%.
   a. There is always a risk.
   b. Too low.
   d. Too high.
   Comprehension/Health Promotion/NA

9. *Correct response: a*
   Fresh fruits and vegetables may be contaminated with organisms and pesticides that can be harmful, if not fatal, to an immunosuppressed child.

b. Children with HIV infection should be encouraged to perform at their optimal level to increase their self-esteem.

c. Families need to learn about transmission modes to prevent the spread of infection and to dispel possible myths.

d. Good hand washing decreases the chance of infecting the immunosuppressed child.

Application/Safe Care/Implementation

10. *Correct response: c*

This is a classic presentation of rubeola or measles.

a. Rubella, German measles, presents with a similar rash but the child does not appear ill.

b. Roseola presents with a mild rash after the child's fever subsides.

d. Varicella, chicken pox, is a multilesion rash.

Application/Physiologic/Analysis (Dx)

11. *Correct response: b*

The pseudomembrane and the characteristic lymphadenitis are seen in diphtheria.

a. Pertussis is whooping cough.

c. Mumps begins with enlarged parotid glands and neck swelling, but there is no pseudomembrane.

d. Tetanus is lockjaw; trismus and other characteristic symptoms are early signs.

Knowledge/Physiologic/Assessment

Respiratory Dysfunction

I. Essential concepts: Respiratory development and function

A. Respiratory tract development

1. Appearance of the laryngotracheal groove around the fourth week of gestation is closely followed by development of the larynx and trachea.

2. Development of the bronchial tree occurs predominantly between weeks 5 and 16 of gestation.

3. In weeks 16 through 12 of gestation, luminal and blood vessel growth occurs in the bronchi and bronchioles.

4. Production of surfactant (a phospholipid protein complex that reduces alveolar surface tension, thereby decreasing the tendency of the alveoli to collapse during expiration) occurs at about 24 weeks of gestation.

5. Two surface tension-reducing substances, lecithin and sphingomyelin, can be detected in amniotic fluid and are useful predictors of lung maturity; a lecithin-sphingomyelin ratio of 2:1 or greater indicates fetal lung maturity.

6. The detection of phosphatidylglycerol in amniotic fluid also indicates fetal lung maturity.

7. At birth, the lungs contain fluid; this is replaced by air as the infant begins respiration.

8. Lungs continue to develop after birth, and new alveoli form until about age 8 years. Therefore, a child with pulmonary damage or disease at birth may regenerate new pulmonary tissue and eventually attain normal respiratory function.

B. Function
The major function of the respiratory system is to deliver oxygen (O_2) to arterial blood and remove carbon dioxide (CO_2) from venous blood, a process known as gas exchange.

2. Normal gas exchange depends on three processes:
    a. Ventilation: movement of gases from the atmosphere to the alveoli
    b. Diffusion: transfer of inhaled gases across the alveolar membrane to the lung
    c. Perfusion: movement of oxygenated blood from the lungs to the tissues
3. Control of respiration involves neural and chemical processes.
    a. The neural system, composed of three parts located in the pons, medulla, and spinal cord, coordinates respiratory rhythm and regulates the depth of respirations.
    b. Chemical processes perform several vital functions, such as:
        (1) Regulating alveolar ventilation by maintaining normal blood gas tension
        (2) Guarding against hypercapnia (excessive CO_2 in the blood) as well as hypoxia (reduced tissue oxygenation caused by decreased arterial oxygen [PaO_2]). An increase in arterial CO_2 ($PaCO_2$) stimulates ventilation; conversely, a decrease in $PaCO_2$ inhibits ventilation.
        (3) Helping to maintain respirations (through peripheral chemoreceptors) when hypoxia occurs
4. The normal functions of gas exchange, O_2 and CO_2 tension, and chemoreceptors are similar in children and adults. However, children respond differently than adults to respiratory disturbances; major areas of difference include:
    a. Poor tolerance of nasal congestion, especially in infants who are obligatory nose breathers up to age 4 months
    b. Increased susceptibility to ear infection due to shorter, broader, and more horizontally positioned eustachian tubes
    c. Increased severity of respiratory symptoms due to smaller airway diameters
    d. A total-body response to respiratory infection, with such symptoms as fever, vomiting and diarrhea

II. Respiratory system overview
A. Assessment

1. The health history should disclose whether the problem is acute or chronic, self-limiting, recurrent, or life-threatening. Other important points include alleviating or exacerbating fac-

tors, effects of previous treatments, a family history of respiratory problems, and other chronic problems such as human immunodeficiency virus (HIV) disease.

    2. The physical assessment should focus on the following:
        a. Alertness, changes in mental status
        b. Activity level and complaints of fatigue
        c. Skin color changes, especially cyanosis
        d. Respiratory rate and pattern, presence of apnea
        e. Intracoastal, suprasternal, sternal and substernal retractions: presence and severity
        f. Quality of breath sounds
        g. Adventitious lung sounds (rales, rhonchi, wheezes)
        h. Cough: productive versus nonproductive and type
        i. Dyspnea, stridor, grunting, nasal flaring
        j. Position that child maintains
        k. Vital signs and temperature; signs of dehydration

B. Laboratory studies and diagnostic tests
    1. Radiologic evaluation may include:
        a. Chest x-ray study to visualize internal structures
        b. Lung scan to visualize pulmonary blood flow
    2. Thoracentesis, which involves puncturing the chest wall with a needle and syringe to obtain a pleural fluid specimen for analysis
    3. Pulmonary function tests to measure ventilatory function
    4. Blood gas analysis, which involves drawing blood for analysis of arterial and venous oxygen and carbon dioxide levels and pH as well

C. Psychosocial implications
    1. Acute respiratory illness is frightening to both the child and the parents and calls for effective crisis intervention by the nurse.
    2. Chronic respiratory illness in children is commonly accompanied by a history of acute crisis episodes and chronic stress.
    3. The respiratory-impaired child's developmental needs can be best met by maintaining optimal exercise and activity levels.

III. Bronchopulmonary dysplasia (BPD)
    A. Description: a chronic pulmonary disease of infancy marked by the need for oxygen therapy beyond 28 days after birth
    B. Etiology and incidence
        1. The cause of BPD is unknown, although several risk factors have been identified. BPD has been attributed to iatrogenic causes (therapies used to treat lung disease).
        2. BPD most commonly affects very low birth weight (VLBW [under 2500 g]) and extremely low birth weight (ELBW [under 1000 g]) infants with lung disorders (*e.g.*,

respiratory distress syndrome, also called hyaline membrane disease, and meconium aspiration). For instance, it occurs in 10% to 30% of VLBW infants treated for respiratory distress syndrome.

3. A premature infant who is mechanically ventilated and receives high concentrations of oxygen is at greatest risk.
4. BPD may also occur after ventilation therapy with meconium aspiration, persistent pulmonary hypertension, and cyanotic heart disease.

C. **Pathophysiology and management**
1. Positive inspiratory pressures and high concentrations of oxygen can injure the alveolar sacules and small airway epithelium and lead to fibrosis of these structures.
2. Areas of cystic foci and atelectasis appear in the lung parenchyma.
3. Airway smooth muscle hypertrophy results in bronchospasm and endothelial cell damage causing interstitial edema.
4. These changes further aggravate airway obstruction and necessitate long-term oxygen therapy.
5. Cor pulmonale is the leading cause of death in infants with BPD.

D. **Clinical assessment findings**
1. Clinical manifestations vary widely based on a continuum of the disease process.
2. Characteristics include cyanosis on room air, tachypnea, retractions, grunting, nasal flaring, increased anteroposterior diameter of the chest, wheeze, rales, and copious secretions.
3. Manifestations of right heart failure may be present, including periorbital edema, hepatomegaly, and jugular vein distention. Pulmonary edema may occur.
4. Usually the child is thin with height and weight in the bottom 50th percentile. Growth and development usually are delayed secondary to poor nutrition and prolonged hospitalization.

E. **Diagnostic assessment findings**
1. Pulmonary function test (PFT) findings: increased airway resistance, decreased compliance (increased lung stiffness) and increased functional residual capacity (FRC).
2. Chest x-ray (CXR) shows characteristic streakiness with areas of hyperinflation and atelectasis.
3. ECG and echocardiogram may show evidence of right-side hypertrophy.

F. **Nursing diagnoses**
1. Activity intolerance
2. Ineffective airway clearance
3. Risk for altered body temperature

4. Ineffective breathing pattern
5. Altered family processes
6. High risk for fluid volume deficit
7. Knowledge deficit
8. Altered nutrition: less than body requirements
9. Pain

G. **Planning and implementation**

1. Give bronchodilators as prescribed. Bronchodilators are used to promote pulmonary smooth muscle relaxation and improve respiratory function.

2. Administer steroidal agents as prescribed. Steroids may be used to decrease respiratory inflammation.

3. Administer antibiotics, as prescribed. Antimicrobial therapy is used to treat acute respiratory illness. Respiratory syncytial virus (RSV) is the major pathogen, requiring ribavirin, given via small particle aerosol generator.

  a. **Keep in mind the general nursing implications for antibiotics.**

    (1) **Obtain all culture and sensitivity (C&S) specimens before giving antibiotics.**

    (2) **Check for allergies.**

    (3) **Check storage of medications.**

    (4) **Monitor client's temperature.**

    (5) **Provide instruction for the client and family, as follows: Advise client to take the antibiotic exactly as prescribed for the full time prescribed. Most prescribed antibiotics do not work for viral infections; most work best on empty stomach. Antibiotics may decrease the effects of oral contraceptives. Fungal superinfections are possible, especially thrush and monilial diaper rash.**

  b. **Keep in mind the nursing implications for specific antibiotics as follows:**

    (1) Penicillin (PCN): give Amoxil with food, child may break out in nonallergic rash between days 7 and 10 day of Amoxil therapy.

    (2) Erythromycin: do not give with fruit juice; do not give intramuscularly (IM); erythromycin increases theophylline levels.

    (3) Tetracycline: limit exposure to sunlight; do not give with antacids or milk, $NaHCO^3$ or iron; contraindicated in children under age 9 and pregnant women because of possible fetal bone growth retardation and irreversible tooth staining.

        (4) Cephalosporins: 15% of all clients who are allergic to penicillin are allergic to cephalosporins.

        (5) Aminoglycosides: assess for ototoxicity and nephrotoxicity; increase fluid intake; monitor intake and output, keep urine alkaline.

        (6) Ribavirin: monitor apical pulse and respirations every 1 to 2 hours; pregnant nurses should not care for these children.

4. Administer diuretics, if prescribed. Diuretics are used for congestive heart failure and cor pulmonale.

5. Provide respiratory support through continuous mechanical ventilation and administration of oxygen via oxygen hood, nasal catheter or cannula.

6. Support safe weaning from oxygen as indicated by clinical manifestations of readiness:

    a. Maintenance of normal arterial blood gas, PaO_2, and $PaCO_2$ levels.

    b. No increase in the work of breathing

    c. Normal growth and development

7. Provide chest physiotherapy (postural drainage with percussion and vibration) consistent with the infant's tolerance level, which can be monitored by transcutaneous oxygen levels at each position change and a determination of the time it takes for oxygen levels to return to pretreatment oxygen saturation levels.

8. Periodically change the infant's position from side to side and front to back to improve bronchial drainage and promote expansion and ventilation of all lung fields.

9. Promote optimal nutrition without overhydration by feeding at appropriate intervals and closely monitoring fluid intake.

10. Protect the compromised infant from infection by maintaining strict asepsis.

11. Teach parents about the disease process, complications, and treatments. Provide answers to their questions and reinforcing information provided by the physician and other members of the health care team.

12. In preparing for home care, encourage parents to become involved in their infant's care in the hospital, as appropriate.

13. Provide the opportunity for parents to express their feelings and concerns.

14. Participate with other members of the health care team in preparing the family for home care.

H. Evaluation

1. The infant's supplemental oxygen requirements are stabilized or supplemental oxygen is no longer required.

        2. Parents verbalize an understanding of diagnosis, treatments, home care, and follow-up visits.

        3. The infant is adequately incorporated into the family unit.

IV. Sudden infant death syndrome (SIDS)

A. Description: sudden, unexpected death of any infant for whom a postmortem examination fails to determine the cause of death. The death usually occurs during sleep.

B. Etiology and incidence

    1. Incidence is 2 per 1000 live births.

    2. **Infants at greatest risk for SIDS include premature infants, infants with apneic episodes, infants with prenatal drug exposure, and siblings of infants who have died of SIDS. Home monitoring is suggested for those infants at risk.**

    3. **Although the cause of SIDS is unknown, it has been related to hypoxemia, apnea, an immature nervous system, and prone positioning. SIDS may also be related to a brain stem abnormality in neuroregulation of cardiorespiratory control.**

    4. Recent findings have suggested an increased incidence of SIDS in infants who sleep in the prone position.

    5. Peak age ranges from 2 to 4 months, with most SIDS cases occurring before 6 months.

    6. Affects male infants more than female infants and usually occurs in winter.

C. Pathophysiology and management

    1. There is no known cause, but autopsies reveal consistent findings, such as pulmonary edema and intrathoracic hemorrhages.

D. Clinical assessment findings

    1. No characteristic finding before death.

    2. Usually parents discover that child has died in his or her sleep.

    3. Typically, the child is found in a disheveled bed, with blankets over head and huddled in a corner; frothy, blood-tinged fluid fills the mouth and nostrils, and the infant may be lying in secretions; the diaper is filled with urine and stool; and the hands may be clutching the sheets. The suddenness and the appearance of the infant add to the horror that the parent faces.

E. Diagnostic assessment findings

    1. There are no specific laboratory tests.

F. Nursing diagnoses

    1. Potential ineffective family coping

    2. Potential dysfunctional grieving

    3. Risk for altered parenting (other children)

4. Powerlessness
5. Guilt
6. Potential for spiritual distress

G. Planning and implementation
1. Evaluate family coping and grieving patterns.
2. Provide anticipatory guidance for typical feelings.
3. Allow parents to verbalize; listen and validate feelings.
4. Refer family for counseling if needed.
5. Refer to appropriate community self-help groups.
6. Monitor children at risk for apnea.
7. **Teach parents proper infant positioning.**

H. Evaluation
1. Parents and other family members can move adequately through the grieving process.

V. Acute otitis media

A. Description: inflammation of the middle ear

B. Etiology and incidence
1. **Usually caused by *Haemophilus influenzae* or *Streptococcus pneumoniae*.**
2. Factors predisposing infants and children to otitis media:
   a. Anatomic features: short, horizontally positioned eustachian tubes
   b. Poorly developed cartilage lining, which makes eustachian tubes more likely to open prematurely
   c. Enlarged lymphoid tissue, which obstructs eustachian tube openings
   d. Immature humoral defense mechanisms, which increases the risk of infection
   e. **Bottle-feeding an infant in the supine position, which allows formula to pool in the pharyngeal cavity.**
   f. **Passive smoking is recognized as a significant factor in acute otitis media.**
3. Acute otitis media is one of the most prevalent diseases of early childhood, with peak incidence occurring between age 6 months and 2 years. Approximately 70% of all children will have had at least one episode of otitis media.
4. Boys are affected more frequently than girls.
5. Breast-fed infants have a lower incidence than formula-fed infants.

C. Pathophysiology and management
1. Eustachian tube dysfunction enables bacterial invasion of the middle ear and obstructs drainage of secretions.

      2. Antibiotic therapy is the main treatment with amoxicillin still the drug of choice. Other antibiotics include sulfamethoxazol-trimethoprim (Bactrim-Septra), erythromycin-sulfisoxazole (Pediazole), and cephalosporins (sometimes the treatment of choice because of their broad-spectrum activity and bactericidal effect on beta lactamase-producing pathogens).

      3. Possible complications include hearing loss, tympanosclerosis (scarring), tympanic perforation, adhesive otitis ("glue-ear"), chronic suppurative otitis media, mastoiditis, meningitis, and cholesteatoma.

      4. Follow-up is needed to evaluate antibiotic effectiveness and to check for complications such as effusion and hearing impairment.

D. **Clinical assessment findings**

      1. Infants characteristically do not localize infections.

      2. Health history and physical assessment data may reveal:
         a. Complaints of ear pain, pulling at the ears
         b. Fever
         c. Irritability
         d. Loss of appetite
         e. Nasal congestion
         f. Cough
         g. Vomiting and diarrhea

      3. Otoscopic findings disclose:
         a. Injected or erythematous tympanic membrane; bulging tympanic membrane with no visible landmarks, including no light reflex; diminished tympanic membrane mobility
         b. Purulent discharge

E. **Diagnostic assessment findings**

      1. Culture and sensitivity tests may be done to identify organism in aural discharge.

      2. Audiometric testing establishes a baseline or detects any hearing loss secondary to recurring infection.

F. **Nursing diagnoses**

      1. Risk for altered body temperature
      2. Ineffective breathing pattern
      3. Risk for fluid volume deficit
      4. Pain
      5. Impaired tissue integrity

G. **Planning and implementation**

      1. Reduce fever by administering antipyretics as prescribed and by having child remove extra clothing (but avoid chilling).

      2. Relieve pain with prescribed analgesics, by offering soft foods to help the child limit chewing, and by applying local heat or warm compresses to affected ear.

3. Facilitate drainage by having the child lie with affected ear in a dependent position.
4. Prevent skin breakdown by keeping external ear clean and dry.
5. Assess for hearing loss and refer for audiologic testing if indicated.
6. Administer prescribed antibiotics—usually amoxicillin for 10 to 14 days; prophylactic antibiotic treatment may be prescribed for children with recurrent infections.
7. Administer prescribed oral decongestants, such as pseudoephedrine hydrochloride, to relieve nasal congestion.
8. Provide preoperative and postoperative care if needed. Occasionally a myringotomy, (incision in the posterior inferior aspect of the tympanic membrane) may be necessary for draining exudate and releasing pressure. Tympanoplasty ventilating tubes or pressure-equalizing tubes may be inserted into the middle ear to create an artificial auditory canal that equalizes pressure on both sides of the tympanic membrane.
9. Provide patient and family teaching:
   a. Explain dosage, administration techniques, and possible side effects of medications.
   b. Emphasize the importance of completing the entire course of antibiotics.
   c. Identify signs of hearing loss and stress the importance of audiologic testing if needed.
   d. Discuss preventive measures, such as holding the child upright for feedings, gentle nose blowing, blowing games, and chewing sugarless gum.
   e. Point out the need for follow-up care, after completing antibiotic therapy to check for persistent infection.
10. If the child requires surgery, provide appropriate preoperative and postoperative teaching. For example, if the child has tympanoplasty with tubes, caution against getting water in the ears because water may be a source of infection.

H. Evaluation
1. The child remains afebrile and without pain, maintains normal hearing, and takes antibiotics as prescribed.
2. Parents verbalize knowledge of diagnosis, treatment, home care, preventive measures, and follow-up care.
3. Following tympanoplasty with tubes, parents verbalize the necessity of preventing water from entering the child's ear to reduce the risk of infection.

VI. Bronchiolitis
A. **Description: inflammation of the bronchioles with tenacious mucus causing varying obstruction leading to air trapping and**

hyperinflation. If enough alveoli collapse, hypercapnia, hypoxemia, and respiratory acidosis may follow.

B. Etiology and incidence

    1. Rare in children over age 2; usually occurs from age 2 months to 12 months; peak at age 6 months.

    2. Usually occurs in winter and spring.

    3. **Respiratory syncytial virus (RSV) is responsible for more than half of all cases. The next most responsible viral causes are adenoviruses and parainfluenza viruses.**

C. Pathophysiology and management

    1. The mucosa of the bronchioles swells with mucus and exudate in the bronciolar lumen.

    2. The walls of the bronchi and bronchioles become infiltrated with inflammatory cells.

    3. Peribronchial interstitial pneumonitis is usually present.

D. Clinical assessment findings

    1. Early: rhinorrhea; pharyngitis; coughing; sneezing; wheezing; diffuse rhonchi, rales, and wheezing; and intermittent fever

    2. As illness progresses: increased coughing and sneezing, air hunger, tachypnea and retractions, and cyanosis

    3. In severe illness: tachypnea >70 breaths per minute, listlessness, apneic spells, poor air exchange, markedly diminished breath sounds

E. Diagnostic assessment findings

    1. Nasal washing may identify RSV by enzyme-linked immunosorbent assay (ELISA).

    2. Chest X-ray shows hyperaeration and areas of consolidation.

F. Nursing diagnoses

    1. Ineffective airway clearance

    2. Risk for aspiration

    3. Risk for altered body temperature

    4. Ineffective breathing pattern

    5. Impaired gas exchange

    6. Anxiety

    7. Potential for fluid volume deficit

G. Planning and implementation

    1. Monitor for respiratory distress; note respiratory rate and rhythm, breath sounds and adventitious sounds, especially wheezing; check skin coloration and monitor hydration status.

    2. Obtain nasal washing for RSV testing as prescribed.

    3. Institute contact isolation.

    4. Administer prescribed bronchodilators and ribavirin; instruct parents on their use and side effects. Recommendations for the use of ribavirin include the following:

    a.   Use for children at high risk for complications caused by other conditions (premature infants, immunosuppressed children, severe RSV infection)

    b.   Consider using for infants at increased risk for progressing from mild to severe disease (less than 6 weeks of age, underlying conditions)

    c.   Nebulize ribavirin via a small-particle aerosol generator (SPAG) into an oxygen hood, tent, or mask for 12 to 20 hours daily for 3 to 5 days.

    d.   Continue contact isolation.

    e.   Observe precautions for health care workers and visitors: provide information about potential but unknown risks of drug; advise pregnant women to avoid giving direct care to infants receiving ribavirin; lower environmental exposure to ribavirin (temporarily stop medication when tent is open, administer drug in well-ventilated rooms).

  5. Ensure high humidity with oxygen as prescribed; increase fluids to maintain adequate hydration, offering small amounts frequently to prevent aspiration (child may need intravenous [IV] fluids if tachypnea imposes risk of aspiration) and ensure rest.

  6. Monitor IV infusion if needed.

  7. As prescribed, administer bronchodilators and corticosteroids.

  8. Maintain proper positioning to promote aeration, usually high Fowler's (an infant may be placed in an infant seat inside the croupette).

  9. Provide humidified oxygen as prescribed via croupette or oxygen hood.

  10. Provide support for parents.

H. **Evaluation**

  1. The child resumes regular breathing pattern without wheezing or using accessory muscles and regains normal respiratory rate and rhythm and color.

  2. The child ingests adequate fluids.

  3. The family experiences decreased anxiety.

VII. Acute laryngotracheobronchitis (LTB)

A. **Description: inflammation and narrowing of the laryngeal and tracheal areas.**

B. **Etiology and incidence**

  1. Cause is usually viral; common agents include parainfluenza viruses, adenoviruses, RSV, influenza viruses, and measles virus. LTB may be of bacterial origin (diphtheria or pertussis).

        2.   There may be some predisposition: genetic, allergic and emotional.

        3.   LTB affects boys more than girls, usually between the ages of 3 months and 8 years.

        4.   Peak incidence is in winter months.

C.   **Pathophysiology and management**

        1.   LTB is usually preceded by an upper respiratory infection, which proceeds to laryngitis and then descends into the trachea and sometimes the bronchi.

        2.   The flexible larynx of a young child is particularly susceptible to spasm, which may cause complete airway obstruction.

        3.   Profound airway edema may lead to obstruction and seriously compromised ventilation.

        4.   Treatment consists of humidity and racemic epinephrine.

D.   **Clinical assessment findings**

        1.   Spasmodic croup: sudden onset, waking at night with barklike cough

        2.   Acute LTB: gradual onset from upper respiratory tract infection, progressing to signs of distress

        3.   Hoarseness, inspiratory stridor, retractions; may have severe respiratory distress

        4.   May have low-grade fever

        5.   Restlessness and irritability

        6.   Pallor or cyanosis

        7.   Wheezing, rales, rhonchi, and localized areas of diminished breath sounds

E.   **Diagnostic assessment findings**

        1.   None

F.   **Nursing diagnoses**

        1.   Ineffective airway clearance

        2.   Anxiety

        3.   Ineffective breathing pattern

        4.   Risk for fluid volume deficit

        5.   Risk for injury

        6.   Altered tissue perfusion

        7.   Fear

        8.   Anxiety

        9.   Knowledge deficit

G.   **Planning and implementation**

        1.   Assess for airway obstruction by evaluating respiratory status: color, respiratory effort, evidence of fatigue, and vital signs.

        2.   Keep emergency equipment (tracheotomy and intubation tray) near the bedside.

3. Administer oxygen and increase atmospheric humidity, as prescribed, usually with a mist tent, to alleviate hypoxia.
4. Administer IV or oral fluids as prescribed to ensure adequate hydration.
5. Administer medications as prescribed. Aerosol racemic epinephrine may be prescribed; the use of corticosteroids is controversial.
6. Reduce the child's anxiety by maintaining a quiet environment, promoting rest and relaxation, and minimizing intrusive procedures. Encourage parent and child interactions and diversion.
7. Provide parental support to reduce anxiety.
8. Provide patient and family teaching:
   a. Explain medication dosages, administration techniques, and possible side effects.
   b. Define symptoms to watch for.
   c. Describe how to manage child at home (*e.g.*, when child awakens with barklike cough, place him or her in the bathroom and run hot water to produce steam; instruct parents to stay in bathroom with child to prevent accidental injury).

H. Evaluation
1. The child maintains normal respiratory function and is afebrile and well hydrated.
2. Parents verbalize understanding of diagnosis, treatment, care and follow-up.

VIII. Epiglottitis
A. Description: acute and severe inflammation of the epiglottis
B. Etiology and incidence
1. **Primarily caused by *H. influenzae*, type B.**
2. Usually affects children between the ages of 1 and 8 years.
C. Pathophysiology and management
1. The soft tissue of the epiglottis becomes inflamed causing *life-threatening* marked obstruction.
2. Progressive obstruction results in hypoxia, hypercapnia, and acidosis, closely followed by decreased muscle tone, altered level of consciousness and, if obstruction becomes complete, sudden death.
3. Endotracheal intubation or tracheotomy usually is considered. IV antibiotics are initiated and steroids may be used for edema.
D. Clinical assessment findings
1. Sudden onset of fever, lethargy, dyspnea
2. Restlessness and anxiety

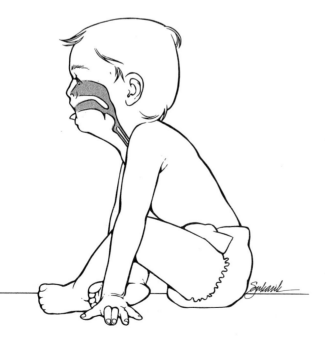

   3.   **Hyperextension of the neck, drooling, severe sore throat with refusal to drink**
4.   **Stridor, hoarseness**
5.   Rapid thready pulse

   6.   **Characteristic "tripod" position: child sitting upright, leaning forward, with chin out thrust, mouth open, and tongue protruding (Fig. 10-1)**
7.   Late signs of hypoxia: listlessness, cyanosis, bradycardia, decreased respiratory rate with decreased aeration
8.   Child's throat red and inflamed with a large, cherry red, edematous epiglottis

   9.   **Note: When epiglottitis is suspected, have an otolaryngologist or other specially trained person examine the throat. Also make sure that emergency equipment (endotracheal intubation tray and tracheotomy tray) is readily available because the throat examination may precipitate complete airway obstruction.**

  E. **Diagnostic assessment findings**
    1.   Lateral neck X-ray film shows epiglottal enlargement, which confirms the diagnosis.
    2.   Elevated white blood cell (WBC) count and increased bands and neutrophils seen on differential count.
    3.   Causative bacteria may be identified by blood cultures.

FIGURE 10-1.
Classic tripod position of a child with epiglottitis: forward sitting, balanced onhands, mouth open, tongue protruding, and head tilted in sniffing position to relieve airway obstruction.

F. Nursing diagnoses
   1. Ineffective airway clearance
   2. Anxiety
   3. Risk for altered body temperature
   4. Risk for fluid volume deficit
   5. Risk for infection
   6. Risk for injury

G. Planning and implementation
   1. Prepare for emergency hospitalization. After diagnosis is confirmed, endotracheal intubation or tracheostomy typically is performed to maintain a patent airway. Swelling usually decreases after 24 hours and the child is generally extubated by the third day.
   2. Administer prescribed steroids and antibiotics. The infection usually is treated with antibiotics (ampicillin and chloramphenicol or cefuroxime) for 7 to 10 days, and an IV line is started to maintain adequate hydration and deliver antibiotics.
   3. Closely monitor respiratory status to ensure airway patency. If the child presents with symptoms of epiglottitis, ensure that throat examination is performed by appropriate personnel and that emergency equipment is at hand.
   4. After the child is intubated, monitor closely and maintain a patent airway. Suction as needed and provide oxygen therapy as prescribed.
   5. Observe closely for signs of respiratory distress after extubation.
   6. Monitor for signs and symptoms of infection.
   7. Ensure adequate hydration by monitoring IV fluids and intake and output.
   8. Help relieve anxiety by maintaining a calm environment, limiting intrusive procedures, encouraging parent-child interactions, providing diversion, assisting the child in finding a comfortable position for breathing before intubation, and administering a sedative, as prescribed, during intubation.
   9. Provide family support to reduce anxiety.
   10. Administer prescribed medications.
   11. Provide client and family teaching:
       a. Outline home care and follow-up
       b. **Recommend that all children receive *H. influenzae* type B (Hib) conjugate vaccine, beginning at age 2 months.**

H. Evaluation
   1. The child displays normal respiratory function and is afebrile and well hydrated.
   2. Parents verbalize an understanding of diagnosis, treatment, home care, and follow-up.

IX. Pneumonia
A. Description
1. Acute inflammation of the lung parenchyma (bronchioles, alveolar ducts and sacs, and alveoli) that impairs gas exchange.
2. Pneumonia is classified according to etiologic agent (see below).
3. Pneumonia may also be classified according to location and extent of pulmonary involvement:
    a. Lobar: involves a large segment of one or more lobes
    b. Bronchopneumonia: begins in the terminal bronchioles and involves the nearby lobules
    c. Interstitial: confined to the alveolar walls and peribronchial and interlobular tissues

B. Etiology and incidence
1. Pneumonia most commonly results from infection with viruses, bacteria, or mycoplasms, or from aspiration of foreign substances. Pneumonia may also be caused by chlamydia, a bacterialike organism,
2. Viral pneumonia is the most common type, with RSV the most common agent, in infants. In older children the most common agents are adenoviruses, influenza, and parainfluenza viruses.
3. The major bacterial agents in infants under age 3 months are pneumococci, streptococci, staphylococci, enteric bacilli, and chlamydia; in children 3 months to 5 years, pneumococci and *H. influenzae* (decreased since vaccine); in children over 5 years, *Mycoplasma pneumonia.*

C. Pathophysiology and management
1. Pneumonia typically begins with a mild upper respiratory tract infection.
2. As the disorder progresses, parenchymal inflammation occurs.
3. Bacterial pneumonia most often causes lobular involvement and sometimes consolidation; viral pneumonia usually causes inflammation of interstitial tissue.

D. Clinical assessment findings
1. Common findings in viral pneumonia include:
    a. Variations ranging from mild fever, slight cough, and malaise to high fever, severe cough, and prostration
    b. Nonproduction or productive cough with whitish sputum
    c. Rhonchi or fine rales
2. Common findings in bacterial pneumonia include:
    a. High fever
    b. Respiratory: cough (unproductive to productive with whitish sputum), tachypnea, rhonchi, rales, dullness on percussion, chest pain, retractions, nasal flaring, pallor or cyanosis (depending on severity)

      c.   Irritability, restlessness, lethargy

      d.   Nausea, vomiting, anorexia, diarrhea, and abdominal pain

E. Diagnostic assessment findings

1. Chest x-ray studies may reveal diffuse or patchy infiltrates, consolidation, disseminated infiltration or patchy clouding depending on type of pneumonia.

2. Blood tests may reveal elevated WBC count.

3. Causative agent may be disclosed by blood culture or Gram stain and culture of sputum.

4. Positive antistreptolysin-O (ASO) titer is diagnostic of streptococcal pneumonia.

F. Nursing diagnoses

1. Ineffective airway clearance

2. Impaired gas exchange

3. Activity intolerance

4. Risk for altered body temperature

5. Ineffective breathing pattern

6. Potential fluid volume deficit

7. Altered nutrition: less than body requirements

8. Pain

G. Planning and implementation

1. Initiate medication interventions as prescribed.

      a. *Viral pneumonia:* Treatment is usually supportive, although antibiotic therapy may be recommended to reduce the risk of a secondary bacterial infection.

      b. *Bacterial pneumonia:* antibiotic therapy is indicated; penicillin G usually is used for pneumococcal and streptococcal pneumonia; a penicillinase-resistant penicillin (methicillin) usually is used for staphylococcal pneumonia.

      c. Humidified oxygen, chest physiotherapy, and suctioning may be required for either kind of pneumonia.

2. Assess for respiratory distress by monitoring vital signs and respiratory status.

3. Ease respiratory effort by:

      a. Administering oxygen and humidity as prescribed

      b. Performing chest physiotherapy

      c. Using incentive spirometry

      d. Suctioning as needed

      e. Changing child's position frequently and elevating the head of the bed

4. Ensure adequate hydration by encouraging oral fluids or by monitoring IV fluids.

5. Promote rest by maintaining bed rest and organizing nursing care to minimize disturbances.

6. Provide support for the family.

7. Administer prescribed medication as scheduled.
8. Provide patient and family teaching:
    a. Discuss home care and follow-up measures.
    b. Recommend the pneumococcal vaccine for children age 2 years and older who are at risk.

H. **Evaluation**
1. The child exhibits normal respiratory function and is afebrile and well hydrated.
2. Parents verbalize an understanding of diagnosis, treatment, home care, and follow-up.

X. Asthma

A. **Description: a chronic, reversible obstructive airway disease, characterized by wheezing, caused by a spasm of the bronchial tubes or the swelling of their mucous membranes, after exposure to various stimuli.**

B. **Etiology and incidence**
1. Most common chronic disease in childhood, with most children experiencing their first symptoms by age 5 years
2. Commonly results from allergic hyperresponsiveness of the trachea and bronchi to irritants
3. Common irritants include viral infections, air pollution, dust, smoke, molds, certain foods, animal danders, rapid changes in environmental temperatures, exercise, and psychological stress
4. Shows familial tendency
5. Before puberty, affects more males than females; at puberty, increased incidence in females
6. More severe in younger children; may decrease in severity with age
7. Incidence greater in urban areas

C. **Pathophysiology and management**
1. Three events contribute to symptoms: bronchial spasm, inflammation and edema of the mucosa, and production of thick mucus, which results in increased airway resistance, premature closure of airways, hyperinflation, increased work of breathing, and impaired gas exchange.
2. If not treated promptly, status asthmaticus—acute, severe, prolonged asthma attack that is unresponsive to the usual treatment—may occur, requiring hospitalization.

D. **Clinical assessment findings**
1. Dyspnea, retractions, and tachypnea with prolonged expiration
2. Cyanosis
3. Wheezing and cough (tight and nonproductive to loose and productive with progression)
4. Fatigue and diaphoresis

E. **Diagnostic assessment findings**

    1. Peak expiratory flow reflects the degree of airway obstruction in the large airways and correlates with the degree of small airway obstruction.

    2. Blood gas values reveal CO_2 retention and acidosis. (See Table 10-1 for normal arterial blood gas values.)

F. **Nursing diagnoses**

    1. Ineffective airway clearance

    2. Activity intolerance

    3. Anxiety

    4. Body image disturbance

    5. Ineffective breathing pattern

    6. Altered family processes

    7. Risk for fluid volume deficit

    8. Altered health seeking behaviors

    9. Risk for infection

    10. Risk for injury

    11. Knowledge deficit

    12. Noncompliance

    13. Self-esteem disturbance

G. **Planning and implementation**

    1. Administer prescribed bronchodilators carefully:

        a. **Monitor vital signs; check for toxicity (nausea and vomiting, tachycardia, seizures); monitor blood gas levels especially when giving methylxanthines, such as**

TABLE 10-1.
Normal Arterial Blood Gas Values by Age

PARAMETER	NORMAL VALUE	
PO_2	Birth:	8–24 mm Hg
	Day 1:	45–95 mm Hg
	Thereafter:	83–108 mm Hg
$PaCO_2$	Neonate:	27–40 mm Hg
	Infant:	27–41 mm Hg
	Thereafter:	
	Male:	35–48 mm Hg
	Female:	32–45 mm Hg
pH	Premature neonate (48 hours after birth):	
		7.35–7.5 mm Hg
	Full-term neonate (at birth): 7.11–7.36	
	Day 1:	7.29–7.45 mm Hg
	Thereafter:	7.35–7.45 mm Hg

        theophylline and aminophylline, to provide bronchodilation for daily maintenance and acute attacks.

    b. **Monitor for paroxysmal bronchospasm and increase fluids when administering sympathomimetics (beta adrenergics), such as albuterol and terbutaline, to promote bronchodilation in daily maintenance and acute attacks.**

2. Administer other prescribed medications (*e.g.,* Cromolyn sodium) administered by inhaler as a prophylactic measure; corticosteroids, usually administered by inhaler to reduce airway inflammation; and antibiotics if the child has an infection.

3. Increase respiratory effectiveness by:
   a. Administering medications as prescribed.
   b. Elevating the head of the bed.
   c. Administering oxygen as prescribed.
   d. Performing chest physiotherapy as prescribed.

4. Assess respiratory status, closely evaluating breathing patterns and monitoring vital signs.

5. Promote rest by scheduling nursing activities so that they do not coincide with rest periods, and encourage activities appropriate to tolerance level.

6. Ensure adequate hydration by encouraging fluids or monitoring IV infusion.

7. Monitor for effectiveness of medication therapy.

8. Help child and family identify potential precipitating factors, and discuss possible ways to avoid them.

9. Explain the possible use of hyposensitization therapy.

10. Help child cope with poor self-esteem by encouraging him or her to ventilate feelings and concerns. Listen actively as child does so, focus on child's strengths, and help him or her to identify the positive and negative aspects of his or her situation.

11. Help alleviate anxiety by remaining calm and by promoting a quiet environment.

12. Provide support for the family.

13. Encourage family members to participate in the child's care.

14. Encourage family members to verbalize their feelings related to acute exacerbations of asthma and their feelings related to the chronicity of the illness.

15. Discuss need for periodic pulmonary function tests to evaluate and guide therapy and to monitor the course of the illness.

16. Provide patient and family teaching:
    a. Detail measures to prevent respiratory infection by avoiding exposure to persons with known infections and by maintaining good hygiene and sound health patterns.
    b. Explain the diagnosis.

   c. Express ways to identify and prevent known attack precipitants.

   d. Define the need for hydration to keep mucous secretions thin.

   e. Discuss ways to perform physical activities commensurate with tolerance level.

   f. Demonstrate and explain rationale for breathing exercises, inhalation therapy, and chest physiotherapy.

   g. Outline dosage, administration, and possible side effects of medications.

   h. Assist child and family to name signs and symptoms of an acute attack and appropriate treatment measures.

  17. Refer family to appropriate community agency for assistance.

  18. Assist the client and family in receiving hyposensitization therapy if needed.

 H. **Evaluation**

  1. The child exhibits a normal breathing pattern with lungs clear on auscultation and remains afebrile and well-hydrated.

  2. The child and parents verbalize an understanding of the diagnosis, treatment, preventive measures, psychosocial care, and follow-up measures.

XI. Cystic fibrosis (CF)

 A. **Description: a chronic inherited disorder of the exocrine glands characterized by abnormally thick pulmonary secretions.**

 B. **Etiology and incidence**

  1. **CF is an autosomal recessive hereditary disorder that affects the pancreas, respiratory system, gastrointestinal tract, salivary glands, and reproductive tract.**

  2. The gene responsible for CF was identified in 1989. The gene is on chromosome 7.

  3. The most common lethal inherited disease affecting Caucasians, CF occurs in about 1 in 1600 live births.

  4. Incidence is equal in both sexes.

  5. About 95% of young people with CF survive until age 16; 50% survive about 28 years.

 C. **Pathophysiology and management**

  1. The underlying defect is thought to be related to a protein or enzyme alteration.

  2. Several mechanisms result in the CF process: exocrine glands become obstructed by thick mucus; electrolyte concentrations in the exocrine secretions are abnormal; the ciliary lining in the respiratory tract moves five to ten times slower than normal; secretions accumulate in respiratory passages, increasing respiratory infections and causing obstruction, air-trapping, and infection (most commonly *Pseudomonas aeruginosa*). Recurrent infections lead to bronchiectasis and fibrosis. The small intestine, bile ducts, salivary glands, and the reproductive system also are affected by thickened secretions.

D. **Clinical assessment findings**

1. Manifestations vary with severity and time of emergence; they may appear at birth or take years to develop.
2. Respiratory signs and symptoms include:
    a. Wheezing, dyspnea, cough, cyanosis
    b. As disease progresses, atelectasis and generalized obstructive emphysema result from mucoid obstruction in small airways, producing the characteristic features of barrel chest and finger clubbing
    c. Chronic sinusitis, bronchitis, bronchopneumonia, or ear, nose, and throat problems
3. Gastrointestinal signs include:

    a. **Meconium ileus at birth**
    b. **Rectal prolapse (most common gastrointestinal (GI) sign)**
    c. Loose, bulky, frothy fatty stools; voracious appetite; weight loss; marked tissue wasting; failure to thrive; distended abdomen; thin extremities; evidence of Vitamin A, D, E, K deficiencies
4. Reproductive signs include:
    a. Females: decreased fertility apparently from increased viscosity of cervical mucus, which blocks the entry of sperm
    b. Males: sterility caused by blockage of the vas deferens with abnormal secretions, which prevents sperm from forming
5. Cardiovascular signs include:
    a. Cor pulmonale, right-sided heart enlargement and congestive heart failure resulting from obstruction of pulmonary blood flow
    b. Signs and symptoms of hyponatremia, necessitating rapid IV electrolyte replacement to prevent circulatory collapse

E. **Diagnostic assessment findings**

1. **Elevated chloride levels on sweat test (iontophoresis with pilocarpine), chloride level is above 60 mEq/L.**
2. Absence of pancreatic enzyme activity, helping to confirm diagnosis.
3. Steatorrhea detected in stool analysis.
4. Evidence of generalized obstructive emphysema on chest radiograph.

F. **Nursing diagnoses**
1. Ineffective airway clearance
2. Ineffective breathing pattern
3. High risk for infection
4. Risk for activity intolerance
5. Altered family process
6. Impaired gas exchange
7. Anticipatory grieving
8. Knowledge deficit
9. Altered nutrition: less than body requirements
10. Sleep pattern disturbance
11. Body image disturbance
12. Self-esteem disturbance
13. Potential for diarrhea

G. **Planning and implementation**
1. Encourage pulmonary hygiene measures to aid sputum expectoration, such as chest physiotherapy, postural drainage, aerosol treatments with bronchodilators, and breathing exercises.
2. Monitor respiratory status by evaluating respiratory pattern and vital signs.
3. Encourage adequate nutrition; serve desirable foods in a pleasant atmosphere. (The prescribed diet typically is high in calories and protein, with fats as tolerated and increased salt intake during hot weather or febrile periods.)
4. Assess nutritional status by maintaining calorie counts, monitoring intake and output, and recording daily weights.
5. Provide family support.
6. **Administer medications as prescribed, including pancreatic enzymes with food. Wipe child's lips and face after administration because the substance is caustic. Maintain airway patency with bronchodilators; control infection with antibiotics primarily targeted toward pseudomonas and staphylococci (aminoglycosides, such as tobramycin and gentamicin cephalosporins). Administer fat-soluble vitamins (A, D, E, K) as prescribed.**
7. Promote growth and development by proving appropriate activities.
8. Monitor for signs of infection; prevent infection by promoting good health and hygiene practices as well as limiting exposure to infected persons.
9. Promote adequate rest by clustering nursing activities and by allowing rest periods.

10. Help child maintain positive self-concept by active listening, encouraging verbalization, identifying strengths.
11. As necessary, assist in arranging for tutor or other help with school work.
12. Allow family and child to verbalize about the chronic nature of the disorder and its long-term implications, including death and dying.
13. Provide client and family teaching:
    a. Review the diagnosis, disease process, long-term implications and chronic nature of the condition.
    b. Highlight the importance of good pulmonary hygiene infection prevention and general well-being.
    c. Explain dosage, administration, and side effects of medication.
    d. Outline special dietary instructions.

H. **Evaluation**
1. The child exhibits improved respiratory status, is afebrile, reports no pain or discomfort, tolerates the prescribed diet and gains or maintains weight.
2. Child and parents verbalize an understanding of the diagnosis, treatment, associated care aspects, psychosocial factors, and follow-up care.
3. The child and family cope with the chronicity of the disorder and with the grieving process.

Bibliography

Alfaro-LeFevre, R., et al. (1992). *Drug Handbook: A Nursing Process Approach.* Redwood City, CA: Addison-Wesley.

Betz, C.L., Hunsberger, M.M. and Wright, S. (1994). *Family Centered Nursing Care of Children,* 2nd ed. Philadelphia: W.B. Saunders.

Bradford, B.J. (1993). Index of suspicion: Acute epiglottitis. *Pediatrics in Review, 14,* 281.

Castiglia, P.T. and Harbin, R.B. (1993). *Child Health Care: Process and Practice.* Philadelphia: J.B. Lippincott.

Jackson, D.B. and Saunders, R.B. (1993). *Child Health Nursing: A Comprehensive Approach to the Care of Children and Their Families.* Philadelphia: J.B. Lippincott.

Modlin, J.F. (1994). Bacterial pneumonia. In Oski, F.A., et al (eds). *Principles and Practice of Pediatrics,* 2nd ed. Philadelphia: J.B. Lippincott.

Wong, D.L. (1993). *Whaley and Wong's Essentials of Pediatric Nursing,* 4th ed. St. Louis: C.V. Mosby.

Wong, D. L. (1995). *Whaley and Wong's Nursing Care of Infants and Children,* 5th ed. St. Louis: C.V. Mosby.

STUDY QUESTIONS

1. When caring for a very low birth weight newborn, the nurse carefully monitors inspiratory pressure and oxygen (O^2) concentration to prevent:
   a. Respiratory distress syndrome (RDS)
   b. Respiratory syncytial virus (RSV)
   c. Bronchopulmonary dysplasia (BPD)
   d. Meconium aspiration syndrome

2. Which of the following infants is least likely to develop SIDS?
   a. An infant who was premature
   b. A sibling of an infant who died of SIDS
   c. An infant with prenatal drug exposure
   d. An infant who sleeps on his or her side

3. Parent teaching for otitis media should include:
   a. Cleaning the ears with cotton swabs
   b. Supine bottle feeding
   c. Avoiding contact with people who have upper respiratory infections
   d. Giving amoxicillin (Amoxcil) on an empty stomach

4. The disorder that results from inflammation of the bronchioles with tenacious mucus causing variable obstruction is:
   a. Bronchiolitis
   b. Bronchitis
   c. Bronchopneumonia
   d. Bronchopulmonary dysplasia

5. Ribavirin is used for:
   a. All cases of bronchiolitis
   b. All cases of RSV bronchiolitis
   c. Severe RSV bronchiolitis
   d. No cases of bronchiolitis

6. Which of the following respiratory conditions is always considered a medical emergency?
   a. Laryngotracheobronchitis
   b. Epiglottitis
   c. Asthma
   d. Cystic fibrosis

7. Immunization of children with the *H. influenzae* type B (Hib) vaccine decreases the incidence of which of the following conditions?
   a. Laryngotracheobronchitis
   b. Epiglottitis
   c. Pneumonia
   d. Bronchiolitis

8. In a child with asthma, methylxanthines such as aminophylline are administered primarily to:
   a. Decrease postnasal drip
   b. Dilate the bronchioles
   c. Reduce airway inflammation
   d. Reduce secondary infections

9. Common findings in older children with pneumococcal pneumonia include:
   a. Bulging fontanel
   b. Mild cough
   c. Slight fever
   d. Chest pain

10. A severe prolonged asthmatic attack is referred to as:
    a. Intrinsic asthma
    b. Status asthmaticus
    c. Reactive airway disease
    d. Extrinsic asthma

11. When teaching an asthmatic child and the family, the nurse should include all of the following except:
    a. Identifying precipitators to prevent attacks
    b. Using bronchodilator inhaler before steroid inhaler
    c. Minimizing exercise and activities to prevent attacks
    d. Increasing fluid intake regularly to thin secretions

12. How is cystic fibrosis transmitted?
    a. Autosomal dominant gene
    b. Autosomal recessive gene
    c. Direct contact
    d. Indirect contact

ANSWER KEY

1. *Correct response: c*
   Bronchopulmonary dysplasia has been related to high inspiratory pressures and oxygen concentrations.
   a. RDS is a disorder caused by lack of surfactant and usually is found in premature infants.
   b. RSV is a group of viruses that cause respiratory infections such as bronchiolitis and pneumonia.
   d. Meconium aspiration syndrome is a respiratory disorder created by the aspiration of meconium in the perinatal period.
   Application/Safe Care/Planning

2. *Correct response: d*
   There has been an association between SIDS and infants who sleep on their abdomens, not their sides.
   a, b, and c. All have been considered risk factors for the development of SIDS.
   Application/Safe Care/Assessment

3. *Correct response: c*
   Otitis media is commonly precipitated by an upper respiratory tract infection; therefore children prone to otitis should avoid persons known to have an upper respiratory tract infection.
   a. Cotton swabs can cause injuries, such as tympanic perforation.
   b. A bottle-fed child should be fed in an upright position; feeding the child supine may actually precipitate otitis by creating pools of formula in the pharyngeal cavity.
   d. Amoxicillin should be given with food to prevent stomach upset.
   Application/Physiologic/Implementation

4. *Correct response: a*
   Bronchiolitis is an inflammation of the bronchioles.
   b. Bronchitis is inflammation of the tracheobronchial tree.
   c. Bronchopneumonia is an acute inflammation of the lungs and bronchioles.
   d. Bronchopulmonary dysplasia is a chronic pulmonary disease of infancy.
   Knowledge/Physiologic/NA

5. *Correct response: c*
   Ribavirin is an antiviral medication used for treating severe RSV infection and for children with RSV who are compromised (such as children with bronchopulmonary dysplasia or heart disease).
   a and b. Ribavirin should be reserved for those noted above and is not used for all children who have bronchiolitis.
   d. Ribavirin is used as noted above.
   Comprehension/Physiologic/Planning

6. *Correct response: b*
   Epiglottitis is always considered an acute medical emergency because it is life-threatening.
   a. Acute LTB requires close observation for airway obstruction, but it is not always an emergency.
   c. Asthma is a chronic disease; however, status asthmaticus and acute attacks require prompt treatment.
   d. Cystic fibrosis is a chronic disease and is not considered an emergency.
   Application/Safe Care/Planning

7. *Correct response: b*
   Epiglottitis is a bacterial infection of the epiglottis primarily caused by *H. influenzae* type B. Administration of the vaccine has decreased the incidence of epiglottitis.
   a. Acute laryngotracheobronchitis is of viral origin.
   c. The most common bacterial organisms causing pneumonia in children are pneumococci, streptococci, and staphylococci.

d. Bronchiolitis is usually caused by RSV.

Application/Health Promotion/ Implementation

8. Correct response: b
Methylxanthines are highly effective bronchodilators.
a. Decongestants may be given for postnasal drip.
c. Corticosteriods may be used for their anti-inflammatory effect.
d. Antibiotics are used to prevent secondary infection.

Application/Physiologic/Assessment

9. Correct response: d
Older children with pneumococcal pneumonia may complain of chest pain.
a. A bulging fontanel may be seen in infants with meningitis.
b. A mild cough may be seen in viral pneumonia.

c. A slight fever is more likely to occur in viral pneumonia.

Application/Physiologic/Assessment

10. Correct response: b
Status asthmaticus is a prolonged, severe asthmatic attack.
b. Intrinsic is a term for internal precipitating factors such as viruses.
c. Reactive airway disease is another general term for asthma.
d. Extrinsic is a term for external precipitating factors such as allergens.

Application/Physiologic/Assessment

11. Correct response: c
Asthmatic children should be encouraged to exercise as tolerated.
a, b, and d. All are measures that should be taught to asthmatic children and their families.

Application/Health Promotion/ Implementation

Gastrointestinal Dysfunction

11

I.   Essential concepts: gastrointestinal (GI) structures and function

  A.   Development

  1.   Development of a primitive digestive system begins during the fourth week of gestation, with the most extensive development occurring in the last few weeks before birth.

  2.   A newborn's stomach capacity is only 10 to 20 mL at birth, and peristalsis is rapid, resulting in frequent regurgitation.

  3.   Normal newborns pass one to six stools per day.

  B.   Function

  1.   Digestion involves physical and chemical breakdown of food into absorbable substances.

  2.   Absorption involves transfer of the end products of digestion across the intestinal wall into the circulation for use by the cells.

II.   GI system overview

  A.   Assessment

  1.   Assessing a child's GI system involves obtaining a complete health history, with emphasis on nutrition and elimination, and performing a physical assessment, particularly of the oral cavity and the abdomen.

  2.   Abnormal findings indicating possible GI dysfunction.

   a.   Growth and development: height and weight below standard age-related normals

   b.   Skin: pallor, jaundice, carotenemia

   c.   Hair: abnormal texture, sparse

   d.   Head: microcephaly, craniotabes

   e.   Mouth: caries, periodontal disease

   f.   Abdomen: distention, depression, umbilical herniation, visible peristaltic waves, tenderness, masses, enlarged liver or spleen, and increased, decreased, or absent bowel sounds

   g.   Anus: rectal bleeding, nonpatency

B. **Laboratory studies and diagnostic tests**
1. Stool cultures
2. Stool sample evaluation for ova and parasites
3. Stool sample evaluation for blood, mucus, fat, urobilogen, trypsin, and leukocytes (Table 11-1)
4. Stool-reducing substances and pH tests
5. Complete blood count with differential
6. Urine specific gravity
7. Bowel studies: upper GI series, barium enema, biopsy, rectosigmoidoscopy
8. Liver and endocrine function tests
9. Abdominal radiographs

C. **Psychosocial implications**
1. **Infants: Oral gratification may be compromised by an infant's inability to suck well owing to a cleft lip or palate, surgery, and alternate feeding methods.**
2. Toddlers: Locomotion is compromised in a child receiving long-term hyperalimentation or drug therapy.
3. Preschoolers: Malnourishment may interfere with development of normal motor skills such as running.

TABLE 11-1.
Stool Analysis

PARAMETER	NORMAL FINDINGS	IMPLICATIONS OF ABNORMAL FINDINGS
Color	Brown (shade varies with diet)	Black: GI bleeding Tan or clay: common bile duct blockage; pancreatic insufficiency Red streaked: lower GI bleeding
Blood	Negative	GI bleeding; ulcerative colitis
Mucus	Negative	Ulcerative colitis; bacillary dysentery
Fat	Fatty acids: 0–6 yr: <2 g/24 h 6 and over: 2–6 g/24 h	Increase: malabsorption syndromes
Urobilogen	30–200 mg/100 g of feces	Increase: hemolytic anemia Decrease: biliary obstruction; severe liver disease; oral antibiotic therapy that alters intestinal flora; disorders causing decreased hemoglobin turnover (*e.g.*, aplastic anemia)
Trypsin	Positive for small amounts in 95% of all children	Absence: pancreatic insufficiency
pH	7.0–7.5	Acid: carbohydrate fermentation Alkaline: protein breakdown
Nitrogen	1–2 g/24 h	Increase (along with high fecal fat); chronic progressive pancreatitis

4.   School-age children and adolescents: Body image and self-concept may be challenged by a child's altered body function and health maintenance needs.

III.   Cleft lip and palate

A.   Description

1.   Cleft lip is a congenital anomaly involving one or more clefts in the upper lip ranging from a slight dimple to a large cleft involving nasal structures.

2.   Cleft palate is a congenital anomaly consisting of a cleft ranging from soft palate involvement alone to a defect including the hard palate and portions of the maxilla in severe cases.

B.   Etiology and incidence

1.   Causes include genetic, environmental, and teratogenic factors.

2.   Cleft lip occurs in approximately 1 of every 800 births, most commonly in boys. Cleft palate occurs in 1 of every 2000 births; incidence in girls is double that of boys.

3.   **Children may have associated dental malformations, speech problems, and frequent otitis media, the latter resulting from improper functioning of the eustachian tubes.**

C.   Pathophysiology and management

1.   These defects occur during embryonic development: the lip between weeks 7 and 8 of gestation; the palate between weeks 7 and 12 of gestation.

2.   Cleft lip results from failure of fusion of lateral and medial tissues forming the upper lip; cleft palate, from failure of fusion of tissues that form the palate.

3.   These defects may occur separately or in combination to produce complete unilateral or bilateral cleft from the lip through the soft palate.

4.   Depending on the defect and the child's general condition, surgical correction of the cleft lip usually occurs at age 1 to 2 months; of the palate, between ages 6 and 18 months. Cleft palate repair may require several stages.

5.   Early correction of cleft lip enables more normal sucking patterns and facilitates bonding. Early correction of cleft palate enables development of more normal speech patterns. Delayed closure or large defects may require the use of orthodontic appliances.

D.   Clinical assessment findings

1.   These defects are readily apparent at birth.

2.   Careful physical assessment should be performed to rule out other midline birth defects.

E.   Diagnostic assessment findings

1.   There are no specific diagnostic assessments.

F. **Nursing diagnoses**
1. Ineffective airway clearance
2. Altered family process
3. Risk for infection
4. Risk for injury
5. Knowledge deficit
6. Altered nutrition: less than body requirements
7. Pain
8. Ineffective infant feeding pattern
9. Altered growth and development

G. **Planning and implementation**
1. Ensure adequate nutrition and prevent aspiration.
   a. Provide special nipples or feeding devices (*e.g.,* soft pliable bottle with soft nipple with enlarged opening) for a child unable to suck adequately on standard nipples.
   b. Hold the child in a semi-upright position; direct the formula away from the cleft and toward the side and back of the mouth to prevent aspiration.
   c. Feed the infant slowly and burp him or her frequently to prevent excessive air swallowing and regurgitation.
2. Support the infant's and parents' emotional and social adjustment. Help facilitate the family's acceptance of the infant by encouraging the parents to express their feelings and concerns and by conveying an attitude of acceptance toward the infant. Reassure parents that reparative surgery usually is successful.
3. Preoperatively
   a. Reinforce physician's explanation of surgical procedures.
   b. Provide mouth care to prevent infection.
4. Postoperatively
   a. Assess airway patency and vital signs; observe for edema and respiratory distress.
   b. Use mist tent, if prescribed, to minimize edema, liquefy secretions, and minimize distress.
   c. **Position the child with cleft lip on his or her back, in an infant seat, or propped on side to avoid injury to the operative site; position child with a cleft palate on abdomen to facilitate drainage.**
   d. Clean suture line and apply antibacterial ointment as prescribed to prevent infection and scarring. Monitor site for signs of infection.
   e. Use elbow restraints to maintain suture line integrity. Remove them every 2 hours for skin care and range of motion exercises.

f. **If used, keep Logan's bow (device used to protect suture line from trauma) in place for children who have undergone cleft lip repairs.**

g. Feed the infant with a rubber-tipped medicine dropper, bulb syringe, Breck feeder, or soft bottle-nipple, as prescribed, to help preserve suture integrity. For older children, diet progresses from clear fluids; they should not use straws or sharp objects.

h. Attempt to keep child from putting tongue up to palate sutures.

i. Manage pain by administering analgesics as prescribed.

4. Provide client and family teaching:
   a. Demonstrate surgical wound care.
   b. Show proper feeding techniques and positions.
   c. Explain that temperature of feeding formulas should be monitored because new palate has no nerve endings; therefore, child can burn self easily.
   d. Explain handling of prosthesis if indicated.
   e. Stress the importance of long-term follow-up, including speech therapy, and preventing or correcting dental abnormalities.
   f. Discuss the need for at least annual hearing evaluations because of the increased susceptibility to recurrent otitis. The child may requires myringotomy and surgical placement of drainage tubes.

H. Evaluation

1. Parents demonstrate acceptance of the child and verbalize an understanding of preoperative and postoperative aspects of care.

2. The child gains weight and is free from infection and signs of respiratory distress.

3. The family is referred for follow-up care from a multidisciplinary health care team that may include a pediatrician, nurse, plastic surgeon, orthodontist, prosthodontist, otolaryngologist, speech therapist, psychiatrist, and social worker.

4. The family is referred to a support group for clients and families with cleft lip and palate.

5. Parents receive genetic counseling if indicated.

IV. Pyloric stenosis

A. Description: narrowing of the pyloric sphincter at the outlet of the stomach.

B. Etiology and incidence

1. The exact cause is unknown; however, heredity may play an important role.

    2. Incidence is 5 of every 1000 males and 1 of every 1000 females. It is more common in Caucasians.

C. **Pathophysiology and management**

    1. The pylorus narrows because of progressive hypertrophy and hyperplasia of the circular pyloric muscle. The muscle may grow to twice its size (Fig. 11-1).

    2. This leads to obstruction of the pyloric sphincter, with subsequent gastric distension, dilatation, and hypertrophy.

    3. Pyloromyotomy (creation of an incision along the anterior pylorus to split the muscle) is commonly performed to relieve obstruction.

D. **Clinical assessment findings**

    1. Usually no abnormal signs in the first weeks after birth

    2. Regurgitation or nonprojectile vomiting beginning by age 3 weeks; emesis is not bile stained and contains only gastric contents but may be blood tinged.

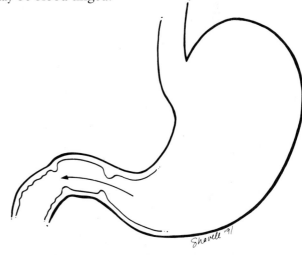

A

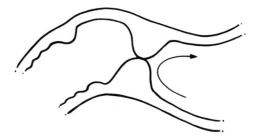

FIGURE 11-1.
Pyloric stenosis. **(A)** *Arrow* represents normal passage through pyloric sphincter. **(B)** *Curved arrow* represents stoppage of flow because of stenotic sphincter.

B

𝑚   3.   **Vomiting increases in frequency and force over the next 1 to 2 weeks until most of ingested food is expelled through projectile vomiting.**

      4.   Good appetite and feeding habits

      5.   No evidence of pain

      6.   Weight loss

      7.   Upper abdominal distention

𝑚   8.   **Palpable olive-shaped mass in the epigastrium just to the right of the umbilicus**

      9.   Visible gastric peristaltic waves moving from left to right across the epigastrium

    10.   Decreased frequency and volume of stools

    11.   Signs of malnutrition and dehydration

   E.   **Diagnostic assessment findings:**

      1.   Ultrasonography and upper GI series revealing delayed gastric emptying and an elongated, thin pylorus

      2.   Increased serum pH and bicarbonate levels, indicating metabolic alkalosis

      3.   Decreased serum chloride, sodium, and potassium levels

      4.   Increased hematocrit and hemoglobin values, reflecting hemoconcentration

   F.   **Nursing diagnoses**

      1.   Risk for aspiration

      2.   Ineffective breathing pattern

      3.   Altered family process

      4.   Risk for fluid volume deficit

      5.   Knowledge deficit

      6.   Altered nutrition: less than body requirements

      7.   Pain

      8.   Risk for altered parenting

      9.   Impaired skin integrity

   G.   **Planning and implementation**

      1.   Monitor feeding pattern and the association between feedings and vomiting.

      2.   Assess the amount, character, and frequency of emesis.

      3.   Monitor hydration status: record intake and output (I&O), weigh the child daily, evaluate urine specific gravity.

      4.   Administer parenteral fluids as prescribed to replenish potassium and correct alkalosis.

      5.   Provide postoperative nutrition as prescribed, typically small amounts of clear liquids 4 to 6 hours postoperatively, advancing to formula as tolerated.

      6.   Feed infant slowly, burp frequently, and position in high Fowler's on the right side after feedings.

7. Promote comfort by providing good oral care and offering a pacifier while the infant is receiving nothing by mouth (NPO), and by encouraging parents to hold infant. Administer analgesics as prescribed.
8. Provide client and family teaching:
    a. Cover all procedures, scheduled surgical procedure, and preoperative and postoperative care measures.
    b. Demonstrate feeding and positioning techniques and surgical wound care as well.

H. **Evaluation**
1. The child appears well hydrated, retains feedings, gains weight, and appears comfortable.
2. Parents verbalize understanding of feeding techniques, wound care, and follow-up appointments.

V. Gastroesophageal reflux (GER)

A. **Description: backflow of gastric contents into the esophagus resulting from relaxation or incompetence of the lower esophageal (cardiac) sphincter.**

B. **Etiology and incidence**
1. The cause is unknown, but GER may result from delayed maturation of lower esophageal neuromuscular function or impaired local hormonal, control mechanisms.
2. GER is the most common esophageal problem in infancy. Some reflux occurs normally in infants, children, and adults. GER is deemed pathologic when it is severe, persists into late infancy, or is associated with complications. Approximately 1 of 300 to 1 of 1000 children have a significant problem with GER.
3. GER is not uncommon in children with tracheoesophageal or esophageal atresia repairs, neurologic disorders, scoliosis, asthma, or cystic fibrosis.

C. **Pathophysiology and management**
1. Inappropriate relaxation or failure of cardiac sphincter contraction leads to increased gastric or abdominal pressure and resultant reflux of gastric contents.
2. Delayed gastric emptying may be a contributing factor in GER.
3. Repeated reflux of acidic gastric contents can damage delicate esophageal mucosa.
4. GER commonly is self-limiting, usually resolving by age 1 year. In more severe cases, the child may require hospitalization and possibly surgery, such as a Nissen fundoplication, in which the gastric fundus is wrapped around the distal esophagus.

D. **Clinical assessment findings**

1. Forceful vomiting, possibly with hematemesis
2. Weight loss
3. Aspiration and recurrent respiratory infections
4. Cyanotic and apneic episodes that may be life-threatening
5. Esophagitis and bleeding from repeated irritation of the esophageal lining with gastric acid
6. Melena
7. Heartburn, abdominal pain, and bitter taste in the mouth

E. **Diagnostic assessment findings**

1. Observation of reflux following barium swallow and absence of gastric or duodenal obstruction on barium swallow and upper GI radiograph
2. Low resting lower esophageal sphincter pressure on esophageal manometry
3. Anemia secondary to blood loss
4. Intraesophageal pH monitoring measuring reflux acid from the stomach
5. Scintigraphy, which detects radiographic substances in the esophagus after feeding a compound to the child

F. **Nursing diagnoses**

1. Ineffective airway clearance
2. Risk for aspiration
3. Fluid volume deficit
4. Altered family process
5. Altered nutrition: less than body requirements
6. Risk for infection
7. Knowledge deficit
8. Pain
9. Impaired tissue integrity

G. **Planning and implementation**

1. Ensure adequate hydration by assessing for signs and symptoms of dehydration, monitoring I&O, and administering intravenous (IV) fluids as prescribed.
2. Assess the amount, frequency, and characteristics of emesis.
3. Assess the relationship between feeding and vomiting and the infant's activity level.
4. **Improve nutritional status through feeding techniques such as formula thickened with cereal, enlarging nipple holes, and burping infant frequently.**
5. **Help prevent reflux and respiratory complications by positioning the infant upright, as prescribed, through feedings and afterwards, in infant seat.**

      6.   Assess breath sounds before and after feedings; keep suctioning equipment at bedside.

      7.   Place infant on cardiac-apnea monitor as prescribed.

      8.   Administer prescribed medications:

         a.   Drugs that promote gastric emptying or pyloric sphincter relaxation, such as bethanecol, metoclopramide, and domperidone.

         b.   Antacids, to neutralize the acidity of refluxed contents and help prevent esophageal tissue damage.

      9.   Provide client and family teaching:

         a.   Demonstrate proper feeding techniques (thickening formula and positioning infant).

         b.   Explain all treatments and procedures.

         c.   Describe problems that may follow surgery (*e.g.*, flatulence, inability to vomit, poor feeding habits, and choking on solid foods).

H.   **Evaluation**

      1.   The child gains weight and eats normally.

      2.   The child maintains balanced fluid and electrolyte status and exhibits decreased vomiting, clear lungs on auscultation, and no signs of respiratory distress.

      3.   Parents verbalize an understanding of and demonstrate proper feeding techniques.

      4.   Parents plan follow-up care to monitor child's weight gain and nutritional status.

VI.   **Celiac disease**

A.   **Description: a chronic inability to tolerate foods containing gluten**

B.   **Etiology and incidence**

      1.   Celiac disease is believed to result from either an inborn error of metabolism or an abnormal immunologic response. Most likely, it is inherited though a dominant gene with incomplete penetrance.

      2.   The incidence is reported to be between 1 in 300 and 1 in 4000, and appears to be declining.

      3.   Celiac disease occurs more frequently in Europe than in the United States and is rarely reported in African-Americans or Asians.

C.   **Pathophysiology and management**

      1.   Intolerance for and inability to digest gluten (specifically the gliadin fraction of gluten found in wheat, barley, rye, and oats) results in the accumulation of the amino acid glutamine, which is toxic to intestinal mucosal cells.

2. As a result, intestinal villi eventually atrophy, which reduces the absorptive surface of the small intestine and affects absorption of ingested nutrients.

3. **The disorder is characterized by episodes of celiac crises, precipitated by infections, prolonged fasting, ingestion of gluten, or exposure to anticholinergic drugs, and characterized by a general flare-up of symptoms.**

4. Celiac crisis may lead to electrolyte imbalance, rapid dehydration, and severe acidosis.

D. Clinical assessment findings

1. Symptoms typically appear within 3 to 6 months after introduction of gluten to the diet.
2. Symptoms from impaired fat absorption:
   a. Steatorrhea
   b. Exceedingly foul smelling stools
3. Symptoms from impaired absorption of nutrients:
   a. Malnutrition (growth failure, weight loss)
   b. Muscle wasting, edema of lower extremities due to hypoproteinemia
   c. Anemia and anorexia
   d. Abdominal distention, vomiting, and abdominal pain
   e. Epistaxis, ecchymosis, or intestinal bleeding from disturbed blood coagulation due to inadequate vitamin K
4. Behavioral changes:
   a. Irritability
   b. Fretfulness
   c. Uncooperativeness
   d. Apathy
5. Symptoms of celiac crisis:
   a. Acute, severe episodes of profuse watery diarrhea
   b. Vomiting
6. For unknown reasons, some children do not exhibit symptoms until after age 5 years; in these cases, growth retardation and delayed sexual maturation are the predominant manifestations.

E. Diagnostic assessment findings

1. Biopsy of the small intestine revealing flat mucosal surface, absence or atrophy of villi, and deep visible crypts. These characteristic lesions return to normal after dietary restriction of gluten, which helps confirm diagnosis.
2. Steatorrhea diagnosed after analysis of 72-hour quantitative fecal fat level
3. Anemia caused by low serum iron and inadequate vitamin B12 and folic acid

   4. Osteoporosis (reduction of bone mass) and osteomalacia (softening of the bone as a result of demineralization) due to impaired calcium absorption related to low levels of vitamin D
   F. **Nursing diagnoses**
      1. Diarrhea
      2. Altered family process
      3. Altered health maintenance
      4. Risk for injury
      5. Risk for infection
      6. Knowledge deficit
      7. Self-esteem disturbance
      8. Risk for fluid volume deficit
   G. **Planning and implementation**
      1. Promote optimal nutrition through education and support regarding dietary restrictions, which should be maintained indefinitely and which typically include:
         a. Gluten-free diet (Table 11-2)
         b. Supplemental vitamins, iron, and folate
         c. Temporary lactose-free diet (eliminating all milk products) for children with severe mucosal damage
         d. Avoidance of high-fiber foods such as nuts, raisins, raw vegetables, and fruits with skin until inflammation subsides
         f. Temporary parenteral hyperalimentation in cases of severe malnourishment
      2. Refer the child and parents for nutritional counseling; ensure that the child's food preferences are taken into account in diet planning.

TABLE 11-2.
Basics of a Gluten-Free Diet

Foods Allowed

Meats: beef, pork, poultry, fish
Eggs
Milk and dairy products: milk, cream, cheese
Fruits and vegetables: all
Grains: rice, corn, gluten-free wheat flour, puffed rice, corn flakes, corn meal, precooked gluten-free cereals

Foods Prohibited

Milk: commercially prepared ice cream, malted milk, prepared puddings
Grains: anything made from wheat, rye, oats, or barley (e.g., bread, rolls, cookies, cakes, crackers, cereal, spaghetti, macaroni, noodles)
Beer and ale

---

3. Prevent infection through good general hygiene and avoiding exposure to persons with infections.
4. If celiac crisis occurs, prepare the child for gastric decompression and fluid and electrolyte replacement therapy, as prescribed.
5. Support the parents and child by encouraging them to express their feelings and concerns. Refer them to the American Celiac Society for additional information and support.
6. Promote a positive self-concept in the child and emphasize positive changes resulting from dietary restrictions that will lead to better adherence to diet.
7. Provide client and family teaching:
   a. Supply information about the disease and the diet.
   b. **Emphasize the importance of adhering to a gluten-free diet even after the symptoms have subsided to prevent reoccurrence. (Ensure that parents and child understand that the restrictions are lifelong.)**
   c. Identify measures to prevent celiac crisis.
   d. Explain the need for infection prevention.

H. **Evaluation**
1. The child maintains adequate nutritional status and avoids celiac crisis.
2. The child and the parents verbalize an understanding of the disease process and its treatment.
3. Parents are referred to the American Celiac Society or similar organization.

VII. **Hirschsprung's disease (congenital aganglionic megacolon)**
    A. **Description: a congenital anomaly resulting in mechanical intestinal obstruction due to inadequate motility in an intestinal segment**
    B. **Etiology and incidence**
       1. Hirschsprung's disease is believed to be a familial, congenital defect.
       2. Incidence is about 1 in 500 births.
       3. It is at least four times more common in males than in females, and is seen more commonly in children with Down's syndrome.
    C. **Pathophysiology and management**
       1. Absence of autonomic parasympathetic ganglion cells in one segment of the colon causes lack of innervation in that segment.
       2. This leads to absence of propulsive movements, causing accumulation of intestinal contents and distention of the bowel proximal to the defect (Fig. 11-2).

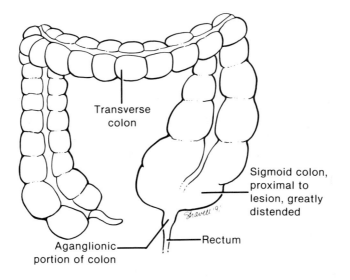

Transverse colon

Sigmoid colon, proximal to lesion, greatly distended

Rectum

Aganglionic portion of colon

FIGURE 11-2.
In Hirschsprung's disease the sigmoid colon is dilated proximal to bowel.

D. Clinical assessment findings:
   1. Clinical manifestations vary with age at time of diagnosis:
      a. Newborns: failure to pass meconium, reluctance to ingest fluids, abdominal distention, bile-stained emesis
      b. Infants: failure to thrive, constipation, abdominal distention, vomiting, episodic diarrhea
      c. Older children: chronic constipation, foul smelling stools, abdominal distension, visible peristalsis, palpable fecal mass, malnourishment, signs of anemia and hypoproteinemia
   2. Rectal examination typically reveals a rectum empty of stool, tight anal sphincter, and stool leakage.
   3. Ominous signs signifying enterocolitis, a life-threatening situation: explosive, watery diarrhea, fever, and severe prostration.
E. Diagnostic assessment findings
   1. Barium enema reveals megacolon.
   2. Absence of ganglionic cells on rectal biopsy confirms diagnosis.
F. Nursing diagnoses
   1. Constipation
   2. Altered family processes
   3. Risk for fluid volume deficit
   4. Altered health maintenance
   5. Knowledge deficit
   6. Risk for self-esteem deficit
   7. Altered nutrition: less than body requirements
   8. Pain

G.   Planning and implementation

1.   Improve nutritional status by providing smaller and more fre-quent feedings.
2.   Assess hydration status by monitoring I&O and daily weights.
3.   Note and record the frequency and characteristics of stools.
4.   Administer enemas, as prescribed, to relieve constipation.
5.   Avoid taking temperatures rectally because of the potential for damaging frail mucosa.
6.   Assess for and promptly report any signs of enterocolitis.
7.   Administer prescribed medications, which may include:
     a.   Systemic antibiotics given with enemas to reduce intesti-nal flora
     b.   Stool softeners to relieve constipation
8.   Carefully assess for altered fluid status in a child who is given nothing by mouth (NPO) and receiving frequent enemas. Administer IV fluids as prescribed.
9.   Periodically measure abdominal girth to assess for increasing distention.
10.   Decrease discomfort due to abdominal distention by elevating the head of the bed and changing the child's position fre-quently; at the same time, assess for any respiratory difficulty associated with distention.
11.   Support the child and parents; encourage them to express their feelings and concerns. Encourage parents to visit and partici-pate in the child's care, as appropriate.
12.   Prepare the child and the parents for procedures and treat-ments, which may include:
     a.   Manual dilatation of the anus, dietary management, and cleansing enemas until the child can tolerate surgery
     b.   Surgery to remove the aganglionic, nonfunctioning seg-ment of the colon, followed by anastomosis in three stages: a temporary colostomy before definitive surgery to allow the bowel to rest and the child to gain weight; reanastomosis by means of an abdominoperineal pull-through about 9 to 12 months later; and closure of the colostomy about 3 months after the pull-through proce-dure.
     c.   In a small percentage of children diagnosed later in childhood with mild symptoms, possibly conservative management with enemas, stool softeners, and a low-residue diet
13.   Educate the client and family:
     a.   Explain procedures and treatments, such as enemas, stool softeners, and a low-residue or low-fiber diet (allowing tender meats, poultry, fish, white bread, clear soups;

omitting highly seasoned foods, fruits and fruit juices, raw vegetables, and whole grain cereals and breads).

    b. Discuss and answer questions about diagnosis, surgery, preoperative and postoperative care, and colostomy care, if applicable.

    14. Arrange for consultation with an ostomy nurse to assist with teaching, as indicated.

H. Evaluation

1. The child exhibits improved nutritional and hydration status, gains weight, has no signs of abdominal distension or respiratory discomfort, and exhibits appropriate elimination patterns after surgery and other treatments.
2. Parents verbalize an understanding of the disorder and the treatment regimen.
3. Child maintains a positive self-image.
4. Parents demonstrate knowledge of ostomy care, if appropriate.
5. Parents verbalize an understanding of the need for medical and surgical follow-up care.

VIII. Intussusception

A. Description: invagination or telescoping of one portion of the intestine into an adjacent portion, causing obstruction.

B. Etiology and incidence

1. In most cases the cause is unknown. It may be associated with viral infections, intestinal polyps, Meckel's diverticulum, or lymphoma.
2. It is one of the most frequent causes of intestinal obstruction in children and typically affects children between the ages of 3 months and 5 years, most commonly between 3 and 12 months.
3. It is twice as common in males as females.

C. Pathophysiology and management

1. Invagination typically begins with hyperperistalsis in an intestinal segment, most often at or near the ileocecal valve.
2. Peristalsis continues to pull the invaginated segment along the bowel; intestinal edema and obstruction occur and blood supply to the area is cut off (Fig. 11-3).
3. Intussusception rarely reduces spontaneously. Initial treatment focuses on reduction through barium enema (hydrostatic reduction); if this proves unsuccessful, surgical reduction is required.
4. If treatment is delayed for longer than 24 hours, bowel strangulation may occur, leading to necrosis, hemorrhage, perforation, peritonitis, and shock. If untreated, intussusception is incompatible with life.

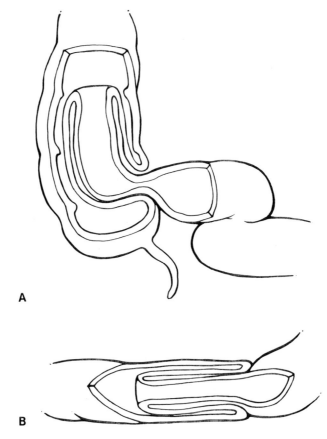

A

B

FIGURE 11-3.
Intussusception: (A) ileocolic variety, (B) ileoileal variety.

D. Clinical assessment findings

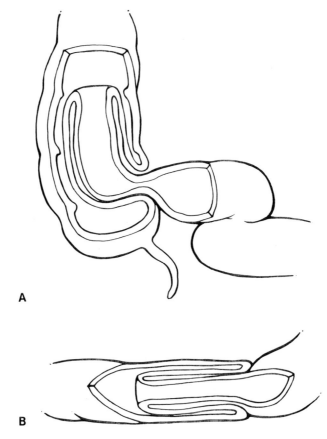 1. Severe paroxysmal abdominal pain, causing the child to scream and draw his or her knees to the abdomen
2. Vomiting of gastric contents

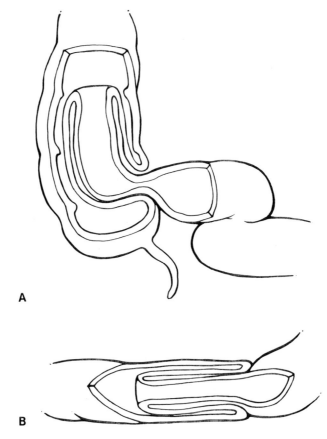 3. Tender, distended abdomen, possibly with a palpable mass
4. With continued obstruction, lethargy, "currant jelly" stools (containing blood and mucus), bile-stained or fecal emesis, and shocklike syndrome, which may progress to death

E. Diagnostic assessment findings: barium enema indicating intestinal telescoping confirms diagnosis.

F. Nursing diagnoses
1. Pain
2. Risk for injury
3. Risk for infection

       4.   Impaired tissue integrity
       5.   Risk for fluid volume deficit
       6.   Knowledge deficit
       7.   Altered family process

G. **Planning and implementation**

       1.   Assess hydration status; evaluate for signs of dehydration and monitor I&O, including IV fluid therapy when patient is NPO. Also monitor nasogastric tube drainage when appropriate.

       2.   Encourage intake of clear liquids after surgery and advance diet as tolerated.

       3.   Monitor bowel elimination status for return to normal function; assess stool amount and characteristics, performing guaiac testing on all stools; observe for abdominal distention; and auscultate for bowel sounds.

       4.   Postoperatively, monitor for infection; assess the surgical wound for redness, swelling, and drainage; and monitor temperature.

       5.   Support the parents by allowing them to verbalize their anxieties and concerns and by encouraging them to participate in the child's care as appropriate.

       6.   Educate the child and family:
           a.   Explain the diagnosis and treatment.
           b.   Discuss preoperative and postoperative care.

H. **Evaluation**

       1.   The child appears comfortable, attains normal hydration status, and demonstrates normal bowel activity.

       2.   Parents verbalize knowledge of follow-up care.

IX. **Hernias and hydroceles**

A. **Description**

       1.   Hernia: protrusion of the bowel through an abnormal opening in the abdominal wall; in children, most commonly at the umbilicus and through the inguinal canal.

       2.   Hydrocele: presence of abdominal fluid in the scrotal sac.

B. **Etiology and incidence**

       1.   These defects most commonly arise from congenital anomalies.

       2.   Inguinal hernias occur most often in males (90%) and account for about 80% of all hernias in general; umbilical hernias are most common in African-American children.

C. **Pathophysiology and management**

       1.   In an umbilical hernia, incomplete closure of the umbilical ring results in protrusion of portions of the omentum and intestine through the opening. The defect usually closes spontaneously by 3 to 4 years; surgical correction is necessary if closure does not occur or if the herniated bowel becomes incarcerated.

2. Inguinal hernias result from incomplete closure of the tube (processus vaginalis) between the abdomen and the scrotum (or uterus in females), leading to descent of an intestinal portion. Incarceration results when the descended portion becomes tightly caught in the hernia sac, which compromises blood supply. An incarcerated hernia is considered a medical emergency requiring immediate surgical repair; a nonincarcerated hernia also necessitates surgical repair.

3. Hydoceles may be communicating or noncommunicating.

    a. In a *noncommunicating hydrocele,* most commonly seen at birth, residual peritoneal fluid is trapped within the lower segment of the processus vaginalis (the tunica vaginalis), with no communication with the peritoneal cavity. The fluid usually is absorbed during the first months after birth and requires no treatment.

    b. A *communicating hydrocele* is commonly associated with a hernia because the processus vaginalis remains open from the scrotum to the abdominal cavity. In most cases, hydrocelectomy is performed if spontaneous resolution does not occur by age 1 year.

D. **Clinical assessment findings**

1. Umbilical hernia: soft swelling or protrusion around the umbilicus, usually reducible with the finger
2. Inguinal hernia: usually a painless swelling in the inguinal area; swelling reducible and possibly subsiding during periods of rest but visible when the infant is crying
3. Incarcerated hernia: irritability, tenderness at the site, anorexia, abdominal distention, and difficulty defecating; may lead to complete intestinal obstruction and gangrene
4. Noncommunicating hydrocele: painless swelling in scrotum that does not change in size or shape with the infant's activities and that is easily transilluminated
5. Communicating hydrocele: inguinal swelling that may vary in size with positioning and that is not reducible

E. **Diagnostic assessment findings**

1. There are no specific diagnostic testings for any of these.

F. **Nursing diagnoses**

1. Risk for injury
2. Risk for fluid volume deficit
3. Pain
4. Knowledge deficit
5. Altered family processes

G. **Planning and implementation**

1. Postoperatively, assess for wound infection by observing the incision for redness or drainage and by monitoring temperature.

2. Maintain good hydration status by administering IV fluids, if prescribed, monitoring I&O, and advancing the child's diet after surgery.

3. Promote comfort by administering analgesics as needed and, in a child who has undergone hydrocelectomy, applying ice bags and using a scrotal support to help relieve pain and swelling, if prescribed.

4. Support parents by allowing them to verbalize their concerns and by encouraging them to participate in the child's care, as appropriate.

5. Educate child and family:
   a. Identify signs and symptoms of incarceration to watch for and report.
   b. Emphasize the need to avoid ineffective and potentially harmful home remedies (*e.g.*, taping a hernia).
   c. Explain and answer questions about surgical procedures, and preoperative and postoperative care.
   d. Discuss the signs and symptoms of wound infection.
   e. List precautions and restrictions (*e.g.*, no tub bath until incision heals, having older child avoid strenuous activity for about 3 weeks).

H. **Evaluation**

1. The child resumes a regular diet and exhibits no signs of infection.

2. Parents verbalize a knowledge of signs of incarceration, infection, home care, and follow-up care.

Bibliography

Betz, C.L., Hunsberger, M.M., and Wright, S. (1994). *Family Centered Nursing Care of Children,* 2nd ed. Philadelphia: W.B. Saunders.

Castiglia, P.T. and Harbin, R.B. (1993). *Child Health Care: Process and Practice.* Philadelphia: J.B. Lippincott.

Jackson, D.B. and Saunders, R.B. (1993). *Child Health Nursing: A Comprehensive Approach to the Care of Children and Their Families.* Philadelphia: J.B. Lippincott.

Malfair, A. (1992). Supporting the child with special needs. *Canadian Nurse, 88,* 17.

Porth, C.M. (1995). *Pathophysiology: Concepts of Altered Health States,* 4th ed. Philadelphia: J.B. Lippincott.

Sizer, F. and Whitney, E. (1994). *Nutrition Concepts and Controversies,* 6th ed. Minneapolis/St. Paul: West Publishing.

Wong, D.L. (1993). *Whaley and Wong's Essentials of Pediatric Nursing,* 4th ed. St. Louis: C.V. Mosby.

Wong, D.L. (1995). *Whaley and Wong's Nursing Care of Infants and Children,* 5th ed. St. Louis: C.V. Mosby.

STUDY QUESTIONS

1. Which of the following will most likely be compromised in a newborn with cleft lip?
   a. The ability to suck
   b. Respiratory status
   c. Locomotion from restraints
   d. Gastrointestinal function

2. Cleft palate is associated with all of the following except:
   a. Frequent otitis media
   b. Gastroesophageal reflux (GER)
   c. Speech problems
   d. Dental malformations

3. When caring for the postoperative cleft palate client, the nurse should position the child:
   a. Supine
   b. Prone
   c. In an infant seat
   d. On the side

4. A clinical manifestation that suggests pyloric stenosis is:
   a. Regurgitation
   b. Steatorrhea
   c. Projectile vomiting
   d. Currant jelly stools

5. All of the following nursing diagnoses are appropriate for an infant with gastroesophageal reflux except:
   a. Fluid volume deficit
   b. Risk for aspiration
   c. Altered nutrition: less than body requirements
   d. Altered oral mucous membranes

6. The nurse should evaluate the effectiveness of thickened feedings for an infant with gastroesophageal reflux by:
   a. Monitoring vomiting
   b. Monitoring stools
   c. Monitoring urine
   d. Monitoring weight

7. Discharge teaching for a child with celiac disease should include avoidance of:
   a. Rice
   b. Milk
   c. Wheat
   d. Chicken

8. A child with celiac disease has an upper respiratory infection. The nurse should primarily monitor the child for:
   a. Respiratory distress
   b. Lethargy
   c. Watery diarrhea
   d. Weight gain

9. The nurse notes that a child with Hirschsprung's disease has a fever and watery explosive diarrhea. What should the nurse do first?
   a. Notify the physician immediately
   b. Administer antidiarrheal medications
   c. Monitor child every half hour
   d. Nothing, this is characteristic of Hirschsprung's disease

10. A newborn's failure to pass meconium within the first 24 hours after birth may indicate:
    a. Hirschsprung's disease
    b. Celiac disease
    c. Intussusception
    d. Abdominal wall defect

11. When assessing a child for possible intussusception, the nurse would perform all of the following except:
    a. Description of stools
    b. Pattern of pain
    c. Family history
    d. Abdominal palpation

12. The defect that results from residual peritoneal fluid trapped within the lower segment of the processus vaginalis is called:
    a. Noncommunicating hydrocele
    b. Communicating hydrocele
    c. Inguinal hernia
    d. Incarcerated hernia

ANSWER KEY

1. **Correct response: a**
   The defect may leave the child unable to form mouth around nipple, thereby requiring special devices to allow for feeding and sucking gratification.
   b. Respiratory status may be compromised if the child is fed improperly or during postoperative period.
   c. Locomotion would be a problem for the older infant.
   d. Gastrointestinal functioning is not compromised in cleft lip.
   Analysis/Physiologic/Planning

2. **Correct response: b**
   There is no association between these two disorders.
   a. Eustachian tube dysfunction leads to frequent otitis media in children with cleft palate.
   c. Speech problems result from defects such as velopharyngeal incompetency.
   d. Dental malformations result from bony structural deformities.
   Comprehension/Health Promotion/Assessment

3. **Correct response: b**
   Postoperatively, children with cleft palate should be placed on their abdomens to facilitate drainage.
   a. If child is supine, he or she may aspirate.
   c. Infant seat does not facilitate drainage.
   d. Side-lying does not facilitate drainage as well as prone positioning.
   Application/Physiologic/Implementation

4. **Correct response: c**
   Projectile vomiting is a key symptom of pyloric stenosis.
   a. Regurgitation is seen more in gastroesophageal reflux.
   b. Steatorrhea occurs in malabsorption disorders such as celiac disease.
   d. Currant jelly stools are characteristic of intussusception.

5. **Correct response: d**
   Gastroesophageal reflux has no effect on the oral mucous membranes.
   a, b, and d. All are appropriate diagnoses.

6. **Correct response: a**
   The purpose of thickened feedings is to stop the vomiting; therefore, the child should be evaluated for same.
   b and c. There is no relationship between feedings and characteristics of stools and urine.
   d. If feedings are ineffective, this should be noted before there is any change in the child's weight.
   Application/Physiologic/Evaluation

7. **Correct response: c**
   Wheat is contraindicated as it contains gluten. Children with celiac disease cannot tolerate or digest gluten.
   a, b, and d. These do not contain gluten.
   Application/Physiologic/Planning

8. **Correct response: c**
   Celiac crisis, characterized by severe watery diarrhea, may be precipitated by an infection.
   a. Respiratory distress is unlikely in a routine upper respiratory infection.
   b. Child is more likely to be irritable.
   d. Weight is more likely to decrease with diarrhea.
   Analysis/Physiologic/Assessment

9. **Correct response: a**
   Fever and explosive diarrhea indicate enterocolitis; therefore, the physician should be notified immediately.
   b. In general, antidiarrheals should not be used in Hirschsprung's disease.
   c. Monitoring would waste time as child is acutely ill.
   d. This is not typical of Hirschsprung's disease, which presents with chronic constipation.
   Application/Safe Care/Implementation

10. Correct response: a

Failure of a newborn to pass meconium is an important diagnostic indicator of Hirschsprung's disease.

  b. This is not associated with celiac disease.

  c. This is not associated with intussusception.

  d. This is not associated with abdominal wall defect.

Application/Physiologic/Analysis (Dx)

11. Correct response: c

Intussusception is not believed to have a familial tendency.

  a. Currant jelly stools, containing blood and mucus, are an indication of intussusception.

  b. Acute, episodic abdominal pain is characteristic of intussusception.

  d. A sausage-shaped mass may be palpated in the right upper quadrant.

Analysis/Physiologic/Assessment

12. Correct response: a

This is the definition of a noncommunicating hydrocele.

  b. A communicating hydrocele usually is associated with an inguinal hernia.

  c. An inguinal hernia arises from the incomplete closure of the processus vaginalis leading to the decent of an intestinal portion.

  d. Incarceration occurs when the hernia becomes tightly caught in the hernia sac.

Comprehension/Physiologic/Assessment

Hematologic Dysfunction

12

I. Hematologic structures and function

A. Hematopoiesis

1. Hematopoiesis is formation and development of blood cells.
2. Hematopoietic activity occurs by the second week of embryonic life, when blood islands arise from the yellow sac and liver.
3. From the second to fifth month of gestation, the liver is the most active site of hematopoiesis.
4. The spleen functions as an erythropoietic organ from the third to the fifth fetal months.
5. Bone marrow becomes active around the fourth fetal month (within 2 to 3 weeks after birth, the bone marrow is the main site of hematopoietic activity).

B. Functions of blood cells and cellular elements

1. Blood consists of liquid plasma and formed elements: erythrocytes, leukocytes, and thrombocytes.
2. Plasma transports formed elements and helps maintain homeostasis.
3. Erythrocytes (red blood cells [RBCs]) primarily transport oxygen to and carbon dioxide from body tissues; this activity relies on hemoglobin, a component of the erythrocytes. Erythrocytes also give blood its red color. Their typical life span is about 120 days.
4. The primary function of leukocytes (white blood cells [WBCs]) is to protect the body against infection. Two types of leukocytes exist: granulocytes (neutrophils, basophils, and eosinophils) and agranulocytes (monocytes and lymphocytes).
5. Thrombocytes (platelets), the smallest blood cells, contain coagulation factors and help regulate hemostasis through a sequence of events known as the coagulation process.

II. Hematologic system overview

A. Assessment

1. The health history should focus on bleeding or bruising tendencies, medication use, and family history of bleeding problems.
2. Inspection and history may disclose possible hematologic problems. Physical assessment focuses on various body structures:
   a. Skin: pallor, flushing, jaundice, purpura, petechiae, ecchymoses, pruritus, cyanosis, brownish discoloration, decreased capillary refill time
   b. Eyes: jaundiced sclera, conjunctival pallor, retinal hemorrhage, blurred vision
   c. Mouth: gingival and mucosal pallor
   d. Lymph nodes: lymphadenopathy, tenderness

      e.   Cardiac: tachycardia, murmurs, signs and symptoms of congestive heart failure, fatigue

      f.   Pulmonary: tachypnea, orthopnea, dyspnea

      g. Neurologic: headache, vertigo, irritability, depression, impaired thought processes, lethargy, sensitivity to cold

      h. Gastrointestinal: anorexia, abdominal tenderness, hepatomegaly, splenomegaly

      i.   Musculoskeletal: weight loss, decreased muscle mass, bone pain, joint swelling and pain

      j.   Genitourinary: blood in urine, abnormal or excessive menstrual bleeding

B. **Laboratory studies and diagnostic tests**

    1.   Complete blood count (CBC) provides a fairly complete picture of the blood's formed elements, which usually includes the following components (Table 12-1):

      a.   RBC count

      b.   WBC count

      c.   Differential WBC count (granulocytes and agranulocytes)

      d.   Hemoglobin (Hgb)

      e.   Hematocrit (Hct)

      f.   Mean corpuscular volume (MCV)

      g. Mean corpuscular hemoglobin (MCH)

      h. Mean corpuscular hemoglobin concentration (MCHC)

      i.   Platelet count

    2.   Bone marrow aspiration findings aid in the diagnosis of aplastic anemia, leukemia, and other disorders.

    3.   Reticulocyte count helps to differentiate between types of anemias.

    4.   Coagulation and hemostasis studies aid in differential diagnosis of hemorrhagic disorders.

C. **Psychosocial implications**

    1.   Children with hematologic dysfunction commonly undergo a multitude of invasive tests, procedures, and treatments, leading to anxiety and stress.

    2.   These children typically depend on others for care and support, and need the opportunity to perform as many self-care activities as possible to develop a normal sense of self-esteem and independence.

III. **Iron deficiency anemia**

    A. **Description: anemia caused by inadequate supply of iron for normal RBC formation, resulting in smaller cells, depleted RBC mass, decreased hemoglobin concentration, and decreased oxygen-carrying capacity of the blood.**

TABLE 12-1.
Normal Peripheral Blood Values

AGE	WBC/mm³	NEUTROPHILS (%)	LYMPHOCYTES (%)	PLATELETS/mm²	HEMOGLOBIN (G/dL)	HEMATOCRIT (%)	MCV (FL)
Birth	9000–30,000	60	30	84,000–478,000	13.5–21	42–65	100–140
1 week	5000–21,000	40	50	84,000–478,000	13.5–21	42–65	95–135
1 month	5000–21,000	35	55	150,000–400,000	10–16	30–48	85–125
6 months	5000–18,000	30	60	150,000–400,000	11–14	33–42	70–84
1 year	5000–15,000	30	60	150,000–400,000	11–14	33–42	70–84
4 years	5000–15,000	50	50	150,000–400,000	11–14	33–42	73–86
8 years	4000–13,000	60	30	150,000–400,000	11.5–14.5	34–44	74–88
12 years	4000–13,000	60	30	150,000–400,000	11.5–15.5	34–47	76–91
Adult male	4000–11,000	60	30	150,000–400,000	14–18	42–54	80–100
Female	(same)	(same)	(same)	(same)	12–16	36–48	(same)

B. Etiology and incidence

1. Iron deficiency anemia is the most prevalent nutritional disorder in the United States. It is prominent in age groups experiencing rapid growth: toddlers, adolescents, and pregnant and lactating women. In the United States, the incidence has decreased owing to improved nutrition and federal programs such as WIC (Women, Infants, and Children).

2. In children, it occurs most often between the ages of 6 months and 3 years; adolescents and premature infants are also at risk.

3. Common causes include inadequate dietary iron intake, iron malabsorption, low iron stores at birth, and significant blood loss.

C. Pathophysiology and management

1. Inadequate supply of iron for normal RBC formation results in formation of microcytic cells.

2. Body stores of iron decrease, as does transferrin, which binds and transports iron.

3. Insufficient body stores of iron lead to depleted RBC mass and eventually to decreased hemoglobin concentration and reduced capacity of blood.

4. The severity of symptoms is directly related to the degree and duration of iron deficiency.

D. Clinical assessment findings

1. May be asymptomatic
2. Pale skin
3. Fatigue
4. Pica (eating nonfood items)
5. Headaches, dizziness, light-headedness
6. Irritability
7. Slowed thought processes, decreased attention span, apathy, and depression

E. Diagnostic assessment findings

1. CBC (RBC: normal to slightly reduced; low hemoglobin and hematocrit; reduced MCV [microcytic]; reduced MCH [hypochromic])

2. Erythrocyte protoporphyrin (EP) level greater than 35

3. Low serum iron capacity (SIC)

4. Elevated total iron binding capacity (TIBC)

5. Reticulocyte count may be obtained 10 days after therapy is initiated to evaluate its effectiveness.

F. **Nursing diagnoses**
  1. Activity intolerance
  2. Fatigue
  3. Altered health maintenance
  4. Risk for infection
  5. Knowledge deficit
  6. Altered nutrition: less than body requirements
  7. Altered peripheral tissue perfusion

G. **Planning and implementation**
  1. Administer medications or therapy as prescribed. Usually treatment aims at correcting the underlying cause, if possible. Options may include:
      a. Oral iron (ferrous sulfate), usually about 5 to 6 mg/kg/d for at least 4 months, is prescribed to create iron stores.
      b. Iron dextran given intravenously (IV) or intramuscularly (IM), parenteral iron and blood transfusions only for severe cases
      c. Supplemental oxygen for severe tissue hypoxia

  2. **Promote an adequate intake of iron-rich foods (iron-fortified formula and cereals, lean meat, fish, dark leafy green vegetables, beans, and whole-grain breads); discourage milk as the predominant food source.**
  3. Provide child and family teaching:
      a. **Emphasize proper administration of oral iron supplements.**
          (1) **Give in two to three divided doses in a small amount of vitamin C-containing liquid (orange juice) before meals to enhance absorption and minimize side effects.**
          (2) **Administer iron with a dropper to an infant or through a straw to an older child.**
          (3) **Brush child's teeth after administration to minimize staining.**
      b. **Explain potential side effects of iron including nausea and vomiting; diarrhea or constipation; dark green or black stools; tooth discoloration.**
      c. Caution about accidental ingestion because iron is toxic when overdosed; also give directions for storing preparation in a safe place out of children's reach.
      d. Discuss infection prevention measures through good hygiene, proper nutrition, and adequate rest.

H. **Evaluation**
  1. Parents verbalize an understanding of iron deficiency anemia, its causes and treatments.

2.   Parents relate the importance of routine medical check-ups and evaluation of hemoglobin level every 6 months to detect recurrence.

IV.   Sickle cell disease

A.   Description: a chronic, severe, hemolytic disease associated with hemoglobin S (HgbS), which transforms RBCs into a sickle (crescent) shape when blood oxygenation is decreased.

B.   Etiology and incidence

1.   Sickle cell disease is an autosomal recessive disorder. Therefore, there is a 25% chance of each child having sickle cell disease when both parents carry the trait.

2.   Hemoglobin SS is the most common form of sickle cell disease.

3.   Sickle cell trait (HgbSA) is autosomal dominant and not usually symptomatic, except under conditions of extreme or prolonged deoxygenation. The sickle cell trait occurs in approximately 8% of African Americans.

4.   Sickle cell disease is found predominantly in blacks. It is the most common hemoglobinopathy in African Americans.

C.   Pathophysiology and management

1.   Abnormal Hgb (HgbS) replaces all or part of normal Hgb; under conditions of increased oxygen tension and lowered pH, RBCs change from round to sickle- or crescent-shaped.

2.   Sickle cells do not slide through vessels as normal cells do. Their angled shape causes clumping, thrombosis, arterial obstruction, increased blood viscosity, hemolysis, and eventually tissue ischemia and necrosis.

3.   As sickling progresses, acute and chronic changes develop in various organs and structures.

D.   Clinical assessment findings

1.   Clinical manifestations are varied; some characteristic signs and symptoms include enlarged spleen from congestion with sickled cells, enlarged and tender liver from blood stasis, hematuria, inability to concentrate urine, enuresis, and occasionally nephrotic syndrome, bone weakness, and dactylitis (symmetric swelling of the hands and feet).

2.   Other problems may include cerebrovascular accident (CVA), myocardial infarction (MI), growth retardation, delayed sexual maturation, decreased fertility, priapism, and recurrent severe infections (especially from pneumococcal and salmonella organisms).

3.   Sickle cell crisis (usually precipitated by infection, but possibly precipitated by dehydration, fever, cold exposure, hypoxia,

strenuous exercise, extreme fatigue, or extreme changes in altitude) may occur in different forms:

   a. **Vaso-occlusive: This is the most common and painful form; sickled cells obstruct blood vessels, causing fever, acute abdominal pain, dactylitis, and arthralgia without exacerbation of anemia. Treatment includes hydration, electrolyte replacement, bedrest, broad-spectrum antibiotics; transfusions and oxygen only for severe cases.**

   b. Splenic sequestration: The spleen pools a large amount of blood causing a severe drop in blood volume and shock; the condition is life-threatening, and symptoms include pallor, irritability, abdominal distention and pain, hypotension, and tachycardia. Treatment includes transfusions and splenectomy.

   c. Aplastic crisis: Occurring infrequently, aplastic crisis features diminished RBC production and is characterized by bone marrow failure. Symptoms include pallor, tachycardia, fever, and congestive heart failure (CHF). Treatment is symptomatic.

   d. Hyperhemolytic crisis: This rare event causes an even greater rate of RBC destruction; the crisis suggests other abnormalities.

E. Diagnostic assessment findings

1. **HgbS is present from conception; however, HgbF (fetal hemoglobin) inhibits sickling, making suspicions equivocal and diagnosis difficult before age 4 months.**

2. Sickledex screen, the most widely used test, may yield false-negative results before the age range of 4 to 6 months.

3. If Sickledex findings are positive, hemoglobin electrophoresis is needed to distinguish between the sickle cell trait and the disease.

4. Accurate prenatal screening is available through chorionic villus sampling (CVS) or by analyzing fetal blood or cells.

5. Hemoglobin electrophoresis should be done at birth on all newborns.

6. Decreased RBC count, elevated WBC and platelet counts, decreased erythrocyte sedimentation rate (ESR), increased serum iron level, decreased serum RBC survival time, and reticulocytosis are all suggestive of sickle cell disease.

F. Nursing diagnoses

1. Altered peripheral tissue perfusion

2. Activity intolerance

3. Risk for fluid volume deficit

4. Risk for infection
5. Pain
6. Body image disturbance
7. Altered family processes
8. Knowledge deficit
9. Altered health maintenance
10. Social isolation

G. Planning and implementation

1. Assess pulse and respiration rates at rest and during activity, and during infections or other indications of decreased tissue perfusion. Also monitor same for signs of CHF.
2. Monitor height, weight, and developmental status because child's growth may be delayed by severe anemia.
3. Assess skin color; in dark children, assess mucous membranes.
4. Implement appropriate therapeutic measures, which may include:

   a. **Provide oral and IV hydration fluids to increase the fluid volume of blood and help prevent sickling and thrombosis.**
   b. Administer electrolyte replacement to counter acidosis caused by hypoxia.
   c. Deliver oxygen therapy to promote adequate oxygenation.
   d. Institute bed rest and careful organization of child's activities to minimize energy expenditure.
   e. Administer and monitor transfusions to treat anemia and reduce the viscosity of the blood.

5. Relieve pain by assessing child's need for pain medication and administering prescribed analgesics (acetaminophen, propoxyphene hydrochloride (Darvon), and codeine-containing compounds for mild pain; meperidine and morphine for severe pain. Patient-controlled analgesia (PCA), by IV infusion pump, may be used in children as young as 5 years and is helpful for managing the severe pain of vaso-occlusive crisis. Monitor the effectiveness of all medications.
6. Position the child for maximal comfort, apply heat to affected areas, as prescribed, and use alternative pain-control techniques, such as relaxation and meditation.
7. Help ensure adequate hydration and a nutritionally balanced diet:
   a. Encourage oral fluid intake.
   b. Monitor IV infusion.
   c. Maintain strict intake and output (I&O) and daily weight records.
   d. Monitor for signs of dehydration and electrolyte imbalance.

8. Monitor for signs of infection and administer antibiotics as prescribed. Help child avoid known sources of infection.

9. Promote tissue oxygenation by helping the child avoid overexertion and emotional stress and by providing passive range-of-motion exercises.

10. Support the child and family by allowing them to verbalize their fears, concerns, anger, and other feelings.

11. Educate the child and family:

   a. Explain the disease process, genetic aspects, and early signs and symptoms of sickling crises.

   b. Discuss home management measures for a mild crisis.

   c. Identify ways to prevent sickling episodes by avoiding factors known to precipitate crises and by recognizing the early signs of infection.

   d. Review the importance of regular health maintenance check-ups, dental check-ups, and eye examinations.

   e. Emphasize the importance of maintaining as normal a lifestyle as possible.

   f. Address the significance of genetic counseling.

   g. Point out the importance of self-esteem and positive body image.

H. Evaluation

1. The child remains free of pain, systemic complications, crisis, and infection.

2. Parents and child verbalize an understanding of the disease process and major management principles.

3. Parents feel comfortable verbalizing any guilt feelings they may have regarding transmission of a potentially fatal, chronic illness.

4. Parents understand the difference between sickle cell trait and actual sickle cell disease.

5. Child exhibits normal growth and development patterns.

V. Aplastic anemia

A. Description: aplastic anemia is characterized by *pancytopenia* (anemia, granulocytopenia, and thrombocytopenia) and bone marrow hypoplasia.

B. Etiology and incidence

1. The incidence is approximately 1 in 100,000. The prognosis is poor with mortality greater than 70%; of those, half die within 6 months.

2. Aplastic anemia may be congenital or acquired.

3. Congenital types include:

   a. **Fanconi's syndrome is inherited as an autosomal re-**

cessive trait, associated with cytopenia and multiple congenital anomalies.

    b.   Blackfan-Diamond syndrome (hypoplastic anemia), a rare condition characterized by destruction of RBCs and a slight decrease in WBCs and platelets; its transmission is unclear.

4.   Common causes of acquired aplastic anemia:

    a.   Half of all cases idiopathic (no known cause)

    b.   Radiation therapy

    c.   **Drugs, such as chloramphenicol, methicillin, sulfonamides, thiazides, and chemotherapeutic agents**

    d.   Toxic agents, such as industrial and household chemicals, including dyes, glue, paint removers, insecticides, petroleum products, and benzenes

    e.   Infections, particularly hepatitis and sepsis

    f.   Immune deficiencies, such as leukemia and lymphoma

5.   Aplastic anemia may run in families and can occur at any age.

C.   **Pathophysiology and management**

1.   In aplastic anemia, the decreased functional capacity of hypoplastic bone marrow results in pancytopenia.

2.   Severe pancytopenia can produce massive bleeding or infection.

3.   The goal of management is to restore functioning of the bone marrow. This may be done by immunosuppressant therapy to remove the presumed immunologic functions that prolong aplasia or by replacement of bone marrow by transplantation.

D.   **Clinical assessment findings**

1.   Whether aplastic anemia results from congenital or acquired factors, assessment findings are related to bone marrow failure as follows:

    a.   Lack of RBCs: pallor, lethargy, tachycardia, shortness of breath on exertion; in children signs of anemia occur only when the hemoglobin levels falls below 5 or 6 g/100 mL.

    b.   Lack of WBCs: recurrent infections, including opportunistic infections

    c.   Lack of platelets: abnormal bleeding, petechiae, bruising

2.   Children with Fanconi's syndrome may have short stature, malformed kidneys and hearts, microcephaly, microphthalmos, dark pigmentation with café-au-lait spots, and congenitally absent radii and thumbs.

E.   **Diagnostic assessment findings**

1.   Pancytopenia on peripheral blood smear.

2.   Bone marrow aspiration and biopsy make definitive diagnosis.

Conversion of red bone marrow to yellow, fatty bone marrow with almost complete absence of hematopoietic activity.

F. **Nursing diagnoses**

1. Activity intolerance
2. Risk for infection
3. Risk for injury
4. Altered oral mucous membrane
5. Knowledge deficit
6. Altered health maintenance
7. Altered family processes

G. **Planning and implementation**

1. Nursing care is similar to that for children with leukemia.
2. Monitor for signs and symptoms of infection; help prevent infection through protective isolation and good hygiene.
3. Assess for abnormal bleeding tendencies (do dipstick test for blood in urine and guaiac test for blood in stools).
4. Provide supportive treatment to prevent or control infection; administer transfusions and steroid or hormone therapy.
5. Provide information regarding bone marrow transplantation procedure and follow-up care. Explain that early bone marrow transplantation is associated with a 3-year survival rate of 80%. (Bone marrow transplantation before blood transfusions decreases the likelihood of rejection.)
6. As prescribed, administer medications and blood products, which may include:
   a. Antilymphocyte globulin (ALG) or antithymocyte globulin (ATG), the treatment of choice, which suppresses T cell-dependent autoimmune responses without causing bone marrow suppression
   b. Androgenic steroids (such as testosterone) used with corticosteroids to stimulate erythropoiesis
   c. Blood products such as RBCs, WBCs, and platelets, as well as antibiotics, used as supportive therapy
7. Explain that response to drug therapy is gradual and that no apparent changes may occur for between 3 and 6 months after beginning therapy.
8. **Monitor for complications of steroid therapy such as gastric irritation, infection, edema, weight gain, and hypertension.**
9. **Monitor for complications of androgen therapy signaled by abnormal liver function test results, weight gain, acne, increased hair growth, and deepening of the voice.**
10. **Monitor for complications of ALG or ATG therapy, including fever, chills, rash, serum sickness, severe thrombocytopenia, and anaphylaxis.**

11. Attempt to eliminate toxic agents from the child's environment.
12. Support the family in coping with procedures and the uncertain prognosis and potential outcome of aplastic anemia.
13. Educate the child and family:
    a. Define the diagnosis and nature of the disorder.
    b. Discuss the diagnostic, therapeutic, and surgical procedures.
    c. Outline possible side effects of therapies.
    d. Explain how to recognize signs of infection and abnormal bleeding.

H. Evaluation
1. The child remains infection free.
2. Bleeding episodes are managed effectively.
3. The child achieves remission.

VI. Thalassemia
A. Description: inherited blood disorders characterized by deficient synthesis of specific globulin chains of the hemoglobin molecule—in the case of beta-thalassemia, the most common type, of beta chains.

B. Etiology and incidence
1. Beta thalassemia is an autosomal recessive disorder.
2. It occurs in two major forms: thalassemia major, the homozygous form, and thalassemia minor, the heterozygous form.
3. **Thalassemia major (beta-thalassemia, Cooley's anemia) is the most severe form and usually is seen in children of Mediterranean (especially Italian and Greek) or Asian origins.**

C. Pathophysiology and management
1. There is a defect in the production of specific globin chains (beta) in hemoglobin.
2. This defect results in compensatory increases in hemoglobin production among other hemoglobin chains that become unbalanced, then disintegrate, and destroy RBC.
3. Compensatory increases in erythropoiesis cannot correct the severe anemia.
4. The object of supportive therapy is to maintain sufficient hemoglobin levels to prevent tissue hypoxia. Transfusions are the foundation of treatment and are administered with desferoxamine (Desferal), an iron chelator, to minimize hemosiderosis (excess iron in tissues).
5. Splenectomy may be necessary to decrease abdominal pressure and increase the life span of cells.
6. Bone marrow transplantation has been used with success.

D. **Clinical assessment findings**

1. Thalassemia minor commonly produces only mild to moderate anemia that may be asymptomatic and often goes undetected.
2. Thalassemia major commonly produces clinical manifestations around age 6 months, when the protective effect of fetal hemoglobin diminishes:
   a. Early signs: insidious onset, anemia, unexplained fever, poor feeding, poor weight gain, and a markedly enlarged spleen
   b. Later signs: chronic hypoxia; damage to liver, spleen, heart, pancreas, and lymph glands from hemochromatosis (damage causing excess iron); slight jaundice or bronze skin color; thick cranial bones with prominent cheeks and a flat nose; growth retardation and delayed sexual development.
3. **Long-term complications result from hemochromatosis with resultant cellular damage leading to:**
   a. **Splenomegaly, usually requiring splenectomy**
   b. **Skeletal complications, such as thickened cranial bones, enlarged head, prominent facial bones, malocclusion of the teeth, and susceptibility to spontaneous fractures**
   c. **Cardiac complications, such as arrhythmias, pericarditis, congestive heart failure, and fibrosis of cardiac muscle fibers**
   d. **Gallbladder disease, including gallstones, possibly needing cholecystectomy (gallbladder removal)**
   e. Liver enlargement leading to cirrhosis
   f. Skin changes such as jaundice and brown pigmentation due to iron deposits
   g. Growth retardation and endocrine complications, such as delayed sexual maturation and diabetes mellitus possibly from endocrine gland sensitivity to iron

E. **Diagnostic assessment findings**

1. CBC: microcytosis, hypochromia, anisocytosis (inequity in size), poikilocytosis (variation in shape), target cells (nonspecific enlarged RBC), and basophilic stippling (spotted staining; decreased hemoglobin and hematocrit values and reticulocyte count
2. Hemoglobin electrophoresis: F and A values will be elevated because these do not depend on beta chains.
3. Marked increase in erythroid precursors in bone marrow
4. Folic acid deficiency
5. Accurate prenatal screening available by CVS (chorionic villus sampling) or by analysis of fetal blood or cells

F. **Nursing diagnoses**
1. Altered tissue perfusion
2. Risk for infection
3. Risk for injury
4. Altered nutrition: less than body requirements
5. Body image disturbance
6. Activity intolerance
7. Altered family processes
8. Altered health maintenance
9. Altered growth and development
10. Knowledge deficit
11. Pain

G. **Planning and implementation**
1. Administer blood transfusions as prescribed, and observe for complications of transfusions; the most common problem is iron overload.
2. **Monitor for iron toxicity related to blood transfusion. Signs and symptoms include abdominal pain, bloody diarrhea, emesis, decreased level of consciousness, shock, metabolic acidosis.**
3. **Implement iron chelation therapy with desferoxamine (20 to 40 mg/kg/d), as prescribed, to eliminate excess iron and its side effects from deposition in tissues. Desferoxamine is administered during transfusion.**
4. **Monitor vital signs, watching for hypotension. Be prepared for allergic reaction; check visual acuity (ocular toxic) and hearing (ototoxic); monitor I&O (drug excreted by kidneys); urine may turn red.**
5. Provide information regarding splenectomy (if warranted) and follow-up care. Explain that prophylactic antibiotics and vaccines are given to prevent complications from splenectomy, and that the child should avoid people with active infections.
6. Administer folic acid as prescribed.
7. Promote infection prevention through good hygiene, avoidance of persons with infections, adequate rest, and good nutrition.
8. Help prevent fractures by encouraging the child to avoid activities that may increase the risk for fractures.
9. Promote adequate rest by coordinating care.
10. Encourage optimal nutrition by taking a dietary history, determining the child's food preferences, and providing a pleasant atmosphere for meals.
11. **Decrease dietary iron as much as possible.**
12. Monitor for signs of hepatitis and iron overload.

13. Help the child cope with the illness by allowing him or her to verbalize concerns, by preparing for procedures, and by assisting him or her to develop coping skills.
14. Support the family by encouraging members to verbalize their feelings, by exploring feelings of guilt regarding the hereditary aspect of the disorder, and by encouraging the child to lead as normal a life as possible.
15. As appropriate, refer to family support groups, such as Cooley's Anemia Foundation.
16. Educate the child and family
    a. Note the nature of the disease and its management.
    b. Identify signs and symptoms of infection, iron overload, and other potential complications to watch for and report.
    c. Provide instructions for home chelation therapy.
    d. Review activity restrictions, including avoidance of activities that increase the risk of fractures.
    e. Outline dietary restrictions.

H. Evaluation
1. The child engages in as normal a life as possible, is free from pain and infection, and copes well with body image changes.
2. Parents verbalize an understanding of their child's illness and treatment measures.

VII. Hemophilia

A. Description: a group of hereditary bleeding disorders characterized by a deficiency in a blood clotting factor.
1. **The two most common forms are factor VIII deficiency (classic hemophilia, hemophilia A) and factor IX deficiency (Christmas disease, hemophilia B). The classic form is the most common.**
2. Hemophilia is classified as mild, moderate, or severe, depending on the level of coagulation involved.

B. Etiology and incidence
1. **Hemophilia is an X-linked recessive disorder transmitted by females. It may also be caused by a gene mutation.**
2. It occurs in about 1 in 10,000 males.

C. Pathophysiology and management
1. In hemophilia A, factor VIII molecule is present but defective in clotting function.
2. Hemophilia B involves a defect or deficiency of factor IX.
3. Clotting factor malfunction causes abnormal bleeding owing to impaired ability to form a fibrin clot.

D. **Clinical assessment findings**
1.   Hemophilia is suspected in a newborn with excessive bleeding from the umbilical cord or after circumcision.
2.   Common manifestations include:
   a.   Easy bruising
   b.   Prolonged bleeding from wounds
   c.   Spontaneous hematuria
   d.   Epistaxis
   e.   Hemarthrosis (hemorrhages in the joints causing pain, swelling, and limited movement
3.   Complications may include:
   a.   Bone changes, osteoporosis, and muscle atrophy, resulting in crippling deformities as a consequence of hemarthrosis
   b.   Intracranial bleeding
   c.   Gastrointestinal (GI) hemorrhage, leading to intestinal obstruction
   d.   Hematomas in the spinal cord, resulting in paralysis
   e.   Airway obstruction due to bleeding into the neck, mouth, or thorax
   f.   Secondary complications from factor replacement such as hepatitis and immunodeficiency (rare after 1985)

E. **Diagnostic assessment findings**
1.   Platelet count, prolonged activated partial thromboplastin time; prothrombin, and thrombin clotting and bleeding time are normal; factor level is low. Blood is drawn for specific assays for factors VII or IX.
2.   Carrier detection and prenatal diagnosis through amniocentesis are possible.

F. **Nursing diagnoses**
1.   Risk for injury
2.   Pain
3.   Activity intolerance
4.   Altered family processes
5.   Knowledge deficit
6.   Self-esteem disturbance

G. **Planning and implementation**
1.   Assess for acute or chronic bleeding: skin, joints, and muscles are assessment priorities. Check vision, hearing, and neurologic development. Also check for hematuria and bleeding from the mouth, lips, gums, rectum.
2.   Prevention is a primary goal. Assess home safety (consider child's developmental level to ask specific safety questions).
3.   Major bleeding requires hospitalization with nursing management. Monitor for bleeding and its consequences; prevent fur-

ther injuries (pad the bed rails, provide knee pads, move carefully) and provide joint care (exercise).

4. Control bleeding by applying pressure and cold to the injury site and elevating and immobilizing the injured area.
5. Observe for swelling and tenderness in the joints, and prevent contractures.
6. Monitor for signs of hypovolemia.
7. Administer medications as prescribed, which may include:
   a. Plasma products
   b. Fresh frozen plasma
   c. Factor VIII cryoprecipitate
   d. Factor VIII concentrate
   e. Factor IX
   f. Corticosteroids to reduce inflammation in affected joints
   g. Acetaminophen with or without codeine for pain management
8. **Avoid analgesics that promote bleeding such as aspirin and aspirin-containing compounds.**
9. Monitor for side effects of therapy such as hepatitis or immunodeficiency.
10. Help prevent crippling effects of joint degeneration by implementing a physical therapy program, including passive range-of-motion exercises, or orthopedic measures such as casts, traction, and joint aspiration.
11. Present information about joint replacement surgery in the event of total disability.
12. Foster child's self-esteem by encouraging him or her to express concerns and feelings and by promoting a positive self-image.
13. Encourage family members to verbalize, especially about any guilt that they may have due to the genetic nature of the disorder and assist their coping efforts by providing information on the disease and its management.
14. Refer the child and family to support groups such as the National Hemophilia Foundation.
15. Initiate child and family teaching:
    a. Explain how to care for and administer factor, as well as how to store and reconstitute it.
    b. Inform the child and family that superficial injuries are treated with ice and pressure.
    c. Identify signs of hemarthrosis and teach parents how to immobilize the joint, pack it in ice, and administer factor.
    d. Assist the child and parents to recognize signs of major bleeding (central nervous system manifestations: head-

ache, blurred vision, vomiting, lethargy, confusion, seizures).

    e.   Discuss injury prevention, including the need for judicious limit setting that allows the child as normal a life as possible.

    f.   Recommend using a soft toothbrush and point out the need for regular dental check-ups.

    g.   Explain the possible side-effects of therapy.

    h.   Demonstrate passive range-of-motion exercises.

    i.   Emphasize avoidance of aspirin and aspirin-containing compounds.

    j.   Provide diet information because weight increases can impose further stress on joints.

H. **Evaluation**

    1.   The child is free from pain and does not exhibit joint deformities.

    2.   The child demonstrates an age-appropriate level of independence.

    3.   Parents verbalize knowledge of disease process and treatment.

    4.   Parents feel free to verbalize any guilt feelings that they may have regarding the genetic aspects of the disease.

VIII. **Idiopathic thrombocytopenic purpura (ITP)**

A. **Description: an acquired hemorrhagic disorder in which the number of circulating platelets is reduced.**

B. **Etiology and incidence**

    1.   May be acute or chronic.

    2.   Occurs most frequently between the ages of 2 and 5 years, but may occur at any age.

    3.   The etiology is unknown, but theories of autoimmune phenomenon are widely accepted.

C. **Pathophysiology and management**

    1.   The number of circulating platelets is reduced as a result of the action of antiplatelet antibody produced in the spleen.

    2.   This autoimmune disease results in bleeding into the tissues (purpura).

    3.   Treatment is supportive as ITP is usually self-limiting; steroids are prescribed for children at high risk for serious bleeding; intravenous immunoglobulin (IVIG) may be used to increase platelet production; splenectomy is performed, if the child is unresponsive to treatment or if bleeding is severe, to remove the source of antiplatelet antibody.

D. **Clinical assessment findings**

    1.   Easy bruising, petechiae

    2.   Bleeding from mucous membranes, blood in stool or urine

   3. Hematomas
   4. Child does not look sick; careful assessment needed to rule out child abuse

E. Diagnostic assessment findings
   1. The platelet count drops below $20,000/mm^3$.
   2. A bone marrow aspiration should be performed to rule out other disorders such as leukemia. In ITP, the aspirate is normal except for a high level of circulating megakaryocytes, the parent cells of platelets.

F. Nursing diagnoses
   1. Risk for injury
   2. Fear
   3. Anxiety
   4. Risk for altered health maintenance

G. Planning and implementation
   1. Observe for bleeding; check daily for new areas of petechiae and bruises.
   2. Focus on safety until platelet count returns to normal. Enforce activity restrictions; **avoid administering aspirin or aspirin-containing products,** rectal temperatures, and IM injections.
   3. **Children on steroids are at increased risk for infection and should be monitored for same and precautions taken.**
   4. Allay family's fears by allowing them to voice their concerns and by explaining diagnosis. Clearly relate that not treating ITP may be the best treatment because the disorder is self-limiting.
   5. Educate the child and family:
      a. Define safety precautions to take to avoid injury and discuss ways to divert child's energy.
      b. Stress that child should avoid aspirin and aspirin-containing products.
      c. Teach parents and child to watch for signs of increased bruising and to notify physician if this occurs.
      d. Stress the importance of follow-up care to monitor child's platelet level, usually every 1 to 2 weeks.

H. Evaluation
   1. Child will not have unexplained bruising or bleeding.
   2. Parents will feel free to verbalize their fears.
   3. Parents will verbalize an understanding of management techniques, especially injury avoidance.

Bibliography

Belkengren, R.P. and Sapala, S. (1993). Pediatric management problems: Iron deficiency anemia. *Pediatric Nursing, 19,* 378.

Betz, C.L., Hunsberger, M.M., and Wright, S. (1994). *Family Centered Nursing Care of Children,* 2nd ed. Philadelphia: W.B. Saunders.

Castiglia, P.T. and Harbin, R.B. (1993). *Child Health Care: Process and Practice.* Philadelphia: J.B. Lippincott.

Jackson, D.B. and Saunders, R.B. (1993). *Child Health Nursing: A Comprehensive Approach to the Care of Children and Their Families.* Philadelphia: J.B. Lippincott.

Sizer, F. and Whitney, E. (1994). *Nutrition Concepts and Controversies,* 6th ed. Minneapolis/St. Paul: West Publishing.

Wong, D.L. (1993). *Whaley and Wong's Essentials of Pediatric Nursing,* 4th ed. St. Louis: C.V. Mosby.

Wong, D.L. (1995). *Whaley and Wong's Nursing Care of Infants and Children,* 5th ed. St. Louis: C.V. Mosby.

STUDY QUESTIONS

1. Iron deficiency anemia is prevalent in all of the following groups except:
   a. Toddlers
   b. Adolescents
   c. Pregnant women
   d. School children

2. Discharge planning for a child with iron deficiency anemia should include stressing all of the following foods except:
   a. Lean meats
   b. Whole-grain breads
   c. Yellow vegetables
   d. Fish

3. In children with sickle cell disease, tissue damage results from:
   a. A general inflammatory response due to an autoimmune reaction from hypoxia.
   b. Air hunger and respiratory alkalosis due to deoxygenated RBC.
   c. Local tissue damage with ischemia and necrosis due to obstructed circulation.
   d. Hypersensitivity of the central nervous system due to elevated serum bilirubin levels.

4. When planning a client education program for sickle cell disease, the nurse should include such topics as:
   a. Proper hand washing and infection avoidance
   b. A high-iron, high-protein diet
   c. Fluid restriction to 1 quart per day
   d. Aerobic exercises to increase oxygenation

5. Which of the following interventions requires safe and effective nursing management of a child with sickle cell disease?
   a. Administration of anticoagulants to prevent sickling
   b. Health teaching to help reduce sickling crises
   c. Observation of imposed fluid restrictions
   d. Avoiding the use of narcotics

6. The long-term complications seen in thalassemia major are related to:

   a. Hemochromatosis
   b. Splenomegaly
   c. Anemia
   d. Growth retardation

7. The physician orders Desferal for a client with thalassemia. Which complaint should alert the nurse to notify the physician?
   a. Decreased hearing
   b. Vomiting
   c. Red urine
   d. Increased blood pressure

8. Which of the following tests is most helpful in diagnosing hemophilia?
   a. Bleeding time
   b. Partial thromboplastin time
   c. Platelet count
   d. Complete blood count

9. All of the following are appropriate nursing actions for bleeding in a child with hemophilia except:
   a. Applying pressure
   b. Applying cold to area
   c. Immobilizing joint
   d. Lowering injured area

10. Which medication should be avoided by children with idiopathic thrombocytopenic purpura?
    a. Aspirin
    b. Acetaminophen
    c. Codeine
    d. Morphine

11. The disorder in which the number of circulating platelets is decreased as a result of antiplatelet antibody is:
    a. Idiopathic thrombocytopenic purpura
    b. Cooley's anemia
    c. Christmas disease
    d. Fanconi's anemia

12. Steroids are prescribed for a child with ITP. What should the nurse monitor for because of the addition of this medication?
    a. Anemia
    b. Bleeding
    c. Bruising
    d. Infection

ANSWER KEY

1. **Correct response: d**
   This is not a period of rapid growth and therefore iron deficiency anemia is not prevalent in schoolagers.
   a, b, and d. All are periods of rapid growth and therefore clients in these groups are more likely to experience iron deficiency anemia. The "picky appetites" of toddlers and adolescents may also predispose them to this condition.
   Comprehension/Health Promotion/ Planning

2. **Correct response: c**
   Yellow vegetables are not good sources of iron.
   a, b, and d. All are good food sources of iron and thus should be encouraged in the diet.
   Comprehension/Health Promotion/ Planning

3. **Correct response: c**
   Characteristic sickle cells tend to clump, which results in poor circulation to tissue and eventual ischemia and necrosis.
   a. Damage is not due to an inflammatory response.
   b. Air hunger and respiratory alkalosis are not present.
   d. Central nervous system effects are due to ischemia.
   Comprehension/Physiologic/Assessment

4. **Correct response: a**
   Prevention of infection is an important measure in the prevention of sickle cell crisis.
   b. This diet has no effect on crisis.
   c. Proper hydration should be encouraged to prevent crisis.
   d. Strenuous exercise and activity should be avoided.
   Application/Health Promotion/Planning

5. **Correct response: b**
   Because there is no cure for sickle cell disease, prevention is one of the main aims of therapeutic management.

   a. Anticoagulants do not prevent sickling.
   c. Fluids are encouraged to increase the fluid volume and prevent sickling.
   d. Narcotics usually are needed for pain control.
   Application/Safe Care/Implementation

6. **Correct response: a**
   Excessive iron deposits collect in the tissues and cause destruction.
   b. Splenomegaly is a result of the disease process.
   c. Anemia is a symptom.
   d. Growth retardation is a symptom.
   Analysis/Physiologic/Evaluation

7. **Correct response: a**
   Desferal causes ototoxicity; therefore, any hearing problem should be promptly reported.
   b. Vomiting is not an emergent issue.
   c. This is an expected occurrence with Desferal.
   d. Blood pressure decreases as a side effect.
   Application/Safe Care/Implementation

8. **Correct response: b**
   Partial thromboplastin time is abnormal in hemophilia.
   a. Bleeding times are normal in hemophilia.
   c. Platelet count is normal in hemophilia.
   d. Hemophilia does not affect the CBC.
   Comprehension/Physiologic/Analysis

9. **Correct response: d**
   The affected area should be elevated, not lowered.
   a, b, and d. All are appropriate measures to take for bleeding.
   Application/Safe Care/Implementation

10. **Correct response: a**
    Aspirin has an antiplatelet action and therefore may increase platelet destruction in ITP.

b, c, and d. These medications are not contraindicated in this disorder.
Comprehensive/Physiologic/Planning

11. *Correct response: a*
This is the definition of idiopathic thrombocytopenic purpura.
  b. Cooley's anemia is thalassemia.
  c. Christmas disease is hemophilia factor IX deficiency.
  d. Fanconi's anemia is a form of aplastic anemia.
Comprehension/Physiologic/NA

12. *Correct response: d*
Steroids may promote immunosuppression, making the child more susceptible to infections.
  a. Anemia is not associated with the disorder or medication.
  b and c. Are due to disorder itself.
Analysis/Physiologic/Evaluation

Cardiovascular Dysfunction

I. Essential concepts: cardiovascular structures and function

A. Development

1. Fetal heart development begins in the first month of gestation. At about 21 days of gestation, the fetal heart begins beating, and blood begins circulating.

2. Between the second and seventh weeks of gestation, the primitive fetal heart undergoes a series of changes that create the four-chambered heart and its great arteries.

3. During gestation, the lungs essentially are nonfunctional and fetal oxygenation occurs via the placenta.

4. Key structures in fetal circulation (Fig. 13-1)

   a. Foramen ovale: opening between the atria that allows blood flow from the right atrium directly to the left atrium.

   b. Ductus arteriosus: conduit between the pulmonary artery and the aorta that shunts blood away from pulmonary circulation.

5. Important circulatory changes occurring during the transition to extrauterine life (Fig. 13-2) include:

   a. Inspired oxygen dilates pulmonary vessels, decreasing pulmonary vascular resistance and increasing pulmonary blood flow, which facilitates lung expansion.

   b. The foramen ovale closes functionally soon after birth owing to the compression of the atrial septum.

   c. The ductus arteriosus closes functionally by 48 hours after birth.

B. Function

1. The cardiovascular system's basic function is to pump oxygenated blood to tissues and remove metabolic waste products from tissues.

2. Valves within the heart and pressure differences between the four heart chambers (the left and right atria and the left and right ventricles) regulate blood flow through the heart into systemic circulation.

3. Blood returns through the heart through the venous system at about 75% oxygenation saturation.

4. As blood passes through the pulmonary capillaries, it loses carbon dioxide (CO_2) and binds oxygen (O_2) from the alveolar air and reaches 97% oxygen saturation.

II. Cardiovascular system overview

A. Assessment

1. Health history findings significant in cardiovascular dysfunction include:

   a. Family history of congenital heart disorders

   b. Presence of murmurs and age at which first noted

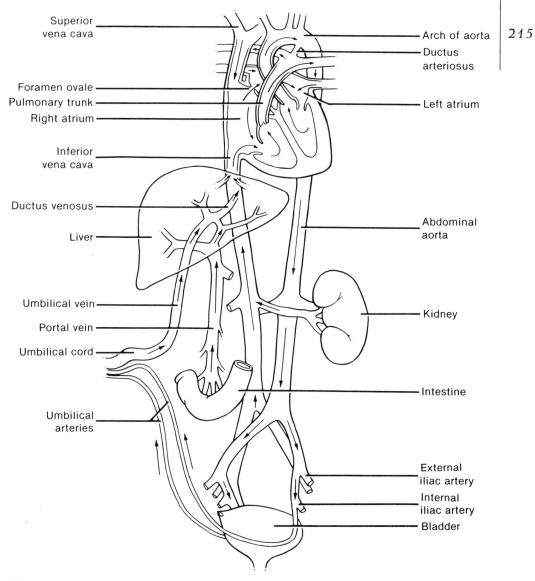

Superior vena cava

Foramen ovale
Pulmonary trunk
Right atrium

Inferior vena cava

Ductus venosus

Liver

Umbilical vein

Portal vein

Umbilical cord

Umbilical arteries

Arch of aorta
Ductus arteriosus

Left atrium

Abdominal aorta

Kidney

Intestine

External iliac artery
Internal iliac artery
Bladder

FIGURE 13-1.
Fetal circulation shortly before birth; *arrows* indicate the course of blood.

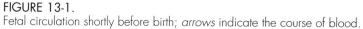

    c. Feeding problems, including fatigue or diaphoresis during feeding, and poor weight gain

    d. Respiratory difficulties, including tachypnea, dyspnea, shortness of breath, cyanosis, and frequent respiratory infections

    e. Chronic fatigue or exercise intolerance

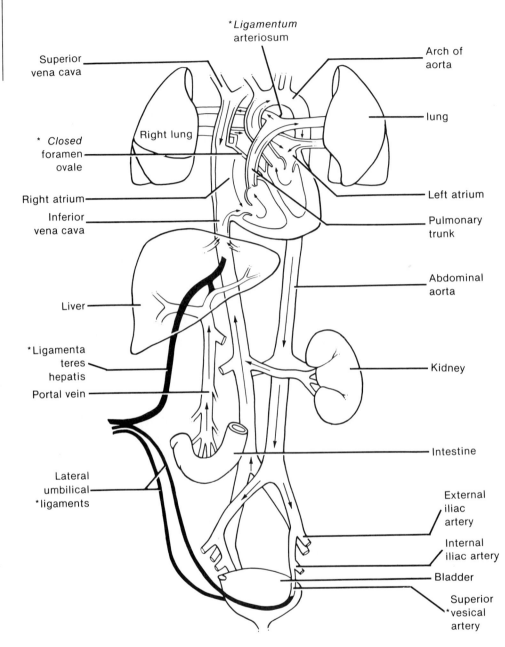

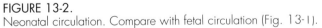

FIGURE 13-2.
Neonatal circulation. Compare with fetal circulation (Fig. 13-1).

2. Significant physical assessment findings may focus on:
   a. Growth abnormalities (failure to thrive)
    b. **Cyanosis**
   c. Clubbing of fingers and toes
   d. Periorbital and peripheral edema
   e. Pulse alterations, including tachycardia or bradycardia, dysrhythmias, diminished peripheral pulses, thready pulse, narrow or wide pulse pressures
   f. **Tachypnea**
   g. Hypotension or unequal blood pressure in arms and legs
   h. Engorged neck veins
   i. **Murmurs, bruits, thrills**
   j. Abdominal distention, hepatomegaly, splenomegaly

B. Laboratory studies and diagnostic tests
   1. Relevant laboratory results may include:
      a. Compensatory increase in hematocrit, hemoglobin, and erythrocyte count (polycythemia)
      b. Altered blood gases
      c. Abnormalities in hemostasis, such as thrombocytopenia; decreased platelet function; low prothrombin level; decreased or absent clotting factors V, VII, or IX
   2. Important diagnostic studies include:
      a. Electrocardiography (ECG), which helps evaluate cardiac musculature, cardiac rate and rhythm, and cardiac impulse conduction (Table 13-1)
      b. Chest radiography, which provides information on the size of the heart and its chambers and on the prominence and distribution of pulmonary blood flow
      c. Echocardiography, which can help assess the thickness of the heart walls, the size of cardiac chambers, the motion of the valves and septa within the heart, and anatomic relationships of great vessels to various intracardiac structures
      d. Cardiac catheterization, which provides information on oxygen saturation within heart chambers, pressures within chambers, changes in cardiac output or stroke volume, and anatomic abnormalities (see section VI for more information)

C. Psychosocial implications
   1. Developmental delays often occur in children with cardiovascular disorders, particularly in those with cyanotic defects.
   2. Allowing the child sufficient time to complete tasks and activities is essential for nurturing a positive self-concept and promoting independence.
   3. Activity limitations may be essential; however, such restrictions

TABLE 13-1.
Commonly Measured ECG Components

COMPONENT	WHAT IT REPRESENTS	CORRELATION WITH CARDIAC CYCLE
P wave	Atrial depolarization	Contraction of the right atrium begins at the peak of the P wave; left atrial contraction follows.
T wave	Ventricular repolarization	Repolarization occurs while the ventricles are still contracting.
P-R interval	Interval between the beginning of the P wave and the beginning of the QRS complex	This is the interval between the onset of atrial depolarization and the onset of ventricular depolarization (*i.e.*, the conduction time between the atria and the ventricles).
Q-T interval	Interval from the beginning of the QRS complex to the end of the T wave	This is the total time of ventricular depolarization and repolarization.
QRS complex	Wave of ventricular depolarization	Left ventricular contraction begins at the peak of the R wave; right ventricular contraction, shortly thereafter.

may be difficult to impose in a child with cardiac disease who has no overt symptoms.

4. With many defects, an older child may be allowed to self-limit activities according to how he or she feels.

5. Parents need support and guidance in setting limits, providing discipline, and meeting their child's emotional needs.

III. Acyanotic heart defects

A. Description: congenital heart defects in which no deoxygenated or poorly oxygenated venous blood enters systemic arterial circulation.

1. Types of acyanotic defects
   a. Left to right shunting through an abnormal opening (*e.g.*, patent ductus arteriosus [PDA], atrial septal defect [ASD], ventricular septal defect [VSD])
   b. Obstructive lesions that restrict ventricular outflow (*e.g.*, aortic valvular stenosis, pulmonic stenosis, and coarctation of the aorta) (Fig. 13-3)

B. Etiology and incidence

1. The incidence of congenital heart defects (CHD) ranges from 4 to 10 of 100 live births. CHD is the second major cause, after prematurity, of death in the first year of life.

2. Children with CHD are more likely to have associated defects such as tracheoesophageal fistula.

3. In greater than 90% of CHD cases, the exact etiology is unknown.

4. Factors associated with increased incidence of CHD include:

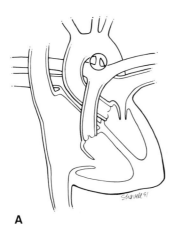

A

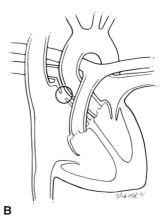

B

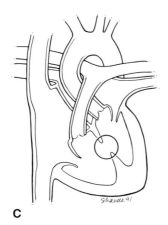

C

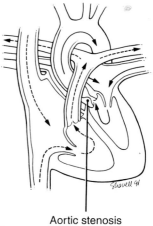

Aortic stenosis

D

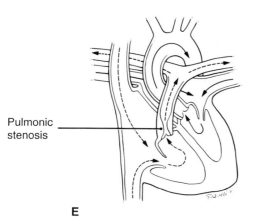

Pulmonic
stenosis

E

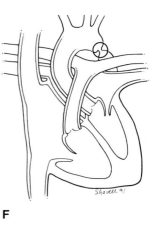

F

FIGURE 13-3.
Acyanotic defects that compromise circulation and tissue perfusion. (A) Patent ductus arteriosus.
(B) Atrial septal defect. (C) Ventricular septal defect. (D) Aortic stenosis. (E) Pulmonic stenosis.
(F) Coarctation of the aorta.

        a.   Fetal and maternal infection during the first trimester, especially rubella

        b.   Maternal alcoholism

        c.   Maternal use of other drugs with teratogenic effects

        d.   Maternal age over 40

        e.   Maternal dietary deficiencies

        f.   Maternal insulin-induced diabetes

        g.   Sibling with CHD

        h.   Parent with CHD

        i.   A chromosomal abnormality such as Down's syndrome

    3.   Incidence of acyanotic heart defects is as follows:

        a.   PDA: occurs more frequently in females and accounts for between 5% and 10% of all congenital cardiac lesions, excluding premature infants

        b.   ASD: occurs more frequently in females and accounts for between 5% to 10% of all CHD

        c.   **VSD: most common CHD in all groups; accounts for 20% to 25% of total cardiac lesions**

        d.   Aortic stenosis: accounts for 5% of all CHD

        e.   Pulmonic stenosis (PS): occurs in 5% to 8% of all cardiac lesions, and many children with PS have other associated cardiac lesions

        f.   Coarctation of the aorta (COA): occurs more frequently in males and accounts for about 8% of CHD

C.   **Pathophysiology and management**

    1.   **Patent ductus arteriosus (PDA)**

        a.   **PDA is failure of the fetal ductus arteriosus to close completely after birth.**

        b.   PDA typically affects preterm infants.

        c.   Blood flows from the aorta through the PDA and back to the pulmonary artery and lungs, causing increased left ventricular work load and increased pulmonary vascular congestion.

    2.   **Atrial septal defect (ASD)**

        a.   **Atrial septal tissue does not fuse properly during embryonic development.**

        b.   In ASD pressure is higher in the left atrium than the right, causing blood to shunt from the left to the right side of the heart.

        c.   The right ventricle and pulmonary artery enlarge because they are handling more blood.

    3.   **Ventricular septal defect (VSD)**

        a.   **The degree of this defect may vary from a pin hole between the right and left ventricles to an absent septum.**

      b. Pressure from the left ventricle causes blood to flow through the defect to the right ventricle, resulting in increased pulmonary vascular resistance and right heart enlargement.

      c. Right ventricular and pulmonary arterial pressures increase, leading eventually to obstructive pulmonary vascular disease.

4. Aortic valvular stenosis

      a. **This defect primarily involves an obstruction to the left ventricular outflow of the valve.**

      b. Left ventricular pressure increases to overcome resistance of the obstructed valve and allow blood to flow into the aorta, eventually producing left ventricular hypertrophy.

      c. Myocardial ischemia may develop as the increased oxygen demands of the hypertrophied left ventricle go unmet.

5. Pulmonic stenosis

      a. **This defect involves obstruction of blood flow from the right ventricle.**

      b. As a result of right ventricular pressure increase, right ventricular hypertrophy may develop.

      c. Eventually, right ventricular failure may result.

6. Coarctation of the aorta

      a. **This defect involves a localized narrowing of the aorta.**

      b. There are three types, depending on location:

          (1) Preductal: proximal to the insertion of the ductus arteriosus

          (2) Postductal: distal to the ductus arteriosus

          (3) Juxtaductal: at the insertion of the ductus arteriosus

      c. There is increased pressure proximal to the defect and decreased pressure distal to it.

      d. Restricted blood flow through the narrowed aorta increases the pressure on the left ventricle and causes dilation of the proximal aorta and left ventricular hypertrophy, which may lead to left ventricular failure.

      e. Eventually, collateral vessels develop to bypass the coarctated segment and supply circulation to the lower extremities.

D. Clinical assessment findings

  1. Clinical manifestations in PDA

      a. **If the defect is small, the child may be asymptomatic.**

      b. **A loud machinelike murmur is characteristic.**

      c. Child may have frequent respiratory infections.

      d. Child may have congestive heart failure (CHF) with poor

feeding, fatigue, hepatosplenomegaly (HSM), poor weight gain, tachypnea, and irritability.

e. Widened pulse pressure and bounding pulse rate may be detected.

2. Clinical manifestations in ASD

a. Most infants tend to be asymptomatic until early childhood and up to 40% of defects close spontaneously by age 5 years.

b. Symptoms vary with the size of the defect; fatigue and dyspnea on exertion are the most common symptoms.

c. Slow weight gain and easy fatigue are also symptoms.

 d. **Frequent respiratory infections may occur.**

e. Systolic ejection murmur may be auscultated, usually most prominent at the second intercostal space.

3. Clinical manifestations in VSD

a. Symptoms vary with the size of the defect, age, and amount of resistance; usually the child is asymptomatic.

b. Identifiable symptoms may be failure to thrive (FTT), excessive sweating, and fatigue.

c. Child may be more susceptible to pulmonary infections.

d. Child may exhibit signs and symptoms of CHF.

4. Clinical manifestations in aortic valvular stenosis

a. Child with severe defect may have faint pulse, hypotension, tachycardia, and poor feeding pattern.

b. Child may experience signs of exercise intolerance, chest pain, and dizziness when standing for long periods.

c. Systolic ejection murmur may be heard best at second intercostal space.

5. Clinical manifestations in pulmonic stenosis

a. Child may be asymptomatic or may have mild cyanosis or CHF.

b. Systolic murmur may be heard over the pulmonic area; a thrill may be heard if stenosis is severe.

c. In severe cases, decreased exercise tolerance, dyspnea, precordial pain, and generalized cyanosis may occur.

 6. **Clinical manifestations in COA**

a. **The child may be asymptomatic or may experience the classic difference in blood pressure and pulse quality between the upper and lower extremities; femoral pulses are weak or absent.**

b. Additional manifestations may include epistaxis, headaches, fainting, and lower leg muscle cramps.

c. Systolic murmur may be heard over the left anterior chest and between the scapula posteriorly.

d. Rib notching may be observed in an older child.

E. Diagnostic assessment findings
1. Specific findings vary according to defect.
2. Chest radiography may reveal cardiac enlargement when present.
3. ECG changes may be noted.
4. ECG may demonstrate enlargement of atria and ventricles, presence of the ductus arteriosus, size of shunts, and levels of obstruction.
5. Cardiac catheterization confirms diagnosis and reveals pressure differences.

F. Nursing diagnoses: depend on specific manifestations of the defect. Refer also to nursing diagnoses for CHF, cardiac catheterization, and cardiac surgery.
1. Activity intolerance
2. Anxiety
3. Altered tissue perfusion
4. Altered family processes
5. Risk for infection
6. Risk for injury
7. Anticipatory grieving
8. Knowledge deficit
9. Altered nutrition: less than body requirements
10. Self-esteem disturbance
11. Altered growth and development

G. Planning and implementation

1. **Observe for and assist in managing hypoxia (marked by manifestations of tachypnea, cyanosis, bradycardia, tachycardia, restlessness, progressive limpness, and syncope) as follows:**
   a. Place child in knee-chest position.
   b. Administer oxygen as prescribed.
   c. Administer medications as prescribed.
   d. Document hypoxic episodes.
2. Observe for and assist in managing respiratory distress (manifested by tachypnea, tachycardia, retractions, grunting, nasal flaring, cough, and cyanosis) as follows:
   a. Administer oxygen as prescribed.
   b. Position child to ease breathing.
3. Help maintain optimal nutritional status, as follows:
   a. Promote a well-balanced diet that is rich in iron and potassium and low in sodium.
   b. Provide small, frequent feedings if child tires easily.
   c. Provide nipples that make it easier for an infant to suck

and limit feedings to 45 minutes or less if infant tires easily.

    d.   Evaluate weight gain daily.

4. Help decrease cardiac workload by organizing care to provide periods of uninterrupted rest, preventing excessive crying in infants, and providing diversional activities that involve only limited energy expenditure in older children.

5. Observe for and assist in managing CHF.

6. Observe for and assist in managing bacterial endocarditis (manifested by fever, pallor, petechiae, anorexia, and fatigue) as follows:

    a.   Ensure administration of prophylactic antibiotics before dental work, surgery, or laceration repair.

    b.   Prevent child's exposure to persons with infections.

7. Monitor for signs and symptoms of thrombosis, such as irritability, restlessness, seizure activity, coma, paralysis, edema, hematuria, oliguria, and anuria. To reduce the risk of thrombosis, prevent dehydration, especially during acute illnesses.

8. **Prevent infection through careful hand washing, avoiding contact with infected persons and immunization, and by providing adequate rest and nutrition.**

9. Prevent hypokalemia secondary to diuretic therapy by maintaining a high-potassium diet and administering potassium supplements when prescribed.

10. Prevent anemia by encouraging an iron-rich diet and by administering iron supplements as prescribed.

11. Enhance the child's self-concept by encouraging him or her to express feelings about the defect, clarifying any misconceptions he or she expresses concerning the defect or its treatment, and supporting positive coping mechanisms.

12. Decrease the child's and family's anxiety and increase their understanding by providing needed information on medical and surgical treatments for the specific defect.

13. Provide the following teaching for PDA:

    a.   Explain that surgery may be performed by age 1 or 2 years, earlier if CHF develops. Ligation of PDA is not open-heart surgery and does not require cardiopulmonary bypass.

    b.   Advise parents that in premature infants, PDA sometimes can be closed using prostaglandin-synthetase inhibitors, such as indomethacin, that stimulate closure of the ductus.

    c.   Some children experience transient unexplained hypertension after repair.

14. Provide the following teaching for ASD:

a. Inform parents that surgical closure by suture or patch requires cardiopulmonary bypass and usually is performed on children between ages 4 and 6 years.

b. Forewarn parents that some children develop arrhythmias despite surgery.

15. Provide the following teaching on VSD:

a. Reassure parent that most defects close spontaneously.

b. As appropriate, explain that early surgery, involving closure with a Dacron patch and requiring cardiopulmonary bypass, is recommended for children with pulmonary arterial hypertension, CHF, recurrent respiratory infections, and failure to thrive.

c. Note that surgery is complex and that pulmonary artery banding may be done as a palliative procedure for infants who are poor surgical candidates.

16. Provide the following teaching on aortic valvular stenosis:

a. Tell parents that if the child's symptoms warrant, surgical aortic valvulotomy or prosthetic valve replacement is necessary.

b. Advise that children with this defect may be restricted from sports and physical exertion.

17. Provide the following teaching on pulmonic stenosis:

a. Explain that in moderate to severe cases, surgical valvulotomy is performed.

b. Also explain that surgery is done immediately in symptomatic newborns and is delayed until excessively high pressure in the right ventricle warrants it in children with mild to moderate stenosis.

18. Provide the following teaching on coarctation of the aorta:

a. Inform parents that emergency management includes the administration of medication (prostaglandin E to dilate the ductus arteriosus and restore blood flow to lower extremities).

b. Discuss how later intervention involves management of CHF and surgical resection between ages 2 and 4 years, unless heart failure or severe hypertension occurs earlier.

c. Explain that postoperatively most children continue to exhibit some degree of hypertension and ECG changes with exercise.

19. Assist the child's family in coping with diagnosis, treatment, and prognosis by:

a. Encouraging family members to express feelings

b. Encouraging the family to provide as normal a life as possible for the child and to stimulate him or her with age-appropriate activities consistent with his or her activity tolerance

20. Educate the child and family, covering:
   a. Nature of the defect, diagnosis, treatment, and potential complications
   b. Infection prevention and control measures
   c. Administration, dosage, and side effects of prescribed medication
   d. The child's nutritional requirements and any special diet information
   e. The child's need for adequate rest periods and any physical or activity limitations
   f. The significance of normal developmental tasks and the importance of avoiding overprotectiveness

H. **Evaluation**
   1. Parents verbalize knowledge of their child's defect, treatments, and potential complications.
   2. The child maintains adequate oxygenation, as evidenced by normal color and improved blood gas values.
   3. The child remains infection-free.
   4. The child's breathing is unlabored.
   5. The child gains or maintains adequate weight.
   6. The child verbalizes age-appropriate understanding of the disorder and its treatment.
   7. Parents verbalize the date and time of the next scheduled follow-up appointment.

IV. **Cyanotic heart defects**
   A. **Description: congenital heart defects in which deoxygenated blood enters the systemic arterial circulation.**
      1. Cyanotic heart defects include:
         a. Tetralogy of Fallot
         b. Transposition of the great vessels
         c. Truncus arteriosus
         d. Hypoplastic left heart syndrome
   B. **Etiology and incidence**
      1. The incidence of congenital heart defects (CHD) is about 4 to 10 of 100 live births. In the first year of life, CHD is the major cause of death, other than prematurity.
      2. Children with CHD are more likely to have associated defects such as tracheoesophageal fistula.
      3. In greater than 90% of CHD, the exact etiology is unknown.
      4. Factors associated with increased incidence of CHD include:
         a. Fetal and maternal infection during the first trimester, especially rubella
         b. Maternal alcoholism
         c. Maternal use of other drugs with teratogenic effects
         d. Maternal age over 40

e. Maternal dietary deficiencies
f. Maternal insulin-induced diabetes
g. Sibling with CHD
h. Parent with CHD
i. A chromosomal abnormality such as Down's syndrome

5. Approximate relative incidence of cyanotic defects is as follows:

a. **Tetralogy of Fallot: the most common cyanotic defect; it accounts for 10% of all CHD**
b. Transposition of the great vessels: second most common heart defect; it accounts for about 5% of all CHD, with a higher incidence in males
c. Truncus arteriosus: relatively rare; it accounts for less than 1% of all CHD
d. Hypoplastic left heart syndrome: consists of 2% of all CHD

C. Pathophysiology and management

1. **In these defects, cyanosis results from right to left shunting of blood through intracardiac communication, mixing of blood in a common heart chamber, or abnormal development of major blood vessels.**

2. The specific disease process and clinical manifestations depend on the severity of the defect and the amount of pulmonary blood flow involved.

3. **Tetralogy of Fallot**
    a. **Consists of four major anomalies:**
        (1) **A ventricular septal defect (VSD)**
        (2) **Right ventricular hypertrophy**
        (3) **Pulmonic stenosis**
        (4) **Aorta overriding the VSD**
    b. Pulmonic stenosis impedes the flow of blood to the lungs, causing increased pressure in the right ventricle, forcing deoxygenated blood through the septal defect to the left ventricle.
    c. The increased workload on the right ventricle causes hypertrophy.
    d. The overriding aorta receives blood from both right and left ventricles.
    e. Manifestations depend on the size of the VSD and the degree of pulmonic stenosis.

4. **Transposition of the great vessels**
    a. **The pulmonary artery leaves the left ventricle and the aorta exits the right ventricle, with no communication between systemic and pulmonary circulations.**

  b. This defect results in two separate circulatory patterns: the right heart manages systemic circulation and the left manages pulmonary circulation.

  c. To sustain life, the child must have an associated defect. Associated defects, such as septal defects or patent ductus, permit the blood to mix but cause increased cardiac workload.

  d. Potential complications include: CHF, infective endocarditis, brain abscess, and cerebral vascular accidents resulting from hypoxia or thrombosis.

5. Truncus arteriosus

  a. **The failure of normal septation and division of the embryonic bulbar trunk into the pulmonary artery and aorta results in a single vessel that overrides both ventricles.**

  b. Blood ejected from ventricles enters the common artery and flows either into the lungs or the aortic arch.

  c. Pressure in both ventricles is high and blood flow to the lungs is markedly increased.

  d. Neonates with this defect typically appear normal; however, as pulmonary vascular resistance decreases after birth, severe pulmonary edema and CHF commonly develop.

6. Hypoplastic left heart syndrome

  a. **This disorder involves various left-sided defects, commonly including severe coarctation of the aorta, severe aortic valvular stenosis or atresia, and severe mitral valve stenosis or atresia.**

  b. The left ventricle, aortic valve, mitral valve, and ascending aorta usually are small or hypoplastic.

  c. Survival is possible only while the ductus arteriosus remains patent, which allows for systemic blood flow.

  d. When the ductus arteriosus closes, pulmonary edema and low cardiac output occur, leading to hypoxia, acidosis, and death. Corrective surgery is not feasible.

D. **Clinical assessment findings**

 1. Tetralogy of Fallot: clinical manifestations and diagnostic findings vary depending on the size of the VSD and the degree of pulmonic stenosis and may include:

  a. Acute episodes of cyanosis ("tet spells") and transient cerebral ischemia

  b. Cyanosis, often observed in the neonate only during crying spells; later in life, as stenosis worsens, occurring even at rest

  c. **Squatting (a characteristic posture of older children** that serves to decrease return of poorly oxygenated venous blood from the lower extremities and to increase systemic vascular resistance, which increases pulmonary blood flow and eases respiratory effort)

    d. Slow weight gain

    e. Clubbing, exertional dyspnea, fainting, or slowness due to hypoxia

    f. Pansystolic murmur heard at mid-lower left sternal border

2. Transposition of the great vessels: produces various clinical manifestations depending on associated defects:

    a. In infants with minimal communication, severe depression and cyanosis at birth

    b. In infants with defects, less cyanosis but may have symptoms of CHF

    c. Easily fatigued

    d. Failure to thrive

    d. No murmur or murmur characteristic of associated defect

3. Truncus arteriosus: assessment findings include:

    a. Marked cyanosis, especially on exertion

    b. Signs and symptoms of CHF

    c. Left ventricular hypertrophy, dyspnea, marked activity intolerance, and retarded growth

    d. Loud systolic murmur best heard at the lower left sternal border and radiating throughout the chest

4. Hypoplastic left heart syndrome: manifestations usually are evident by the first 2 weeks after birth and typically include:

    a. Signs and symptoms of CHF and pulmonary edema

    b. Single S_2

    c. Soft systolic ejection murmur

E. **Diagnostic assessment findings**

  1. Chest radiography may reveal cardiac enlargement when present.

  2. ECG changes may be noted.

  3. ECG may demonstrate enlargement of atria and ventricles, presence of the ductus arteriosus, size of shunts, and levels of obstruction.

  4. Cardiac catheterization confirms diagnoses and reveals pressure differences.

  5. Polycythemia and thrombocytopenia.

F. **Nursing diagnoses: Nursing diagnoses depend on specific manifestations of the defect. Refer also to nursing diagnoses for CHF, cardiac catheterization, and cardiac surgery.**

  1. Activity intolerance

  2. Anxiety

3. Altered tissue perfusion
4. Altered family processes
5. Risk for infection
6. Risk for injury
7. Anticipatory grieving
8. Knowledge deficit
9. Altered nutrition: less than body requirements
10. Self-esteem disturbance
11. Altered growth and development

G. **Planning and implementation**

1. Nursing interventions for infants and children with cyanotic defects are similar to those for patients with acyanotic defects, with the exception of child and family teaching about specific defects and their management.

2. Help decrease the child's and family's anxiety and increase their understanding by providing needed information on medical and surgical treatments for the specific defect.

3. For tetralogy of Fallot, cover the following teaching points:
   a. Intervention is based on symptomatology.
   b. Early cyanosis requires a palliative procedure to increase blood flow to the lungs, such as the Blalock-Taussig shunt or Waterson shunt.
   c. Complete surgical repair usually is performed on the infant between the ages of 18 and 36 months; the procedure, which requires cardiopulmonary bypass, involves patch closure of the VSD and relief of the pulmonary stenosis.
   d. Potential complications include heart block, residual VSD or pulmonary stenosis, and pulmonary valve regurgitation.

4. For transposition of the great vessels, cover the following teaching points:
   a. Prostaglandin E is administered to maintain a patent ductus arteriosus while further evaluation is done.
   b. Enlargement of the interatrial communication by balloon septostomy during cardiac catheterization (the Rashkind procedure) maintains adequate mixing of oxygenated and unoxygenated blood.
   c. The Blalock-Hanlon surgical procedure may be performed to enlarge the foramen ovale.
   d. Infants with massive pulmonary flow and intractable heart failure require early surgical intervention usually by placing a band around the pulmonary artery and reducing flow to the lungs, which relieves the congestive failure until the child is old enough for definitive repair.

    e. Surgical procedures for total repair include the Mustard, the Senning, and the arterial switch procedures.

    f. Potential complications of surgery include superior vena cava or inferior vena cava obstruction, arrhythmias, tricuspid regurgitation, and pulmonary venous obstruction.

    g. Without treatment, 90% of infants with this defect die within the first year of life.

  5. For truncus arteriosus, cover the following teaching points:

    a. CHF is treated medically.

    b. Palliative surgery involves pulmonary arterial banding.

    c. Corrective surgery, usually performed before age 2 years, consists of closing the VSD, removing the pulmonary arteries from the truncus arteriosus, and interposing a conduit between the right ventricle and pulmonary artery.

    d. Possible complications of surgery include residual VSD, truncal valve regurgitation, conduit obstruction, and pulmonary vascular disease.

  6. For hypoplastic left heart syndrome, cover the following teaching points:

    a. Without surgery, about 95% of infants die before age 1 month.

    b. Palliative procedures have had limited success at extending life. Some cardiac transplantation has ben performed.

    c. Many parents may take their infants home to die; these families may welcome referral to community hospice programs for support.

 H. Evaluation: See evaluation considerations for acyanotic defects, section III, G.

V. Congestive heart failure (CHF)

 A. Description: severe circulatory congestion due to decreased myocardial contractility resulting in the heart's inability to pump sufficient blood to meet the body's needs.

 B. Etiology and incidence

  1. The primary cause of CHF in the first 3 years of life is congenital heart disease.

  2. Other causes in children include:

    a. Other myocardial disorders, such as cardiomyopathies, arrhythmias and hypertension

    b. Pulmonary embolism or chronic lung disease

    c. Severe hemorrhage or anemia

    d. Adverse effects of anesthesia or surgery

    e. Adverse effects of transfusions or infusions

    f. Increased body demands resulting from conditions such as fever, infection, and arteriovenous fistula

        g.   Adverse effects of drugs, such as doxorubicin

        h.   Severe physical or emotional stress

        i.   Excessive sodium intake

   3.   About 80% of CHF cases occur before age 1 year.

C. **Pathophysiology and management**

   1.   Right ventricular failure: Because the right ventricle is unable to pump, less blood is oxygenated and pressure increases in the right atrium and systemic venous circulation, which results in edema of the extremities.

   2.   Left ventricular failure: Because the left ventricle is unable to pump blood into systemic circulation, pressure increases in the left atrium and pulmonary veins; then the lungs become congested with blood causing elevated pulmonary pressure and pulmonary edema.

D. **Clinical assessment findings**

   1.   **Clinically difficult to differentiate right from left ventricular failure**

   2.   Weakness, fatigue

   3.   Poor feeding

   4.   Irritability

   5.   Pallor, cyanosis

   6.   Dyspnea, tachypnea, orthopnea, wheezing, cough, weak cry, grunting

   7.   Tachycardia, cardiomegaly, gallop rhythm

   8.   Hepatomegaly

   9.   Weight gain from edema, ascites, pleural effusions

  10.   Distended neck and peripheral veins, sweating

E. **Diagnostic assessment findings**

   1.   Chest radiography reveals cardiomegaly and pulmonary congestion.

   2.   Laboratory study results commonly reveal dilution hyponatremia, hypochloremia, and hyperkalemia.

F. **Nursing diagnoses**

   1.   Altered tissue perfusion

   2.   Risk for infection

   3.   Risk for injury

   4.   Decreased cardiac output

   5.   Ineffective breathing pattern

   6.   Activity intolerance

   7.   Anxiety

   8.   Fluid volume excess

   9.   Altered family process

  10.   Altered nutrition: less than body requirements

G.   Planning and implementation

1.   Monitor for signs of respiratory distress. Provide pulmonary hygiene as needed, administer oxygen as prescribed, keep the head of the bed elevated, and monitor arterial blood gas values.

2.   Monitor for signs of altered cardiac output; pulmonary edema; arrhythmias, including extreme tachycardia and bradycardia; and characteristic ECG and heart sound changes.

3.   Evaluate fluid status by maintaining strict intake and output (I&O) measurements, monitoring daily weights, assessing for edema and severe diaphoresis, and monitoring electrolyte values and hematocrit level. Maintain fluid restrictions, as prescribed.

4.   **Help prevent infection by performing scrupulous hand washing and limiting the child's exposure to persons with infections.**

5.   Reduce cardiac demands by keeping the child warm and by scheduling nursing interventions to allow for rest. Do not allow an infant to feed for more than 45 minutes at a time; provide gavage feeding if the infant becomes fatigued before ingesting an adequate amount.

6.   Help ensure adequate nutrition. As necessary, provide small, frequent meals. Maintain a high-calorie, low-sodium diet, as prescribed.

7.   Help decrease anxiety by providing developmentally appropriate explanations, encouraging expression of feelings and concerns, and encouraging parental involvement in the child's care, as appropriate.

8.   Administer medications, as prescribed, which may include:
   a.   Digoxin, to increase cardiac performance
   b.   Diuretics, such as furosemide, hydrochlorothiazide, and spironolactone, to reduce venous and systemic congestion
   c.   Iron and folic acid supplements, to improve nutritional status

9.   **Monitor for medication side effects, such as:**
   a.   **Digitalis toxicity: Specific serum levels of digitalis and extreme bradycardia are cardinal signs of toxicity; withhold digoxin if the child's heart rate falls below the normal range for age (see Table 13-2), unless the physician specifies otherwise.**
   b.   **Hypokalemia, due to diuretic therapy: Monitor potassium level closely and administer supplemental potassium as prescribed.**

TABLE 13-2.
Selected Clinical Signs of Digitalis Toxicity in Children

AGE	HEART RATE	DRUG-BLOOD LEVEL
Newborn	< 100 beats/min	> 4 nl/mL
Infants: 1 month to 1 year	< 100 beats/min	> 3 nl/mL
Infants: more than 1 year	< 100 beats/min	> 2 nl/mL
Young children	< 80 beats/min	> 2 nl/mL
Older children	< 60 beats/min	> 2 nl/mL

10. As appropriate, refer the family to a community health nurse for follow-up care after discharge.
11. Provide patient and family teaching, covering the following teaching points:
   a. Signs and symptoms of CHF to watch for
   b. Diet and fluid restrictions
   c. Dosage, administration, and side effects of prescribed medications

H. Evaluation
1. The child exhibits improved cardiac output, as evidenced by clinical condition and laboratory values.
2. The child has normal fluid and electrolyte values and decreased edema.
3. The child exhibits improved oxygenation, as evidenced by normal coloration and blood gas values within normal ranges.
4. The child maintains adequate nutrition for normal weight.
5. Parents verbalize an understanding of signs and symptoms of CHF and possible complications, correct dosage and administration of medications, and necessary follow-up care.
6. The family is referred to a community health nurse for follow-up as appropriate.

VI. Rheumatic fever (RF)
   A. Description: systemic inflammatory disease that occurs as a result of naturally acquired immunity to group A beta-hemolytic streptococcal infection, with carditis occurring in about 50% of cases.
   B. Etiology and incidence
   1. RF is the most common cause of acquired heart disease in children worldwide, but its incidence has sharply decreased in the United States during this century.
   2. RF usually occurs in children between ages 6 and 15 years, with peak incidence at 8 years.

3. There are more frequent outbreaks in late winter and early spring when streptococcal infections are most common.

4. The onset of RF usually occurs 3 weeks after an untreated upper respiratory infection with group A beta-hemolytic streptococcus. It is believed that a genetic susceptibility to RF is associated with a state of immune hyperreactivity to the streptococcal antigens.

5. The exact etiology of RF is unknown.

C. Pathophysiology and management

1. The child becomes infected with group A beta-hemolytic streptococcal bacteria.

2. Antibodies formed against these bacteria begin to attack the connective tissue of the body, producing inflammation, which affects the heart, joints, central nervous system (CNS), and subcutaneous tissue.

3. In carditis, the characteristic lesion is Aschoff's body—a proliferating, fibrinlike plaque that forms on the heart valve causing edema and inflammation. When the healed area becomes fibrous and scarred, the valve leaflets fuse (stenosis) causing inefficiency and leakage. The mitral and aortic valves are affected most often.

4. Diagnosis is made according to the Jones criteria (need two major or one major and two minor characteristics, and evidence of a preceding streptococcal infection for a diagnosis of RF).

   a. Major characteristics: carditis, polyarthritis, chorea, erythema marginatum, subcutaneous nodules

   b. Minor characteristics: clinical features (fever, arthralgia); laboratory findings include elevated erythrocyte sedimentation rate (ESR), elevated C-reactive protein (CRP)

   c. Supportive evidence of streptococcal infection: positive throat culture or rapid streptococcal antigen test; elevated or rising streptococcal antibody titer

5. Treatment usually consists of eradicating the streptococcal infection with antibiotics, usually penicillin; preventing permanent cardiac damage through rest, palliative therapy, and avoidance of disease recurrences through long-term antibiotic therapy.

D. Clinical assessment findings

1. Clinical findings are variable and depend on the site of involvement, the severity of the attack, and the stage at which the child is first examined.

2. The principal symptoms are noted in the heart, joints, skin, and central nervous system.

3. *Carditis:* tachycardia (higher than would be expected for fever),

cardiomegaly, murmur, muffled heart sounds, precordial friction rub, precordial pain, prolonged PR interval. Carditis can lead to CHF, pericardial friction rubs, cardiomegaly, and aortic or mitral valve regurgitation.

4. *Polyarthritis:* swollen, hot, painful joints; favors large joints. Polyarthritis is the most common presenting symptom and it occurs in about 75% of all cases of RF.

5. *Chorea* (also called Sydenham's chorea or St. Vitus dance): sudden aimless, irregular movements of the extremities; involuntary facial grimaces; speech disturbances; emotional lability; muscle weakness; increased movements with stress, decreased with rest; occurring in about 10% of all cases.

6. *Erythema marginatum:* clear-centered macules, with defined border, transitory, nonpruritic, and noted mostly on trunk and proximal extremities, occurring in about 5% of all cases.

7. *Subcutaneous nodules:* nontender; may persist, then resolve; located over bony prominences; occurring in about 10% of all cases.

8. *Other characteristics:* fever, arthralgia, history of RF or rheumatic heart disease, weight loss, fatigue, abdominal pain, and unexplained epistaxis.

E. Diagnostic assessment findings

1. Because no single laboratory test can confirm RF, Jones criteria are used.

2. Complete blood count (CBC) (transient anemia, elevated white blood count [WBC].

3. ESR is elevated (normal male, 1 to 15; normal female, 1 to 20).

4. C-reactive protein is positive (normal is negative).

5. Throat culture findings may be positive for streptococcal infection and antistreptolysin-O (ASO) titer may be elevated (normal is 0 to 120 Todd units; >333 Todd units indicates recent streptococcal infection in children).

6. Chest x-ray studies may disclose cardiac enlargement.

7. ECG may reveal prolonged PR interval.

F. Nursing diagnoses

1. Risk for injury
2. Pain
3. Risk for impaired skin integrity
4. Risk for infection
5. Risk for altered nutrition: less than body requirements
6. Altered growth and development
7. Diversional activity deficit
8. Altered family processes
9. Knowledge deficit
10. Altered health maintenance

G. Planning and implementation

1. Assess and monitor cardiac, joint, skin, and neurologic status. Note and report any changes. Monitor for signs of CHF and provide interventions as appropriate (see section V, D and G).

2. **Promote compliance with bed rest and activity restrictions by planning low-activity diversions. Allow child some autonomy in selecting activities. Inform child and family that although he or she may feel well, the body has not yet healed adequately.**

3. Promote rest by organizing nursing care to allow for adequate rest periods.

4. Alleviate discomfort of fever and arthralgia by administering medications as prescribed; utilizing alternative pain relief methods such as relaxation and meditation when appropriate; using bed cradles and soft linens to decrease pressure on joints; being careful and supportive when moving affected joints. Manipulation, heat, cold, and massage may aggravate joint pain.

5. Prevent skin breakdown by providing good skin care and by protecting bony prominences.

6. Promote optimal nutrition by assessing child's preferences, providing a diet rich in protein and adequate calories, and conferring with the nutritionist.

7. Promote normal development by encouraging the parent to treat the child as normally as possible within limitations and by encouraging the child to continue with schoolwork when appropriate.

8. Promote diversional activities appropriate for age.

9. Support family coping by encouraging the child and family to verbalize their concerns and feelings, by explaining all procedures and treatments, by stressing that chorea is self-limiting, and by promoting successful coping mechanisms.

10. Provide child and family teaching. Topics to cover include:
    a. The disease and its treatment
    b. The relationship of exercise to cardiac workload
    c. Rationale, side effects, and dosage of prescribed medications, for example:
        (1) Child may receive monthly injections of benzathine penicillin (1.2 million U), two daily oral doses of penicillin (200,000 U), or one daily dose of sulfadiazine (1 g) to prevent recurrent streptococcal infections (duration of long-term prophylaxis is uncertain).
        (2) Aspirin and corticosteroids may be used to minimize inflammation. Side effects of aspirin therapy include

gastrointestinal (GI) disturbance, decreased platelet count, tinnitus, and headaches. Side effects of steroidal therapy include fluid retention, edema, hypokalemia, GI irritation, hyperglycemia, altered growth patterns, and Cushing's syndrome.

   (3) Digoxin may be added to therapy to slow the heart rate and strengthen myocardial contractility. The child should be monitored for signs of toxicity.

   d. How to promote compliance with bed rest

   e. Psychological and physical preparation for procedures

   f. Minimizing contact with infected persons and of hand washing

   g. Recognizing signs of recurrent streptococcal infection and promptly seeking medical attention for a sore throat

11. **Promote prevention of RF by encouraging proper evaluation and treatment of streptococcal infections.**

H. Evaluation

   1. The child experiences little to no discomfort related to carditis, fever, and arthralgia.

   2. The child complies with bed rest restrictions and has adequate diversional activity.

   3. The child with chorea remains injury-free.

   4. The child returns to full range of motion of the extremities.

   5. The child and family comply with long-term antibiotic therapy.

   6. The child and family feel free to verbalize frustrations.

   7. The child and family develop adequate coping mechanisms.

   8. The child and family verbalize an understanding of the teaching points.

VII. Cardiac catheterization

   A. Description: an invasive procedure, in which a radiopaque catheter is introduced into a peripheral blood vessel and advanced into the heart chambers—commonly through a percutaneous puncture into the femoral vein guided by fluoroscopy. May also involve injecting radiopaque contrast material through the catheter into the heart to provide more diagnostic information.

   B. Purpose: The cardiac catheterization procedure may be diagnostic (to provide information concerning oxygen saturation, pressures in the chambers, changes in cardiac or stroke volume, and anatomic abnormalities); interventional (as an alternative to surgery in some types of congenital heart diseases); or electrophysiologic (to evaluate and correct arrhythmias).

C. **Clinical assessment**
1. Assess general health status, including activity level and current infections, history of allergies (many contrast agents are iodine-based and may trigger an allergic response), and history of acute illness.
2. Take and record vital signs.
3. Measure accurate height (to select correct catheter size) and weight.
4. Obtain and review CBC, clotting studies, and urinalysis.
5. Perform a physical examination, including assessing and marking of lower extremity pulses to ease postoperative evaluation.

D. **Nursing diagnoses**
1. Before procedure
   a. Fear
   b. Risk for fluid volume deficit
   c. Knowledge deficit
   d. Altered cardiopulmonary tissue perfusion
2. After procedure
   a. Decreased cardiac output
   b. Pain
   c. Impaired skin integrity
   d. Altered cardiopulmonary tissue perfusion

E. **Planning and implementation**
1. Before procedure
   a. Using developmentally appropriate explanations, prepare the child and family for the procedure.
   b. Help alleviate the child's fears by encouraging him or her to talk about the procedure and ask questions and express concerns. As appropriate, initiate therapeutic play to help identify and relieve the child's fears and misconceptions; allow the child to have a security object.
   c. Support family members by reinforcing and clarifying information provided by the physician.
   d. Maintain oral food and fluid restrictions (NPO status) as prescribed before the procedure, and monitor intravenous (IV) fluids, if prescribed; the child may be sedated before catheterization to minimize pain and trauma.
2. After procedure
   a. Prevent injury by observing the puncture site for bleeding, swelling, and hematoma formation. If hemorrhage occurs, apply pressure above the site and notify the physician.
   b. Maintain the child on bed rest with the affected limb straight, as prescribed, usually 4 to 6 hours after venous

catheterization, and 6 to 8 hours after arterial catheterization.

   c. Keep the child quiet, and frequently evaluate extremity color, temperature, capillary refill time, sensation, and pedal pulses.

   d. Monitor vital signs, especially blood pressure for hypotension that may indicate hemorrhage from the cardiac perforation or from the catheterization site. Assess for cardiac arrhythmias by auscultating the apical pulse for a full minute to detect irregularities. Report abnormalities to the physician.

3. Assess hydration status by monitoring I&O, evaluating urine specific gravity, and observing for signs of dehydration. Encourage oral fluid intake. Infants are at risk for hypoglycemia and should receive IV fluids containing dextrose; monitor blood glucose levels.

4. Assess for pain, and administer analgesics as prescribed.

5. Explore parental feelings about the procedure, its results and its implications.

6. Provide patient and family teaching, covering topics such as:

   a. Signs and symptoms to watch for and report (*e.g.*, any bleeding or swelling at the catheter site).

   b. Home care measures, including bathing: older children may shower; infants and young children should be given sponge baths for the first 3 days.

   c. Catheterization site care: change the bandage over insertion site daily for 3 days and observe for inflammation or excessive tenderness.

F. **Evaluation**

1. The skin at the site remains intact and not inflamed.

2. The child exhibits adequate hydration status, maintains stable vital signs, and remains calm.

3. The child and family state an understanding of and demonstrate proper care of the catheterization site.

4. Parents state dates and times of scheduled appointments for follow-up care.

VIII. **Cardiac surgery**

A. **Description**

1. **Open-heart surgery: involves incision of the myocardium to repair intracardiac structures; requires cardiopulmonary bypass.**

2. **Closed-heart surgery: involves structures related to the heart but not the heart muscle itself; usually can be performed without cardiopulmonary bypass.**

B. Purpose: an emergency or a planned procedure to correct defects or provide symptomatic relief.

C. Clinical assessment

1. The preoperative nursing assessment should include a health history of cardiac, pulmonary, renal, hepatic, hematologic, and metabolic disorders and a medication history that includes allergies and adverse reactions

2. Baseline assessments of:
   a. Height and weight
   b. Vital signs
   c. Sleep-wake patterns
   d. Elimination patterns
   e. Fluid intake

3. Laboratory studies:
   a. Complete blood count
   b. Serum electrolyte levels
   c. Clotting studies
   d. Urinalysis
   e. Nose, throat, and sputum cultures
   f. Antibody screen
   g. Renal and hepatic function tests

4. Radiographic and other diagnostic studies:
   a. Chest radiograph
   b. ECG
   c. Echocardiogram
   d. Cardiac catheterization

D. Nursing diagnoses

1. Activity intolerance
2. Anxiety
3. Ineffective breathing patterns
4. Decreased cardiac output
5. Altered family processes
6. Fear
7. Fluid volume deficit
8. Altered growth and development
9. Altered health maintenance
10. Risk for infection
11. Risk for injury
12. Pain
13. Sensory and perceptual alterations
14. Impaired skin integrity.
    (Note: Also see the nursing diagnoses for specific cardiac anomalies that necessitate surgery.)

E. Planning and implementation

1. Before surgery

      a.   Reinforce and clarify information provided to the child and family as necessary.

      b.   Reduce child's and family's anxiety by:

          (1) Thorough preoperative preparation; include a visit to the intensive care unit and explanations of what to expect before, during, and after surgery.

          (2) Offering developmentally appropriate explanations.

          (3) Allowing and encouraging expression of feelings and questions.

      c.   Carefully assess vital signs and notify surgeon of any signs of infection that may contraindicate surgery.

      d.   Prepare skin preoperatively as prescribed.

      e.   Institute NPO status as prescribed.

      f.   Administer preoperative medications as prescribed, which may include sedatives and antibiotics.

2.   After surgery

      a.   Maintain optimal respiratory status by monitoring respirations and providing good pulmonary hygiene. If the child is intubated, monitor chest tube drainage and patency, monitor blood gas values, and observe for signs of respiratory distress.

      b.   Monitor cardiac status:

          (1) Heart rate and rhythm (count rate for full minute and compare with ECG monitor; document activity)

          (2) Blood pressure, including intra-arterial monitoring

          (3) Central venous pressure (CVP) and other hemodynamic parameters

          (4) Heart sounds

          (5) Peripheral pulses

          (6) Blood chemistry values

      c.   Monitor lung sounds (decreased breath sounds may indicate atelectasis); suction only when needed (avoid vagal stimulation); monitor chest tubes and ventilator settings.

      d.   Prevent postoperative hypothermia by providing external warmth. Monitor for hyperthermia associated with infection.

      e.   Closely monitor I&O, and assess for signs of fluid overload, such as edema. Maintain fluid restrictions, as prescribed. Monitor IV lines: peripheral line for fluids, venous pressure line, and atrial line.

      f.   Promote comfort by assessing for pain and by medicating as needed.

      g.   Maintain skin integrity by inspecting all incision sites frequently, changing child's position, providing skin care, changing dressings as prescribed, and observing for infection.

      h.   Monitor for surgical complications: hypoxia, acidosis, thromboembolism, electrolyte imbalance, and poor systemic perfusion.

      i.   Prevent problems of sensory overload by orienting child to time, place, and person; by preparing him or her for all procedures; and by providing developmentally appropriate explanations. Ensure adequate rest periods and observe for psychic disturbances and sleep deprivation.

      j.   During recovery, provide tactile stimulation for infants and diversions for older children.

      k.   Provide emotional support for children and parents by addressing concerns.

      l.   Refer family for community health nurse visits.

      m.   Provide patient and family teaching, covering topics such as:

          (1) Activity restrictions

          (2) Incision site care

          (3) Dosage, administration, and possible side effects of medications

          (4) Diet and fluid restrictions

          (5) Possible regressive behaviors and psychological distress related to the trauma of surgery and hospitalization

          (6) Physiologic complications to watch for and report, such as tachycardia, fever, severe or persistent chest pain, labored breathing or tachypnea, feeding difficulties, and persistent swelling

F. Evaluation

1. The child maintains adequate oxygenation and exhibits nonlabored respiration.
2. The child maintains adequate cardiac output, as evidenced by normal heart rate and blood pressure, adequate urine output, and good peripheral perfusion.
3. The child maintains fluid and electrolyte balance, as evidenced by normal electrolyte values, absence of edema, and clear lungs on auscultation.
4. The child is well oriented and displays normal psychologic function.
5. The child is free of life-threatening complications of surgery.
6. The child reports minimal to no discomfort.
7. Family members verbalize knowledge of follow-up visits, home care measures, and proper administration and possible side effects of medications.
8. The family is referred to a community health nurse, as needed.

Bibliography

Alfaro-LeFevre, R., et al. (1992). *Drug Handbook: A Nursing Process Approach*. Redwood City, CA: Addison-Wesley.

Alyn, I.B. and Baker, L.K. (1992). Cardiovascular anatomy and physiology of the fetus, neonate, infant, child, and adolescent. *Journal of Cardiovascular Nursing*, 6, 1.

Betz, C.L., Hunsberger, M.M., and Wright, S. (1994). *Family Centered Nursing Care of Children*, 2nd ed. Philadelphia: W.B. Saunders.

Castiglia, P.T. and Harbin, R.B. (1993). *Child Health Care: Process and Practice*. Philadelphia: J.B. Lippincott.

Hardingham, K., et al. (1993). Nursing grand rounds: The pediatric cardiovascular surgery patient: A case study. *Journal of Cardiovascular Nursing*, 7, 80.

Jackson, D.B. and Saunders, R.B. (1993). *Child Health Nursing: A Comprehensive Approach to the Care of Children and Their Families*. Philadelphia: J.B. Lippincott.

Wolfe, R., Boucek, M., Schaeffer, M., and Wiggins, J. (1995). Cardiovascular diseases. In Hay, W., Groothuis, J, Hayward, A., and Levin, M. (Eds.) *Current Pediatric Diagnosis and Treatment*, 12th ed. Norwalk, CT: Appleton & Lange.

Wong, D.L. (1993). *Whaley and Wong's Essentials of Pediatric Nursing*, 4th ed. St. Louis: C.V. Mosby.

Wong, D.L. (1995). *Whaley and Wong's Nursing Care of Infants and Children*, 5th ed. St. Louis: C.V. Mosby.

STUDY QUESTIONS

1. Deoxygenated blood enters the systemic arterial circulation in which of the following disorders:
   a. Patent ductus arteriosus
   b. Tetralogy of Fallot
   c. Coarctation of the aorta
   c. Atrial stenosis

2. While assessing a child with coarctation of the aorta, the nurse would expect to find:
   a. Absent or diminished femoral pulses
   b. Cyanotic ("tet") episodes
   c. Squatting posture
   d. Severe cyanosis at birth

3. A nursing action that promotes optimal nutrition in an infant with congenital heart disease is:
   a. Offering sodium-rich formula
   b. Providing large feedings every 4 hours
   c. Using easy-to-suck nipples
   d. Allowing child to feed for long periods

4. Pulmonary stenosis involves:
   a. Return of blood to the heart without entry into the left atrium
   b. Obstruction of blood flow from the right ventricle
   c. Obstruction of blood from the left ventricle
   d. A single vessel arising from both ventricles

5. Which of the following represents an effective nursing intervention to reduce cardiac demands and decrease cardiac workload?
   a. Scheduling care to provide for uninterrupted rest periods
   b. Developing and implementing a consistent plan of care
   c. Feeding the infant over long periods
   d. Allowing the infant to have his or her way to avoid conflict

6. The defects associated with tetralogy of Fallot are:
   a. Coarctation of the aorta, aortic valve stenosis, mitral valve stenosis
   b. Ventricular septal defect, overriding aorta, pulmonic stenosis, and right ventricular hypertrophy
   c. Tricuspid valve atresia, atrial septal defect, and hypoplastic right ventricle
   d. Origin of the aorta from the right ventricle and of the pulmonary artery from the left ventricle

7. A child with congestive heart failure is receiving digoxin. Which manifestation is a cardinal sign of digoxin toxicity?
   a. Respiratory distress
   b. Extreme bradycardia
   c. Constipation
   d. Headache

8. Which of the following observations indicates that a child with CHF is carefully following the prescribed medical regimen?
   a. The child exhibits an elevated RBC count.
   b. The child exhibits normal weight for age.
   c. The child's pulse rate is under 50.
   d. The child takes daily antibiotics.

9. Prevention of rheumatic fever (RF) can best be done by:
   a. Treating all sore throats with penicillin
   b. Treating streptococcal throat infections with antibiotics
   c. Providing antibiotics before dental work
   d. Administering penicillin to patients with RF

10. All of the following should be taught to the parents of a child with Sydenham's chorea except:
    a. It is progressive and untreatable.
    b. It is manifested by involuntary movements.
    c. It is a symptom of RF.
    d. It decreases with rest and increases with stress.

ANSWER KEY

1. **Correct response: b**
   This is the definition of cyanotic heart disease; tetralogy of Fallot is the only cyanotic heart disease listed.
   a, c, and d. All are acyanotic heart diseases; no deoxygenated or poorly oxygenated blood enters the systemic arterial circulation.
   Comprehension/Physiologic/Assessment

2. **Correct response: a**
   Absent or diminished femoral pulse is a classic characteristic of coarctation of the aorta.
   b. Tet episodes are characteristic of tetralogy of Fallot.
   c. Squatting is characteristic of tetralogy of Fallot.
   d. Severe cyanosis at birth is seen in defects such as transposition of the great vessels.
   Application/Physiologic/Assessment

3. **Correct response: c**
   The infant may easily tire with regular nipples and thus would not be able to suck adequately.
   a. Decreased sodium may be needed.
   b. The child should have small frequent feedings to prevent tiring.
   d. Feedings should last no more than 45 minutes to prevent tiring.
   Application/Health Promotion/ Implementation

4. **Correct response: b**
   Pulmonic stenosis refers to an obstruction of blood flow from the right ventricle.
   a and c. These describe total anomalous pulmonary venous communications.
   d. This describes truncus arteriosus.
   Knowledge/Physiologic/Assessment

5. **Correct response: a**
   Organizing nursing care to provide for uninterrupted periods of sleep reduces cardiac demands.

   b. Developing a consistent plan of care can be important, but it is not related to decreasing cardiac demands or workload.
   c. Feeding time should be restricted to a maximal 45 minutes or discontinued sooner if the infant tires.
   d. Excessive crying should be limited; however, appropriate limit setting should still be observed.
   Analysis/Physiologic/Evaluation

6. **Correct response: b**
   These are the defects associated with tetralogy of Fallot.
   a. These are the defects associated with tricuspid atresia.
   c. These are the defects associated with hypoplastic left heart syndrome.
   d. These are the defects associated with transposition of the great vessels.
   Knowledge/Physiologic/Assessment

7. **Correct response: b**
   Extreme bradycardia is a cardinal symptom of digoxin toxicity.
   a, c, and d. These are not related to digoxin toxicity.
   Application/Physiologic/Assessment

8. **Correct response: b**
   Adequate weight for height demonstrates adequate nutritional intake and lack of edema.
   a. Elevated RBC count demonstrates polycythemia.
   c. Bradycardia probably indicates digoxin toxicity.
   d. Daily antibiotics are not indicated in CHF.
   Application/Health Promotion/ Evaluation

9. **Correct response: b**
   Rheumatic fever (RF) results from improperly treated group A beta-hemolytic streptococcal infections, usually pharyngitis.

a. Not all sore throats are streptococcal.
c. Prophylactic antibiotics are given to children with cardiac disease to prevent carditis.
d. Initial prevention is not possible once the child has RF; however, the child will be treated to prevent recurrence of streptococcal infections.

Analysis/Health Promotion/Planning

10. *Correct response: a*
Sydenham's chorea is a self-limiting problem.
b, c, and d. All are characteristic of Sydenham's chorea.

Analysis/Physiologic/Implementation

Genitourinary Dysfunction

14

I. Essential concepts: renal system structures and function

A. Development

1. Kidney development begins during the first few weeks of gestation but is not complete until the end of the first year after birth.

2. Infants are unable to excrete water at the same rate as older children and adults; glomerular filtration and absorption do not reach adult capabilities until between ages 1 and 2 years.

3. Newborns are more prone to develop severe acidosis.

4. Sodium excretion is also reduced during infancy, and the kidneys are less adaptable to sodium deficiency or excess.

B. Function

1. The kidney's functional unit, the nephron, is composed of:

    a. Glomeruli, which filter water and solutes from blood

    b. Tubules, which reabsorb needed substances (water, protein, electrolytes, glucose, amino acids) from filtrate and allow unneeded substances to leave the body in urine

2. Kidney functions include:

    a. Maintaining body fluid volume and composition by responding appropriately to alterations in internal environment caused by variations in dietary intake and external losses of water and solutes

    b. Secreting hormones, such as erythropoietic stimulating factor (ESF), which stimulates production of red blood cells (RBCs), and renin, which stimulates production of angiotensin, causing arteriolar constriction and blood pressure elevation and aldosterone

3. Urine is formed in the nephron, then passes into the renal pelvis, through the ureter, into the bladder, and out of the body through the urethra.

II. Renal system overview

A. Assessment

1. Health history findings that suggest renal dysfunction include:

    a. Neonate: poor feeding, failure to thrive, frequent urination, crying on urination, dehydration, convulsions, fever

    b. Infant: same as neonate, plus persistent diaper rash, foul-smelling urine, straining on urination

    c. Older children: poor appetite, vomiting, excessive thirst, enuresis, incontinence, frequent urination, urgency, dysuria, bloody urine, foul-smelling urine, fatigue, fever, and flank, abdominal, or back pain

    d. Family history: renal disease, hypertension, and other problems related to renal dysfunction

2. Physical assessment findings may include:

    a. Abnormal rate and depth of respiration

    b. Hypertension

    c. Fever

    d. Growth retardation

    e. Signs of circulatory congestion: peripheral cyanosis, slow capillary refill time, pallor, and peripheral edema

    f. Abdominal distention

    g. Early signs of uremic encephalopathy: lethargy, poor concentration, confusion

    h. Signs of congenital anomalies, such as hypospadias, epispadias, ear abnormalities (ears and kidneys form at the same time in utero), prominent epicanthal folds, beaklike nose, and small chin

B.   **Laboratory studies and diagnostic tests**

    1. Urinalysis is the most valuable laboratory test for determining renal function (Table 14-1).

    2. **Blood urea nitrogen (BUN) and creatinine are common blood tests for assessing renal function:**

        a. BUN represents a gross index of glomerular filtration rate; impaired renal function and rapid protein catabolism result in elevated BUN levels.

        b. Creatinine is a by-product of energy metabolism. As long as muscle mass remains constant, creatinine levels are constant; renal disorders reducing creatinine excretion result in increased serum creatinine levels.

        c. Creatinine generally is a more sensitive indicator of acute renal failure than is BUN.

    3. Tests performed to identify anatomic abnormalities that contribute to developing infection may include:

TABLE 14-1.
Routine Urinalysis (UA) and Related Tests: Normal Values

GENERAL CHARACTERISTICS AND MEASUREMENTS	CHEMICAL DETERMINATIONS	MICROSCOPIC EXAMINATION OF SEDIMENT
Color: pale yellow to amber	Glucose: negative	Casts: negative (occasional hyaline casts)
Turbidity: clear to slightly hazy	Ketones: negative	
Specific gravity: 1.015–1.025 with a normal fluid intake	Blood: negative	Red blood cells: negative or rare
	Protein: negative	White blood cells: negative or rare
pH: 4.5–8.0: average person has a pH of about 5 or 6	Bilirubin: negative	Epithelial cells: few
	Urobilogen: 0.1–1.0	
	Nitrate for bacteria: negative	
	Leukocyte esterase: negative	

(Fischbach, F. [1996]. Manual of Laboratory and Diagnostic Tests, 5th ed. Philadelphia: Lippincott-Raven Publishers)

a. Ultrasonography: nonradiographic, noninvasive examination of the urinary tract using ultrasonic technology

b. Voiding cystourethrography: serial x-rays of the bladder and urethra after intravesicular infusion of an iodine-bound contrast medium

c. Intravenous pyelography (IVP): intravenous injection of a radiopaque contrast medium followed by x-ray imaging of the kidneys and ureters as the contrast agent passes through them

d. Cystoscopy: evaluation of the urinary tract using direct visualization via a metal tube or flexible sheath and fiber optic technology

C. Psychosocial implications

1. Infants: After threatening procedures, the infant needs comforting and acceptance by family members to promote the development of a positive body image.

2. Toddlers: Problems of immobilization frustrate the toddler's drive for independence. Allowing the toddler to participate in care, as appropriate, may be helpful.

3. Preschoolers: Body image awareness is heightened, and the child's natural curiosity about the body may be stimulated by physical examinations. The child's rich fantasy life can contribute to fear of the simplest procedures; castration fears also are prominent at this age and may be heightened by procedures related to genitourinary problems.

4. Schoolagers: Appearing different from peers is extremely anxiety producing, as are prohibitions on diet, sports, and other activities that focus on the child's differences from peers.

5. Adolescents: Because of the increased need for independence by adolescents, the enforced dependence imposed by rigorous therapeutic regimens can increase feelings of resentment and rebelliousness. Body image and sexuality concerns may also be heightened because of genitourinary diagnoses, procedures, and treatment.

III. Urinary tract infections (UTIs)

A. Description: inflammation, usually of bacterial origin, of the urethra (urethritis), bladder (cystitis), ureters (ureteritis), or kidneys (pyelonephritis).

B. Etiology and incidence

1. *Escherichia coli* **and other gram-negative organisms account for most UTIs.**

2. Other pathogens causing UTIs include *Proteus, Pseudomonas, Klebsiella, Staphylococcus aureus, Haemophilus,* and coagulase-negative staphylococcus.

3. In the neonate, the urinary tract may be infected via the blood-

stream; in older children bacteria ascends the urethra, creating an increased incidence in females.

4. Contributing factors include:
    a. Urinary stasis
    b. Urinary reflux
    c. Poor perineal hygiene
    d. Constipation
    e. Pregnancy
    f. Noncircumcision
    g. Indwelling catheter placement
    h. Antimicrobial agents that alter normal urinary tract flora
    i. Tight clothes or diapers
    j. Bubble baths
    k. Local inflammation (*e.g.*, from vaginitis), which increases the risk of ascending infection
    l. Sexual intercourse; improper use of diaphragm
5. Peak incidence occurs between 2 and 6 years, with increased incidence also noted in adolescents who are sexually active.
6. **Females have a 10 to 30 times greater risk of developing UTIs than males (except in neonates) because of their shorter urethral structure, which provides a quick pathway for organisms.**

C. Pathophysiology and management
    1. Inflammation usually is confined to the lower urinary tract in uncomplicated UTI. Recurrent cystitis, however, may produce anatomic changes in the ureter that lead to vesicoureteral valve incompetence and resultant urine reflux, which provide organisms with access to the upper urinary tract.
    2. Pyelonephritis usually results from an ascending infection from the lower urinary tract and can lead to acute and chronic inflammatory changes in the pelvis and medulla, with scarring and loss of renal tissue.
    3. Recurrent or chronic infection results in increased fibrotic tissue and kidney contraction.
    4. Management, for the most part, consists of administering medication to treat infection.

D. Clinical assessment findings
    1. Characteristics vary with age and location of infection.
    2. Infants may exhibit:
        a. Fever
        b. Weight loss
        c. Failure to thrive (FTT)
        d. Vomiting
        e. Diarrhea
    3. In older children, symptoms may include:

a. Lower UTIs: dysuria, frequency, urgency, incontinence, foul-smelling urine, abdominal pain, and possibly hematuria

b. Pyelonephritis: fever, chills, flank pain, costovertebral abdominal (CVA) tenderness

4. About 40% of UTIs are asymptomatic.

E. **Diagnostic assessment findings**

1. Urinalysis may disclose hematuria, proteinuria, and pyuria. Urine may have a foul odor and appear cloudy with strands of mucus.

2. Diagnosis is confirmed by detection of bacteria in urine culture.

F. **Nursing diagnoses**

1. Risk for altered body temperature
2. Risk for infection
3. Pain
4. Altered patterns of urinary elimination
5. Impaired tissue integrity
6. Knowledge deficit
7. Potential for altered growth and development
8. Potential for altered family processes

G. **Planning and implementation**

1. Assess urinary status by observing the appearance and odor of urine, and noting signs and symptoms such as frequency, burning, enuresis, urinary retention, or flank pain.

2. Administer prescribed medications, which may include:

a. Antibiotic agents, such as amoxicillin and sulfamethoxazole-trimethoprim, to treat current disease or to provide prophylaxis

b. Urinary antiseptic agents such as nitrofurantoin

c. Aminoglycoside antibiotics such as gentamicin or tobramycin to treat nosocomial infections

d. Cefaclor to treat resistant UTIs

3. Help prevent infection by maintaining sterile technique when performing urinary catheterization.

4. Provide comfort measures: promote rest; administer analgesics as needed and antipyretics as prescribed; and encourage increased fluid intake to reduce fever and dilute urine.

5. Provide emotional support to all family members and explain all tests and treatments.

6. Provide child and family teaching:

a. Review medication instructions (dosage, administration, and side effects).

b. Explain surgical correction of anatomic abnormalities, if necessary, to prevent recurrent disease.

c. Point out the need for performing follow-up cultures, typically at monthly intervals for 3 months, then at 3-month intervals for the next 6 months.

       d.   Detail preventive measures, such as providing good perineal hygiene (*e.g.*, cleaning a girl from the urethra back toward the anus); avoiding irritants such as bubble bath and tight clothing; wearing cotton underwear instead of synthetics such as nylon; maintaining adequate fluid intake; voiding regularly and completely emptying the bladder with each urination; and maintaining acidic urine by drinking beverages such as cranberry juice.

       e.   Emphasize the importance of voiding both before and after sexual intercourse (for the sexually active adolescent).

H.   Evaluation

    1.   The child voids in a normal pattern and remains asymptomatic.

    2.   Parents verbalize knowledge of rest, fluid intake, medications, prevention of recurrence, and follow-up care, including the schedule for obtaining urine specimens.

IV. Vesicoureteral reflux (VUR)

A.   Description: the backward flow of urine in the urinary tract when voiding.

B.   Etiology and incidence

    1.   Primary reflux results from congenital abnormalities in insertion of ureters into the bladder.

    2.   Secondary reflux results from infection and ureterovesicular junction incompetency related to edema; it may also be related to neurogenic bladder or result from progressive dilation of ureters following surgical urinary diversion.

    3.   The prevalence of VUR in healthy children is estimated at less than 1%; however, it is found in 29% to 50% of children following UTIs and is the most common radiographic abnormality associated with UTIs in children.

    4.   Development of VUR may in part be genetic; siblings are 10 times more likely to develop it than other children.

C.   Pathophysiology and management

    1.   VUR occurs when urine flows from the bladder back into the ureters and the renal pelvis, usually a result of an incompetent valvular mechanism at the ureterovesicular junction.

    2.   VUR is graded according to the degree of reflux:

       a.   Grade I: reflux into lower ureter only

       b.   Grade II: ureteral and pelvic filling without calyceal dilation

       c.   Grade III: ureteral and pelvic filling with mild calyceal dilation

       d.   Grade IV: marked distention of pelvis, calyces, and ureter

        e.   Grade V: massive reflux associated with severe hydro-nephrosis
- 3. VUR is a major cause of renal damage; refluxed urine ascending into the collecting tubules of nephrons gives microorganisms access to the renal parenchyma, initiating renal scarring.
- 4. If the amount of refluxed urine is large, the child feels an urge to void shortly after having voided. If the amount is small, it may remain in the bladder, causing urinary stasis and predisposing the child to infection.

D. Clinical assessment findings
1. Dysuria
2. Urinary frequency, urgency, and hesitancy
3. Urine retention
4. Cloudy, dark, or blood-tinged urine

E. Diagnostic assessment findings
1. Urinalysis may reveal RBCs or pyuria.
2. Structural abnormalities may be detected by IVP, voiding cystourethrography, and cystoscopy.

F. Nursing diagnoses
1. Altered urinary elimination
2. Urinary retention
3. Pain
4. Potential for infection
5. Knowledge deficit
6. Altered family processes
7. Risk for injury (at surgical site)

G. Planning and implementation
1. Administer or teach parents to administer prescribed medications, such as continuous low-dose antibiotics, usually given as nitrofurantoin or trimethoprim-sulfamethoxazole.
2. Instruct the child to take a liberal amount of fluids to dilute urine and to develop a regular (3-hour) voiding plan.
3. Prevent and relieve constipation with high-fiber diet to facilitate muscular relaxation, thereby helping to reduce residual urine.
4. Provide support to the family by answering questions and providing information about diagnosis, tests, and treatments. As appropriate, explain that antireflux surgery, involving reimplantation of ureters, is indicated to prevent renal damage secondary to recurrent infections.
5. Provide preoperative and postoperative care after antireflux surgery:
    a.   Monitor quantity and quality of urine output.
    b.   Observe and protect urinary drainage tubes (*e.g.*, indwelling catheter, suprapubic catheter, ureteral stents).

   c. Administer analgesics for pain and antispasmodics for bladder spasms, as prescribed.

   d. Provide routine postoperative care (*e.g.*, dressing changes, vital signs monitoring, progressive diet, ambulation).

  6. Provide child and family teaching, covering:

   a. Medications (dosage, administration, and side effects)

   b. **Discuss preventive measures, such as practicing good perineal hygiene (*e.g.*, cleaning a girl from the urethra back toward the anus); avoiding irritants such as bubble bath and tight clothing; wearing cotton underwear instead of synthetic fabrics such as nylon; maintaining adequate fluid intake; voiding regularly and completely emptying the bladder with each urination; maintaining acidic urine by drinking beverages such as cranberry juice.**

   c. **Note the importance of voiding both before and after sexual intercourse (for the sexually active adolescent).**

 H. Evaluation

  1. The child voids in a normal pattern and is asymptomatic.

  2. Parents verbalize a knowledge of rest, fluid intake, medications, prevention of recurrence, and follow-up care, including scheduled intervals for obtaining urine specimens.

V. Nephrotic syndrome

 A. **Description: a symptom complex characterized by proteinuria, hypoalbuminemia, hyperlipidemia, altered immunity, and edema; it is of idiopathic origin 95% of the time; prognosis usually is good for the most common type of nephrotic syndrome, which is self-limiting and usually responds to steroidal therapy.**

 B. Etiology and incidence

  1. **Minimal change nephrotic syndrome (MCNS) accounts for 80% of all cases in children ages 2 to 6 years. It is idiopathic in origin.**

  2. Secondary nephrotic syndrome usually occurs after glomerular damage of known or presumed etiology (systemic lupus erythematosus, diabetes mellitus, sickle cell disease).

  3. Congenital nephrotic syndrome (Finnish-type) is caused by an autosomal recessive gene. This rare disorder does not respond to usual therapy and the infant usually dies in the first or second year of life.

  4. Incidence is more common in boys than in girls.

 C. Pathophysiology and management

  1. The pathogenesis in MCNS is not clear, but there is increased permeability to protein, exceeding 2 g/d.

2. Proteins leak through the glomerular membrane resulting in protein, especially albumin, in the urine.
3. Once the albumin is lost, colloidal osmotic pressure decreases, permitting fluid to escape from the intravascular spaces to the interstitial spaces.
4. The volume decrease stimulates antidiuretic hormone (ADH) to reabsorb water.

D. **Clinical assessment findings**

1. **Characteristic findings include periorbital, pedal and pretibial edema to generalized edema (anasarca), weight increase, ascites, pleural effusion, decreased urine output, pallor, anorexia, fatigue, abdominal pain, and diarrhea. With marked edema, the child may appear pale and have respiratory distress.**
2. Blood pressure may be normal or slightly decreased.
3. **Children are more prone to infection from altered immunity.**

E. **Diagnostic assessment findings**

1. Urinalysis shows marked proteinuria, hyaline casts, few RBCs, and high urine specific gravity.
2. Serum protein level is markedly decreased, especially albumin level.
3. Renal biopsy may be performed.

F. **Nursing diagnoses**

1. Risk for infection
2. Altered nutrition: less than body requirements
3. Risk for fluid volume deficit
4. Impaired tissue integrity
5. Activity intolerance
6. Body image disturbance
7. Altered family processes
8. Altered growth and development
9. Knowledge deficit

G. **Planning and implementation**

1. Assess for fluid volume deficit by monitoring for increased edema and by measuring abdominal girth, weight, intake and output (I&O), blood pressure, and pulse rate. Test urine for protein and specific gravity.
2. **Monitor for signs of infection, and take precautions to prevent infection (the child is susceptible to secondary infection because immunoglobulin is lost in the urine).**
3. Administer treatment as prescribed: diuretics and sodium restriction to manage edema; possibly, plasma expanders, such as

salt-poor albumin, to manage severe edema; corticosteroids as the treatment of choice; and, in some cases, immunosuppressant therapy.

4. Administer prescribed medications, which may include:

    a. **Prednisone at a dose of 2 mg/kg/d to reduce proteinuria.**

    b. Immunosuppressant therapy (usually cyclophosphamide) for the child who fails to respond to steroids.

    c. Spironolactone in combination with hydrochlorothiazide to treat severe edema.

    d. A broad-spectrum antimicrobial agent to reduce the risk of infection.

5. Promote skin integrity by checking areas of edema for skin breakdown, ensuring frequent position changes, using scrotal supports for boys, and providing good skin care.

6. Maintain or improve nutritional status by providing a high-protein, high-calorie diet without added salt. Offer small frequent meals of preferred foods in a pleasant atmosphere.

7. Conserve the child's energy by enforcing bed rest and encouraging quiet activities.

8. Help improve the child's self-concept by providing positive feedback, emphasizing strengths, and encouraging social interaction and pursuit of interests.

9. Support the family by answering questions and providing information on diagnosis, tests, and treatment.

10. Provide child and family teaching, covering:

    a. Signs and symptoms of relapse to watch for and report

    b. Urine testing for albumin

    c. Medications (dosage schedule, administration techniques, and side effects)

    d. Special dietary instructions

    e. Infection prevention measures

    f. Skin care

H. Evaluation

1. The child exhibits reduced edema and ascites, absence of skin breakdown and infection, and urine output within acceptable range.

2. Parents verbalize knowledge of the disorder, treatments, medications, home monitoring, diet instructions, and follow-up care.

3. The child resumes or maintains age-appropriate development and participates in age-appropriate activities as tolerated.

VI. Acute glomerulonephritis (AGN)

A. Description: an immune complex disease that results from immune injury, once thought to be secondary to streptococcus, now

other organisms are involved, including pneumococci and viruses. Recovery occurs in about 95% of cases.

B. Etiology and incidence

1. **Acute poststreptococcal glomerulonephritis (APSGN) is the most common form.**
2. APSGN can occur at any age but is usually seen in schoolagers, with peak age 6 to 7 years.
3. The incidence in males is twice that of females.
4. **Most streptococcal infections do not cause AGN. A latent period of 10 to 14 days occurs between the infection, usually of the skin or upper respiratory tract, and the onset of clinical manifestations.**

C. Pathophysiology and management

1. Antibodies interact with antigens that remain in the glomeruli, leading to immune complex formation and tissue injury, filtration decreases, and excretion of less sodium and water.
2. High blood pressure, edema, and heart failure may result.
3. Management usually includes medications to control hypertension, reduce fluid overload, and treat infection and circulatory overload; dialysis in severe AGN or with heart failure; and increased caloric intake to decrease protein breakdown. The occurrence of diuresis indicates beginning resolution and recovery.

D. Clinical assessment findings

1. **Characteristic findings include high blood pressure, pallor, irritability, fatigue, lethargy, periorbital and generalized edema, weight gain, electrolyte imbalance, oliguria and hematuria (urine is brown—cola or tea colored—and cloudy), costovertebral tenderness (CVA), and anorexia.**
2. Child or parents may report history of infection about 10 to 14 days before onset of symptoms.

E. Diagnostic assessment findings

1. Urinalysis: urine contains RBCs, casts, WBCs, and protein. Diuresis indicates resolution; child usually recovers in 2 weeks.
2. Serum chemistry values reveal elevated BUN and creatinine levels; erythrocyte sedimentation rate (ESR) is elevated, and antistreptolysin-O (ASO) titer is elevated if child was exposed to streptococci.
3. Renal biopsy may be performed.

F. Nursing diagnoses

1. Fluid volume excess
2. Risk for infection
3. Altered nutrition: less than body requirements
4. Diversional activity deficit

5. Altered family processes
6. Knowledge deficit
7. Risk for impaired skin integrity

G.   Planning and implementation

1. Assess fluid status by monitoring I&O, taking and recording daily weights, and observing for edema.
2. Ensure early detection of complications by closely monitoring blood pressure and respiratory rate.
3. Administer medications, as prescribed, for example:
   a. For severe hypertension: intravenous (IV) diazoxide (Hyperstat) and furosemide (Lasix)
   b. For moderate hypertension: methyldopa or hydralazine, usually in conjunction with reserpine or furosemide
   c. For mild hypertension: oral hydrochlorothiazide (Hydrodiuril)
   d. Diuretics and sodium and fluid restrictions to manage fluid overload
   e. Antibiotics to treat existing streptococcal infection
   f. Digitalis to combat circulatory overload
4. Administer other treatments as prescribed, for example:
   a. Dialysis to manage severe AGN or heart failure
   b. Increase caloric intake to decrease protein breakdown.
5. Stimulate the child by providing quiet, ambulatory play activities.
6. Maintain adequate caloric intake and nutrition by planning meals around the child's dietary preferences and by serving meals in a pleasant atmosphere.
7. Impose sodium, potassium, or fluid restrictions, as prescribed.
8. Support the child and parents by explaining and answering questions about diagnosis, treatment, and home care.
9. Refer the child and family to a community health nurse for home visits, as needed, to help them adjust to home management.
10. Provide child and family teaching, covering:
    a. The need for medical evaluation and tissue culture of all sore throats
    b. Home care measures, including urine testing, blood pressure monitoring, activity and diet instructions, infection-prevention measures, and signs and symptoms of potential complications to watch for and report (the child will require monthly urinalysis and blood pressure monitoring for 6 months and then every 3 to 6 months until he or she has been symptom-free for 1 year)
    c. Medications (dosage, administration, and side effects)

    d. The possible need for peritoneal dialysis or hemodialysis if renal failure occurs

H. **Evaluation**

  1. The child demonstrates improved urine output, maintains weight, adheres to dietary restrictions, and is free from life-threatening complications.

  2. Parents verbalize knowledge of treatment, home care, and follow-up.

VII. Hypospadias

A. **Description: a condition in which the urethral opening is located below the glans penis or anywhere along the ventral surface (underside) of the penile shaft.**

B. **Etiology and incidence**

  1. Occurs in approximately 1 of 500 newborns.

  2. Testes are undescended in approximately 10% of boys with hypospadias and inguinal hernias are common.

  3. In very mild cases, the meatus is just below the tip; in the most severe cases, the meatus is located on the perineum between the halves of the scrotum.

  4. Chordee (ventral curve of the penis) results from the replacement of normal skin with a fibrotic band and usually accompanies more severe forms of hypospadias.

C. **Pathophysiology and management**

  1. The abnormality results from a failure of the urethral folds to fuse completely over the urethral groove.

  2. The ventral foreskin is lacking, and the distal portion gives an appearance of a hood.

  3. Surgical repair is performed to improve the child's ability to stand when urinating; to improve the appearance of the penis; and to preserve sexual adequacy.

D. **Clinical assessment findings**

  1. Inappropriate placement of meatus should be evident at birth.

  2. Severe hypospadias with undescended testes must be differentiated from ambiguous genitalia.

E. **Diagnostic assessment findings: none, unless ambiguous genitalia need to be ruled out or in cases when other abnormalities are suspected.**

F. **Nursing diagnoses**

  1. Body image disturbance

  2. Altered urinary elimination

  3. Pain (postoperatively)

  4. Risk for infection (postoperatively)

G.   Planning and implementation

1.   Inform parents that early recognition is important so that circumcision is avoided; the foreskin is used for the surgical repair.

2.   Allow parents to verbalize their feelings about the child's structural problem.

3.   Prepare parents and child for the expected surgical procedures and expected cosmetic result; the parents and child may feel great disappointment about this physical imperfection.

4.   Monitor I&O and urinary pattern; encourage fluids; maintain patency and observe infection-prevention measures if child is catheterized.

5.   Prepare parents and child for urinary diversion, if necessary, while new meatus is being constructed.

6.   Teach parents how to care for an indwelling catheter if needed.

H.   Evaluation

1.   Parents and child verbalize an understanding of the disorder and the expected results of surgery.

2.   Parents and child verbalize feelings regarding the disorder.

3.   The child remains free of infection and other complications.

Bibliography

Belkengren, R.P. and Sapala, S. (1993). Pediatric management problems: Urinary tract infection. *Pediatric Nursing, 19,* 184.

Betz, C.L., Hunsberger, M.M., and Wright, S. (1994). *Family Centered Nursing Care of Children,* 2nd ed. Philadelphia: W.B. Saunders.

Castiglia, P.T. and Harbin, R.B. (1993). *Child Health Care: Process and Practice.* Philadelphia: J.B. Lippincott.

Jackson, D.B. and Saunders, R.B. (1993). *Child Health Nursing: A Comprehensive Approach to the Care of Children and Their Families.* Philadelphia: J.B. Lippincott.

Lewy, J.E. (1990). Nephrology, fluids and electrolytes. In Behrman, R.E. and Kliegman, R. (Eds). *Nelson Essentials of Pediatrics.* Philadelphia: W.B. Saunders.

Sizer, F. and Whitney, E. (1994). *Nutrition Concepts and Controversies,* 6th ed. Minneapolis/St. Paul: West Publishing.

Walker, R.D. (1994). Vesicoureteral reflux update: Effect of prospective studies on current management. *Urology, 43,* 270.

Wong, D.L. (1993). *Whaley and Wong's Essentials of Pediatric Nursing,* 4th ed. St. Louis: C.V. Mosby.

Wong, D. L. (1995). *Whaley and Wong's Nursing care of Infants and Children,* 5th ed. St. Louis: C.V. Mosby.

STUDY QUESTIONS

1. Procedures related to genitourinary problems are especially stressful for which age group?
   a. Infants
   b. Toddlers
   c. Preshoolers
   d. Schoolagers

2. Factors that contribute to the development of urinary tract infections (UTIs) include all of the following except:
   a. Urinary stasis
   b. Circumcision
   c. Bubble baths
   d. Indwelling catheters

3. Characteristics of cystitis include:
   a. High fever
   b. Flank pain
   c. Costovertebral tenderness
   d. Dysuria

4. Preventive teaching for UTIs includes:
   a. Wiping back to front
   b. Wearing nylon underwear
   c. Avoiding urinating before intercourse
   d. Drinking acidic juices

5. Secondary vesicoureteral reflux (VUR) usually results from:
   a. Congenital defects
   b. Infection
   c. Acidic urine
   d. Hydronephrosis

6. Which of the following organisms is the most common cause of UTI in children?
   a. *Staphylococcus*
   b. *Klebsiella*
   c. *Pseudomonas*
   d. *Escherichia coli*

7. Which of the following signs and symptoms are characteristic of minimal change nephrotic syndrome?
   a. Gross hematuria, proteinuria, fever
   b. Hypertension, edema, hematuria
   c. Poor appetite, proteinuria, edema
   d. Hypertension, edema, proteinuria

8. For a child with recurring nephrotic syndrome, which of the following areas of potential disturbance should be a prime consideration when planning ongoing nursing care?
   a. Muscle coordination
   b. Sexual maturation
   c. Intellectual development
   d. Body image

9. When teaching parents about known antecedent infections in acute glomerulonephritis, which of the following should the nurse cover?
   a. Herpes simplex
   b. Scabies
   c. Varicella
   d. Impetigo

ANSWER KEY

1. **Correct response: c**
   Preschoolers have more fears in general owing to their fantasies and they also have castration fears, which would make genitourinary procedures extremely stressful for them.
   a, b, and d. Genitourinary procedures do not create greater stress in these age groups.
   Analysis/Psychosocial/Planning

2. **Correct response: b**
   Noncircumcised children are at greater risk for UTIs if they are not properly cleaned.
   a. Urinary stasis creates a medium for growth.
   c. Bubble baths cause irritation.
   d. Indwelling catheters create a route for organisms.
   Comprehension/Physiologic/Evaluation

3. **Correct response: d**
   Dysuria is a symptom of a lower urinary tract infection.
   a, b, and c. All are symptoms of pyelonephritis, which is an upper urinary tract infection.
   Comprehension/Physiologic/Assessment

4. **Correct response: d**
   Drinking acidic juices, such as cranberry juice, helps keep the urine at its desired acid pH and decreases the chance of infection.
   a. The client should wipe from front to back.
   b. The client should wear cotton underwear.
   c. The client should void before intercourse.
   Application/Health Promotion/Implementation

5. **Correct response: b**
   Infection is the most common cause of secondary VUR.
   a. Congenital defects cause primary VUR.

   c. Acidic urine is normal and helps to prevent infection.
   d. Hydronephrosis may result from VUR.
   Knowledge/Physiologic/NA

6. **Correct response: d**
   This is the most common organism associated with UTI.
   a, b, and c. Each of these may cause UTIs, but none is the most common cause.
   Knowledge/Physiologic/Assessment

7. **Correct response: c**
   Clinical manifestations of nephrotic syndrome include loss of appetite due to edema of intestinal mucosa, proteinuria, and edema.
   a. Gross hematuria is not associated with nephrotic syndrome. Fever would occur only if infection also existed.
   b. Hypertension and hematuria are associated with glomerulonephritis.
   d. Hypertension is associated with glomerulonephritis.
   Analysis/Physiologic/Assessment

8. **Correct response: d**
   Potential self-concept and body image disturbances related to changes in appearance and social isolation should be considered.
   a. Muscle coordination is not affected.
   b. Sexual maturation is not affected.
   c. Intellectual function is not affected.
   Application/Psychosocial/Planning

9. **Correct response: d**
   Impetigo, a bacterial infection of the skin, may be caused by streptococci and may precede acute glomerulonephritis.
   a, b, and c. None of these has been associated with acute glomerulonephritis.
   Knowledge/Physiologic/Planning

Musculoskeletal and Neuromuscular Dysfunction

I. Essential concepts: musculoskeletal structures and function

A. Development

1. The musculoskeletal system arises from the embryonic meso-
dermal layer, which appears during the second week of gestation.

2. By the eighth week of gestation, all major bones are present in
the cartilaginous skeleton.

3. Bone formation occurs by ossification, which begins as early as
the eighth week of gestation and continues throughout gestation and childhood.

4. Bone growth occurs in two dimensions: diameter and length.
Growth in length occurs at the epiphyseal plate, a vascular area
of active cell division. These cells are highly sensitive to the influence of growth hormone, estrogen, and testosterone.

5. Sometime in adolescence the epiphyseal plate turns to bone
and growth stops.

B. Function

1. Several significant differences in musculoskeletal function between children and adults have important implications for
nursing care.

2. The epiphyseal plate in children represents an area of bone
weakness that is susceptible to injury through fracture, crush-
ing, or slippage. Damage to the epiphyseal plate can disrupt
bone growth.

3. Because a child is still growing, some bony deformities due to
injury can be remodeled or straightened over time; conversely,
this can also cause some deformities to progress with growth.

4. Because a child's bones are more plastic than an adult's, more
force is required to fracture a bone and specific forces may produce different types of fractures.

5. A child's bones generally heal much faster than those of an
adult, often greatly reducing the time required for immobilization after injury.

II. Musculoskeletal system overview
A. Assessment
1. The complete health history should focus on:
    a. Trauma
    b. Delayed walking or other motor developmental abnormalities
    c. Pain
    d. Structural abnormalities (*e.g.*, clubfoot, hip dysplasia, leg length discrepancy, scoliosis)
    e. Any physical limitation or lifestyle alterations imposed by the problem
    f. Mobility aids used
2. Physical assessment should include examination of:
    a. Posture and gait
    b. Structural abnormalities, including asymmetric limb lengths and spinal deformities
    c. Range of motion in all joints
    d. Muscle symmetry, mass, tone, and strength
    e. Color, temperature, sensation, motion, pain, pulses, capillary filling, and edema of each extremity

B. Laboratory studies and diagnostic tests
1. Radiologic and other imaging studies to assess bones and joints include:
    a. Radiographs (the most common study to assess injury and healing)
    b. Computed tomographic (CT) scan
    c. Bone scan
2. Other important procedures include:
    a. Arthrography
    b. Arthroscopy
    c. Joint aspiration
    d. Electromyography (EMG)

C. Psychosocial implications
1. Treatment for musculoskeletal problems often requires immobilization (casts, traction, body frames), which can be frightening and painful. The impact on the child depends in large part on the child's developmental level.
2. Play, social interaction, and self-care help the immobilized child gain self-esteem and independence and promote normal growth and development.

III. Immobilization
A. Description: therapeutic restriction of motion for a specified time at a site of disrupted muscle or bone integrity.

B. **Etiology and incidence**
1. A child may be immobilized as part of the treatment designed to keep body structures at physiologic rest and in proper alignment or as the result of physical limitations of disease or disability.
2. Common precursors to immobility include:
    a. Congenital defects
    b. Degenerative neurologic disorders
    c. Integumentary disorders
    d. Musculoskeletal trauma
    e. Imposed bed rest to assist healing and restoration
    f. Mechanical restraint as part of therapy
C. **Pathophysiology and management**
1. Restricted movement can cause functional and metabolic responses in most body systems.
2. Most of the changes arise from decreased muscle strength and mass, decreased metabolism, and bone demineralization.
3. Some problems are primary and produce a direct effect (bone demineralization leading to osteoporosis); some are secondary and indirect (pathologic fractures).
4. Physical activity is essential for growth and development; therefore, immobilization may have a serious psychologic effect on children.
D. **Clinical assessment findings**
1. Joint contracture and pain
2. Muscular atony and weakness
3. Fatigue
4. Diminished reflexes
5. Delayed healing
6. Orthostatic hypotension
7. Signs and symptoms of thrombus formation
8. Shallow respirations
9. Anorexia and constipation
10. Renal calculi
11. Urinary incontinence or signs of urinary infection
12. Skin breakdown and pressure ulcers
13. Sensory changes
E. **Diagnostic assessment findings**
1. Hypercalcemia
2. Elevated urinary nitrogen level
3. Anemia
F. **Nursing diagnoses**
1. Impaired mobility
2. Risk for injury

3. Risk for infection
4. Activity intolerance
5. Anxiety
6. Ineffective breathing pattern
7. Decreased cardiac output
8. Constipation
9. Risk for fluid volume deficit
10. Altered growth and development
11. Knowledge deficit
12. Altered nutrition: less or more than body requirements
13. Altered role performance
14. Sensory and perceptual alterations
15. Impaired skin integrity
16. Sleep pattern disturbance
17. Social isolation
18. Altered urinary elimination

G. Planning and implementation
1. Protect skin integrity by turning the child frequently and inspecting for early signs of breakdown.
2. Promote adequate hydration by offering child's favorite juices.
3. Promote good nutrition by offering high-protein, high-calorie foods in small, frequent amounts in a pleasant atmosphere.
4. Promote natural bowel elimination by encouraging fluids and a high-fiber diet. Administer stool softeners as prescribed.
5. Promote urinary elimination by encouraging fluids, monitoring intake and output (I&O), and by checking for bladder distention.
6. Promote as much normal activity as possible and provide age-appropriate diversions.
7. Prevent respiratory complications by keeping the child well hydrated, changing child's position frequently, and encouraging deep-breathing exercises.
8. Help maintain adequate cardiac output by changing the child's position frequently and by providing active and passive range-of-motion (ROM) exercises.
9. Protect the child from injury by moving and positioning the child carefully, and by monitoring physical activities closely; syncope and falling may result if child resumes normal activities too quickly.
10. Help prevent urinary tract infections by keeping the child well hydrated; promoting frequent voiding; providing acid-ash foods such as cereals, fish, poultry, cranberry or apple juice, and meats; limiting calcium intake.
11. Prevent contractures by maintaining proper body alignment and providing ROM exercises.

12. Promote normal growth and development by encouraging self-care and providing regular social contact and age-appropriate activities.
13. Promote effective coping by encouraging verbaization, and by providing play therapy and necessary teaching of procedures and treatments.
14. Administer prescribed medications, which may include:
    a. Antibiotics to treat infection
    b. Diuretics to remove high levels of calcium
    c. Calcium-mobilizing drugs
    d. Anticoagulants to prevent clot formation
    e. Stool softeners to prevent constipation
15. Explain to parents that the child (preschooler) may view immobilization as punishment. Encourage parents to listen for and correct any misconceptions that the child may have.
16. Provide child and family teaching, covering:
    a. The action and purpose of restraining devices, such as a cast or traction
    b. Home care: holding techniques, moving, feeding, care of restrictive devices, and signs and symptoms of complications (*e.g.*, increased temperature, pain or blood on voiding, difficulty breathing)

H. Evaluation
1. The child maintains normal skin integrity, elimination patterns, and respiratory patterns.
2. The child remains well hydrated and well nourished.
3. The child maintains age-appropriate autonomy, interacts with peers and family, and expresses fears and concerns.
4. The child remains free of injury.
5. Family members verbalize an understanding of the home care measures, signs and symptoms of complications, and follow-up care.

IV. Congenital hip dysplasia (CHD)
A. Description: congenital abnormalities of the hip joints, including subluxations and dislocations; types include preluxation, subluxation, and dislocation.
   1. **Of the types of congenital hip abnormalities, subluxation is the most common.**
B. Etiology and incidence
   1. The etiology of CHD is unknown but may result from the effect of maternal estrogen on the fetus causing relaxing of ligaments, from positioning in utero, or from genetic factors.
   2. Incidence is about 1 of 500 to 1 of 100 births.
   3. Occurs seven times more frequently in females than males.

4. CHD occurs 25 to 30 times more often in first-degree relatives than in the general population.
5. About 25% of cases involve both hips; when one hip is involved, it is usually the left.
6. CHD typically is seen with other problems such as neural tube disorders.

C. Pathophysiology and management
1. Preluxation (acetabular dysplasia): There is an apparent delay in acetabular development, but the femoral head remains in the acetabulum.
2. Subluxation: There is incomplete dislocation; the femoral head remains in contact with the acetabulum, but a stretched capsule and ligament tears cause the head of the femur to be partially displaced.
3. Dislocation: The femoral head loses contact with the acetabulum and is displaced posteriorly and superiorly over the fibrocartilaginous rim.
4. **Uncorrected subluxation or dislocation may lead to permanent disability.**
5. Treatment is initiated as soon as the diagnosis is made; it varies with the age of the child and the degree of dysplasia.
   a. Newborn to 6 months: The infant usually is placed in a *Pavlik harness*. This device centers the femoral head into the acetabulum in an attitude of flexion and deepens the acetabulum by pressure. The device is worn until the hip joint is clinically and radiographically stable. Usually by 3 to 6 months, the child may be transferred to a protective abduction brace.
   b. **Infants, 6 to 18 months: *Traction* is used for gradual reduction, followed by cast immobilization until the joint is stable. If soft tissue obstructs reduction, an *open reduction* is performed, followed by a spica cast for 4 to 6 months (Fig. 15-1); this is then replaced with an abduction splint.**
   c. Older child: Correction is difficult because secondary changes create complications. Surgical reduction is required. Successful reduction after 4 years is difficult; it is inadvisable after 6 years.

D. Clinical assessment findings
1. Characteristics vary with age.
2. **Newborn: Ortolani's sign, Barlow's sign, asymmetric gluteal folds, limited abduction of affected hip, Galeazzi's sign.**
3. **Older children: limp, Trendelenburg's sign.**

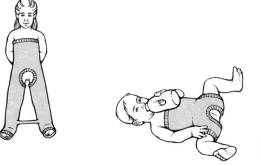

FIGURE 15-1.
Hip spica casts.

E. **Diagnostic assessment findings**
1. Radiographic examination does not yield reliable data until after ossification of the femoral head when the infant is between 3 and 6 months of age.
2. Ultrasonography may be helpful in the newborn.

F. **Nursing diagnoses (also see section III, F)**
1. Altered tissue perfusion
2. Risk for injury
3. Risk for impaired skin integrity
4. Pain
5. Altered growth and development
6. Altered family processes
7. Knowledge deficit

G. **Planning and implementation**

1. **Help prevent circulatory and neurologic impairment caused by cast or device as follows:**
   a. Monitor neurovascular status (color, temperature, capillary refill, sensation, mobility).
   b. Elevate casted extremities.
2. Help prevent skin breakdown as follows:
   a. Petal cast edges.
   b. Provide a sheepskin or alternate pressure mattress.
   c. Provide skin care.
   d. Change child's position frequently.
3. Prevent complications of immobility as follows:
   a. Assess for and report signs and symptoms of the complications of immobility (see section III, D).
   b. Ensure correct use of devices.
   c. Perform interventions suggested for the immobilized child (see section III, G).
4. Maintain cast integrity (when applicable) by promoting complete drying and by protecting the cast and rim.
5. Promote growth and development by encouraging self-care

and providing diversional activities appropriate for the child's age and condition.

6. Ensure comfort by administering pain medications as prescribed, by changing the child's position frequently, and by using pads and pillows for support.

7. Support the child's family by providing information on the child's defect and treatment plan and helping them modify clothing, supportive devices, and means of transportation.

8. Provide child and family teaching, as follows:
   a. Explain signs and symptoms of circulatory impairment and infection, as well as complications of immobilization, to watch for and report.

   b. **Demonstrate how to care for the cast and the child in the cast. Show how to use correct body mechanics when lifting the child, how to avoid using the abduction bar for moving the child, which measures to implement to prevent physical and developmental deficits, and how to keep the cast clean and dry (*e.g.*, tucking a disposable diaper beneath the entire perineal opening in the cast). Also point out the importance of restraining child when moving him or her.**

   c. Offer feeding tips and techniques for an infant or small child in a cast: positioning the child so thaf he or she feels safe; using pillows for support; cuddling the child in the arms; supporting the child in a "football" hold or fashioning a tilt table, depending on infant's size.

   d. Discuss planning family activities to include the child; a child confined in a cast or brace can be held and transported to areas of activity.

   e. Show parents ways to nurture the infant or young child through stroking, holding, and maintaining physical closeness.

H. Evaluation

1. The child's hip(s) remain in desired position with the corrective device in proper position.

2. The child remains free of complications from the device or from immobility (*e.g.*, skin breakdown or circulatory impairment).

3. The child and family adjust to coping with the limitations imposed by the device.

4. Family members verbalize an understanding of the child's defect, treatment plan, home care, and follow-up.

V. Cerebral palsy (CP)

A. **Description: a group of disabilities caused by injury or insult to the brain either before or during birth or in early infancy; the most common permanent disability in childhood.**

B. Etiology and incidence

 1. **Risk factors include prematurity, asphyxia, ischemia, perinatal trauma, congenital and perinatal infections, and perinatal metabolic problems such as hyperbilirubinemia and hypoglycemia.**

2. Infection, trauma, and tumors can cause CP in early infancy and some cases remain unexplained.

3. Estimated occurrence is 1.2 to 2 of every 1000 births.

C. Pathophysiology and management

1. Disabilities usually result from injury to the cerebellum, the basal ganglia, or the motor cortex.

2. CP is nonprogressive but may become more apparent as the child grows older.

3. It is difficult to establish the precise location of neurologic lesions because there is no typical pathologic picture. In some cases, the brain has gross malformations; in others, vascular occlusion, atrophy, loss of neurons, and degeneration may be evident.

4. Classification of CP

   a. **Spastic CP: most common, may involve one of both sides; hallmarks include hypertonicity with poor control of posture, balance, and coordinated movement; impairment of fine and gross motor skills; active attempts at motion increase abnormal postures and overflow of movement to other parts of the body.**

   b. Dyskinetic: abnormal involuntary movements that disappear in sleep and increase in stress; major manifestation is athetosis (wormlike movement), dyskinetic movement of mouth, drooling, dysarthria, and choreiform (jerky) movements.

   c. Ataxic: wide-based gait, rapid repetitive movements performed poorly, disintegration of movements of the upper extremities when the child reaches for objects.

   d. Mixed type: combination of spasticity and athetosis.

   e. Rigid, tremor, and atonic types: uncommon.

5. Although there is no cure, the child can be assisted to reach his or her highest potential. Therapeutic goals include:

   a. To establish locomotion, communication, and self-help

   b. To gain optimal appearance and integration of motor functions

   c. To correct associated defects as effectively as possible

   d. To provide educational opportunities based on the individual's needs and capabilities

6. Successful therapy relies on a multidisciplinary approach and

collaboration among health care team members to manage various aspects of treatment, such as:

    a. Braces to help prevent or reduce deformities, increase energy of gait, and control alignment

    b. Motorized devices to permit self-propulsion

    c. Orthopedic surgery to correct deformities and decrease spasticity (drugs are not helpful for spasticity)

    d. Medications to control possible seizure activity or attention deficit disorder

    e. Speech therapy and physical therapy

D. Clinical assessment findings

1. **The most common clinical manifestation is delayed gross motor development (universal, delay in all motor accomplishments, increases as growth advances).**

2. Additional typical manifestations include abnormal motor performance (early dominant hand preference, abnormal and asymmetric crawl, poor sucking, feeding problems, persistent tongue thrust); alterations of muscle tone (increased or decreased resistance to passive movements, feels stiff when handling or dressing, difficulty in diapering, opisthotonos); abnormal postures (scissoring legs, persistent infantile posturing); and reflex abnormalities (persistent primitive reflexes such as tonic neck, hyperreflexia).

3. Associated disabilities include mental retardation, seizures, attention deficit disorder, and sensory impairment.

E. Diagnostic assessment findings

1. There are no specific diagnostic findings and no specific test to diagnose CP.

2. Severe cases may be observed at birth; mild and moderate cases usually are not detected until age 1 or 2 years.

3. Failure to achieve milestones may be the first sign.

4. Diagnosis is based on prenatal, birth, and postnatal history; neurologic examination; assessment of muscle tone, behavior, and abilities. Other disorders such as degenerative disorders need to be ruled out. All infants should receive periodic developmental evaluations, especially those who are at risk.

F. Nursing diagnoses

1. Activity intolerance

2. Body image disturbance

3. Impaired verbal communication

4. Altered family processes

5. Risk for injury

6. Impaired physical mobility

7. Altered nutrition: less than body requirements

8. Altered role performance
9. Self-esteem disturbance

G. Planning and implementation

1. **Prevent physical injury by providing the child with a safe environment, appropriate toys, and protective gear (helmet, knee pads), if needed.**
2. **Prevent physical deformity by ensuring correct use of prescribed braces and other devices and by providing ROM exercises.**
3. **Promote mobility by encouraging the child to perform age- and condition-appropriate motor activities.**
4. Ensure adequate nutrition by providing a high-protein, high-calorie diet.
5. Foster relaxation and general health by providing rest periods.
6. Administer prescribed medications, which may include:
   a. Sedatives
   b. Muscle relaxants
   c. Anticonvulsants
   d. **Methylphenidate (Ritalin) or dextroamphetamine (Dexedrine) (for attention deficit disorder); nursing implications include no caffeine, monitor attention span, monitor blood pressure.**
7. **Encourage self-care by urging the child to participate in activities of daily living (ADLs), using utensils and implements that are appropriate for the child's age and condition.**
8. Facilitate communication by talking to the child deliberately and slowly, using pictures to reinforce speech. Encourage early speech therapy to prevent poor or maladaptive communication habits and provide a means of articulate speech; technology, such as computer use, may help children with severe articulation problems.
9. As necessary, seek referrals for corrective lenses and hearing devices to decrease sensory deprivation related to vision and hearing losses.
10. Help promote a positive self-image in the child by praising his or her accomplishments, setting realistic and attainable goals, encouraging an appealing physical appearance, and encouraging his or her involvement with age- and condition-appropriate peer group activities.
11. Promote optimal family functioning by encouraging members to express anxieties, frustrations, and concerns and to explore support networks. Provide emotional support and help with problem solving, as necessary. Refer the family to support organizations such as the United Cerebral Palsy Association.

> 12. Prepare the child and family for procedures, treatments, appliances, and surgeries, if needed.
> 13. Inform parents that child will need considerable help and patience in accomplishing each new task. Encourage them not to focus solely on the child's inability to accomplish certain tasks; urge them to relax and demonstrate patience, and to provide positive feedback.
> 14. Encourage the family to seek appropriate functional, adaptive, and vocational training for the child.
> 15. Encourage family members to achieve balance in their lives between caring for disabled child and other family and personal matters.

H. Evaluation

> 1. The child achieves locomotion within capabilities.
> 2. The child engages in self-help and ADLs within capabilities.
> 3. The child is free of injury.
> 4. The child can communicate needs to caregivers.
> 5. The child receives optimal nutrition, activity, and rest, and maintains optimal general health.
> 6. The child demonstrates a positive self-image.
> 7. The child and family receive adequate support and understand the diagnosis, treatment, and follow-up care.

VI. Duchenne muscular dystrophy (MD)

A. Description: most common form of MD in children; from a group of disorders that cause progressive degeneration and weakness of skeletal muscles.

B. Etiology and incidence

> 1. Half of all cases are X-linked and males are almost exclusively affected.
> 2. Muscle weakness is progressive and leads to death, usually in adolescence, from infection or cardiopulmonary failure.
> 3. Incidence is 1 of 3500 births.

C. Pathophysiology and management

> 1. Dystrophin, a protein product in skeletal muscle, is absent in the muscles of children with MD.
> 2. There is a gradual degeneration of muscle fibers characterized by progressive weakness and muscle wasting.
> 3. Therapy is supportive to minimize deformity, prolong ambulation, and assist with activities of daily living. Therapeutic measures also involve symptomatic treatment of complications.

D. Clinical assessment findings

> 1. Symptoms begin between ages 3 and 5 years.
> 2. MD starts with weakness in the pelvic girdle; there are de-

lays in motor development; difficulties in running, riding a bicycle, and climbing stairs are among the first symptoms reported.

3. Later, abnormal gait becomes apparent.

4. **Gower's sign (from a supine position, the child roles over, kneels, and presses his or her hands against the ankles, shins knees, thighs in a "climbing" action to rise to a standing position)**

5. Pseudohypertrophy of calf muscles
6. Cardiac problems
7. Possibly, delayed or impaired development

E. Diagnostic assessment findings

1. Increased creatinine phosphokinase (CPK)
2. Muscle biopsy discloses degeneration of muscle fibers.
3. Electrocardiograph (EKG) and pulmonary function tests (PFTs) establish compromise of heart and lungs.
4. Electromyography (EMG) findings show a decrease in amplitude and duration of motor unit potentials.

F. Nursing diagnoses

1. Impaired mobility
2. Risk for injury
3. Ineffective breathing pattern
4. Body image disturbance
5. Risk for caregiver role strain
6. Fatigue
7. Altered nutrition: less than body requirements
8. Altered growth and development
9. Altered family processes
10. Knowledge deficit
11. Social isolation
12. Altered role performance

G. Planning and implementation

1. **Maintain optimal physical mobility by facilitating the maximal level of activity that the child can manage, by changing position every 2 hours, by ensuring proper body alignment, and by providing ROM exericses.**

2. **Support child and family in coping with this progressive disorder. Encourage family to verbalize concerns. Assist them in developing coping strategies. Encourage participation in the child's care.**

3. Further assist family coping by referring members to support agencies such as the Muscular Dystrophy Association.

4. Compensate for disuse syndrome by positioning child, providing skin care, assessing for breakdown, encouraging fluids,

providing pulmonary toilet, and assisting in developing a bowel routine.

5. Monitor temperature because children with Duchenne type MD are at risk for malignant hyperthermia, a potential complication of anesthesia.

6. Teach family and child about diagnosis, treatment, devices, complications, and prognosis.

7. Assist the family in obtaining genetic counseling.

H. Evaluation

1. The child and family cope with the progressive, incapacitating, and fatal nature of the disorder.

2. The child experiences as much independence as possible.

3. The child experiences as few complications as possible.

4. The child and the family cope with the limitations the disease places on their daily lives.

VII. **Scoliosis**

A. Description: lateral curvature of the spine that may result from leg length discrepancy, hip or knee contractures, pain, neuromuscular disorders, or congenital malformations, but usually is idiopathic (IS).

B. Etiology and incidence

1. **Scoliosis usually is of unknown etiology and usually is seen in females.**

2. Evidence points to a probable genetic autosomal dominant trait with incomplete penetrance; or to multifactorial causes.

3. **The most common spinal deformity, scoliosis affects 3% to 5% of all children.**

C. Pathophysiology and management

1. Deformity progresses during periods of growth (adolescent growth spurt) and stabilizes when vertebral growth ceases.

2. As the spine grows and the lateral curve develops, the vertebrae rotate, causing the ribs and spine to rotate toward the convex part of the spine. Spinous processes rotate toward the concavity of the curve.

3. The child attempts to maintain an erect posture, resulting in a compensatory curve.

4. Vertebrae become wedge-shaped and vertebral disks undergo degenerative changes.

5. Muscles and ligaments either shorten and thicken or lengthen and atrophy, depending on the concavity or convexity of the curve. A hump forms from the ribs rotating backward on the convex side of the curve.

6. The thoracic cavity becomes asymmetric, leading to severe

ventilatory compensation. If scoliosis goes uncorrected, respiratory function is compromised and vital capacity is reduced; eventually, pulmonary hypertension, cor pulmonale, and respiratory acidosis may develop.

7. Treatment may involve one or more of the following:
   a. Exercise may help postural scoliosis.
   b. Bracing: Milwaukee brace, a steel and leather brace that extends from a chin cup and neck pads to the pelvis; low profile brace, numerous varieties for lumbar curves. Braces are used for minimal curves and are worn 23 hours a day.
   c. Electrical stimulation is used for mild to moderate curves. An electrical pulse is transmitted to muscles on the convex side of the curve to cause the muscle to contract at regular intervals, thus possibly straightening the spine.
   d. Surgery may be required for spinal realignment and straightening by external or internal fixation and instrumentation combined with bony fusion of the realigned spine. Several techniques are available. Many instrument systems available, such as Harrington, Dwyer, Zielke, Luque, Cotrel-Dubousset, Isola, and Texas Scottish Rite Hospital (TSRH); posterior or anterior approaches can be used.

D. Clinical assessment findings
   1. Scoliosis is asymptomatic most of the time and goes unrecognized until there is some degree of deformity.
   2. Presence of curve, asymmetry of scapula and extremities, unequal distance between arms and waist.

E. Diagnostic assessment findings
   1. Radiographic examination reveals the degree and location of the curvature.

F. Nursing diagnoses
   1. General and preoperative
      a. Risk for injury
      b. Body image disturbance
      c. Ineffective breathing pattern
      d. Altered family processes
      e. Knowledge deficit
      f. Impaired physical mobility
      g. Risk for impaired skin integrity
      h. Social isolation
   2. Postoperative
      a. High risk for injury
      b. Impaired gas exchange
      c. Pain
      d. Constipation

      e. Fear

      f. Altered nutrition: less than body requirements

      g. Altered role performance

      h. Sensory and perceptual alterations

      i. Impaired skin integrity

      j. Altered tissue perfusion

G. **Planning and implementation**

   1. General and preoperative

      a. Protect the child from injury by assessing for and eliminating or minimizing environmental hazards.

      b. Promote adequate air exchange by keeping the child well hydrated and encouraging periodic deep breathing.

      c. Help maintain skin integrity by properly applying braces and implement corrective action to prevent and treat skin breakdown.

      d. Promote mobility by encouraging the child to be up and out of bed and to walk two or three times a day.

      e. Promote a positive self-concept by encouraging verbalization of concerns and feelings, assisting child in clothing selection to conceal brace, and assisting child and family in developing coping skills.

      f. Promote normal growth and development by encouraging self-care activities and peer socialization.

      g. Provide family support by referring parents to social services or an appropriate support group.

   2. Postoperative

      a. Help prevent neurologic deficit by monitoring motor, sensory, and neurologic status, particularly in extremities; prompt identification of neurologic deficit and correction can prevent permanent damage.

      b. Maintain comfort by administering analgesic and muscle relaxants, as prescribed.

      c. Detect impending hypoxia by monitoring blood gas values; notify physician of abnormalities.

      d. Assess for hypotension by monitoring I&O (will most likely have indwelling catheter) and vital signs, and observing skin color to assess tissue perfusion.

      e. Prevent constipation by keeping the child well hydrated, assessing bowel sounds, and offering high-fiber diet when appropriate.

      f. Help child maintain a feeling of control by explaining all procedures and listening to the child as he or she vents fears.

      g. Help prevent skin breakdown by turning child frequently, maintaining alignment, and by providing good skin care.

      h.   Promote adequate nutrition by maintaining intravenous (IV) therapy until oral feedings are allowed; then provide small, well-liked meals.

      i.   Help prevent injury by keeping needed items within reach and by using proper technique when turning.

      j.   Encourage self-care by arranging grooming and food items within easy reach.

      k.   Promote comfort by administering analgesics as prescribed and by proper positioning.

      l.   Provide child and family with information about scoliosis and its treatment, including equipment.

      m.   Provide support by allowing verbalization and by assisting with coping skills.

      n.   Evaluate child's acceptance of prescribed brace and exercise to determine compliance level and need for reinforced teaching. Encourage positive aspects of wearing the brace, including improved posture and symptom relief.

H.   **Evaluation**

      1.   The child is free of neurologic deficit.

      2.   The child remains free of injury and associated complications.

      3.   The child engages in normal activities and verbalizes fears and concerns.

      4.   The child complies with prescribed treatment.

      5.   The child and family verbalize an understanding of the disorder, prescribed treatments, and follow-up care.

VIII.   **Fractures**

A.   **Description: a break in the continuity of the bone; depending on the type of break and its location, repair (by realignment or reduction) may be made by closed or open reduction followed by immobilization with a splint, traction, or a cast.**

B.   **Etiology and incidence**

      1.   **Fractures in children usually are the result of trauma from motor vehicle accidents, falls, or child abuse.**

      2.   Owing to the resilience of the soft tissue of children, fractures occur more often than soft tissue injuries.

C.   **Pathophysiology and management**

      1.   Fractures occur when the resistance of bone against the stress being exerted yields to the stress force.

      2.   Fractures most commonly seen in children include:

          a.   **Bend: bone bends to the breaking point and will not straighten without intervention**

      b.   Buckle: results from compression failure of the bone, with the bone telescoping on itself

      c.   Greenstick: bone does not fracture completely

  3.   Common sites include: clavicle, humerus (in supracondylar fractures, which occur when child falls backward on hands with elbows straight, there is a high incidence of neurovascular complications due to the anatomic relationship of brachial artery and nerves to fracture site), radius and ulna, femur (often associated with child abuse), and epiphyseal plates (potential for growth deformity).

  4.   Precautions must be taken to prevent complications such as cast syndrome, infections, and compartment syndrome.

D. Clinical assessment findings

  1.   Characteristics include the five "ps": pain, pulse, pallor, paresthesia, paralysis.

  2.   Other characteristic findings include: deformity, swelling, bruising, muscle spasms, tenderness, pain, impaired sensation, loss of function, abnormal mobility, crepitus, shock, refusal to walk (in small children).

E. Diagnostic assessment findings: x-ray examination reveals initial injury and subsequent healing progress.

F. Nursing diagnoses: See section III, F.

G. Planning and implementation

  1.   Emergency management:

      a.   Assess the "five ps."

      b.   Determine the mechanism of injury.

      c.   Immobilize the part.

      d.   Move injured parts as little as possible.

      e.   Reassess the "five ps."

      f.   Apply traction if circulatory compromise is present.

      g.   Elevate injured limb if possible.

      h.   Apply cold to injured area.

      i.   Call emergency medical services.

  2.   Routine management

      a.   See section III, G.

      b.   Provide meticulous routine cast care:

          (1) Assess for circulatory impairment (cyanosis, coldness, mottling, decreased peripheral pulses, positive blanch sign, edema not relieved by elevation, pain, or cramping).

          (2) Assess for neurologic impairment (lack of sensation or movement, pain or tenderness, numbness and tingling).

        (3) Use bed board or firm surface to support cast; place cast on pillows to decrease edema and assist drying; turn wet cast with palms not fingertips to prevent creating pressure points; splint upper extremity casts when dry; check cast for wetness (after drying: gray, cold, musty, and dull to percussion), petal cast when dry.

        (4) Inspect skin below cast (foul odor, complaints of burning pain, or "hot spots" on cast, may indicate infection); to prevent infection, keep cast clean and dry, no crumbs or toys under casts.

    c. Initiate additional care for special casts, such as a spica cast:

        (1) Never use the abduction bar as a handle to turn the child and never place plastic wrap around genital area.

        (2) Place only diapers over genitalia (can use a perineal or bladder pad), and keep perineum clean.

        (3) Turn the child every 2 hours when cast is drying.

        (4) Institute measures to preserve the child's modesty.

        (5) Use a Bradford frame.

    d. Teach child and parents how to care for the cast. Also tell them what to expect when cast is removed (noise, dry skin, slight muscle atrophy).

    f. For open reductions, demonstrate skin and wound care and pin care if applicable. Review infection prevention measures.

H. Evaluation

    1. The child will experience no complications from fracture and treatment.

    2. The child's affected extremity will remain in alignment.

    3. The child will be comfortable and injury free.

    4. The child and the parents verbalize an understanding of post-fracture care and follow-up.

Bibliography

Betz, C.L., Hunsberger, M.M., and Wright, S. (1994). *Family Centered Nursing Care of Children*, 2nd ed. Philadelphia: W.B. Saunders.

Castiglia, P.T. and Harbin, R.B. (1993). *Child Health Care: Process and Practice.* Philadelphia: J.B. Lippincott.

Jackson, D.B. and Saunders, R.B. (1993). *Child Health Nursing: A Comprehensive Approach to the Care of Children and Their Families.* Philadelphia: J.B. Lippincott.

McConnell, E.A. (1993). Providing cast care. *Nursing, 23,* 19.

Sizer, F. and Whitney, E. (1994). *Nutrition Concepts and Controversies*, 6th ed. Minneapolis/St. Paul: West Publishing.

Staheli, L.T. (1993). *Fundamentals of Pediatric Orthopedics*. New York: Raven Press.

Wong, D.L. (1993). *Whaley and Wong's Essentials of Pediatric Nursing*, 4th ed. St. Louis: C.V. Mosby.

Wong. D.L. (1995). *Whaley and Wong's Nursing Care of Infants and Children*, 5th ed. St. Louis: C.V. Mosby.

STUDY QUESTIONS

1. When a child injures the epiphyseal plate, the damage may result in:
   a. Bone growth disruption
   b. Rheumatoid arthritis
   c. Permanent nerve damage
   d. Osteomyelitis

2. A 14-year-old girl wears a Milwaukee brace for structural scoliosis. She verbalizes effective use of the brace when she states:
   a. "I wonder if I can take the brace off when I go to the home-coming dance."
   b. "I'll look forward to taking this thing off to take my bath every day."
   c. "I sure am glad that I only have to wear this awful thing at night."
   d. "I'm really glad that I can take this thing off whenever I get tired."

3. Which of the following is the most common form of congenital hip dysplasia?
   a. Preluxation
   b. Subluxation
   c. Acetabular dysplasia
   d. Dislocation

4. When assessing a newborn for congenital hip dysplasia, the nurse would expect to find:
   a. Symmetrical gluteal folds
   b. Trendelenburg's sign
   c. Ortolani's sign
   d. Characteristic limp

5. To best assess a mother's understanding of and ability to apply a Pavlik harness, the nurse would:
   a. Have the mother verbalize the purpose of the device
   b. Request a home health nurse visit after discharge
   c. Have the mother remove and reapply the harness before discharge
   d. Demonstrate to the mother how to remove and reapply the device

6. The priority nursing action for a child in a fresh spica cast:
   a. Neurovascular checks
   b. Elevate the cast
   c. Cover perineal area
   d. Keep cast clean and dry

7. Which of the following is the most common permanent disability in childhood?
   a. Congenital hip dysplasia
   b. Cerebral palsy
   c. Muscular dystrophy
   d. Scoliosis

8. Which of the following statements made by the mother of a 4-month-old would indicate that the child may have cerebral palsy?
   a. "I'm very worried because my baby has not rolled all the way over yet."
   b. "My baby's left hip tilts when I pull him to a standing position."
   c. "My baby won't lift her head up and look at me; she's so floppy."
   d. "He holds his left leg so stiff that I have a hard time putting on his diapers."

9. Which of the following usually is the first indication of Duchenne type muscular dystrophy?
   a. Inability to suck in the newborn
   b. Lateness in walking in the toddler
   c. Difficulty running in the preschooler
   d. Decreasing coordination in the schoolager

10. Besides assessing neurologic status immediately after Harrington rod instrumentation and spinal fusion for scoliosis, the nurse should be concerned with which of the following factors?
    a. The adolescent's understanding of the procedure
    b. The adolescent's comfort level
    c. The adolescent's physical therapy needs
    d. The adolescent's dietary tolerance

ANSWER KEY

1. *Correct response: a*
   The epiphyseal plate is an important area of bone growth; disruption may result in limb shortening.
   - **b.** Rheumatoid arthritis is a collagen disease with an autoimmune component; there is no relationship to fractures.
   - **c and d.** Nerve damage and osteomyelitis may occur with any fracture, but growth disruption is a primary concern at the epiphyseal plate.

   Comprehension/Physiologic/Planning

2. *Correct response: b*
   The brace should be removed for only 1 of every 24 hours for hygiene and skin care.
   - **a.** Although physical appearance and social activities with peers are important, the brace should not be removed except for hygiene and skin care.
   - **c.** This statement is true only after radiologic studies indicate the spine has bone marrow maturity and the adolescent has been weaned from the brace over 1 to 2 years.
   - **d.** This statement indicates poor understanding of the Milwaukee brace.

   Application/Health Promotion/ Evaluation

3. *Correct response: b*
   Subluxation is the most common form of congenital hip dysplasia.
   - **a.** Preluxation is the mildest form.
   - **c.** Acetabular dysplasia is another name for preluxation.
   - **d.** Dislocation is complete displacement of the femoral head out of the acetabulum.

   Knowledge/Physiologic/Assessment

4. *Correct response: c*
   Ortolani's sign is felt and heard when the young infant's hip is flexed and abducted.
   - **a.** Asymmetrical gluteal folds would be noted in congenital hip dysplasia.
   - **b.** Trendelenburg's sign is noted in the weight-bearing child when the child stands on the affected hip and the pelvis tilts downward on normal side instead of upward.
   - **d.** A characteristic limp would be noted in the ambulatory child.

   Application/Physiologic/Assessment

5. *Correct response: c*
   This allows the nurse to directly observe the mother's technique and comfort level.
   - **a.** Verbalization allows the nurse to assess understanding but not psychomotor skills.
   - **b.** Requesting a home visit is further means of evaluation, but it does not provide immediate feedback.
   - **d.** Although the nurse's demonstration is a good teaching technique, it does not permit evaluation of the mother's technique.

   Application/Safe Care/Implementation

6. *Correct response: a*
   Neurovascular assessment is always a priority in the assessment of a freshly applied cast.
   - **b, c, and d.** Cast elevation to prevent or minimize edema, covering the perineal area to prevent wetness, and keeping the cast dry and clean are all important, but not priority nursing implementations.

   Application/Safe Care/Implementation

7. *Correct response: b*
   Cerebral palsy is the most common cause of permanent disability in childhood, occurring in 1.2 to 2 of every 1000 births.
   - **a.** Congenital hip dysplasia is not (should not be) a permanent disability.

c. Muscular dystrophy occurs in 1 of 3500 births.

d. Functional scoliosis should not result in permanent disability.

Knowledge/Physiologic/NA

8. **Correct response: c**

Infant lifts head to a 90-degree angle by 4 months; only partial head lag by 2 months; hypotonia or floppy infant is an early manifestation.

a. This does not occur until 6 months.

b. This is an indication of congenital hip dysplasia.

d. Although rigidity and tenseness are possible signs of cerebral palsy, a limitation in one leg indicates hip dysplasia.

Analysis/Physiologic/Evaluation

9. **Correct response: c**

Starts with pelvic girdle weakness with signs and symptoms noticed between the ages of 3 and 5 years.

a and b. Duchenne muscular dystrophy usually is not diagnosed this early and sucking is not affected.

d. Diminished coordination is not the first sign of Duchenne muscular dystrophy.

Application/Physiologic/Assessment

10. **Correct response: b**

Instrumentation and spinal fusion cause considerable pain; the adolescent needs vigorous pain management, which involves assessment, administration of pain medication, and evaluation of response.

a. Immediately postoperatively, the child is conscious of sensation and surroundings; assessment of understanding of procedure is a preoperative nursing responsibility.

c. Physical therapy is not an immediate postoperative goal.

d. The adolescent will not be receiving anything by mouth.

Knowledge/Physiologic/Assessment

Neurologic and Cognitive Dysfunction

I. Essential concepts: nervous system structures and function

A. Development

1. The *central nervous system (CNS)* arises from the neural tube during embryonic development. By the fourth week of gestation, the neural tube has developed; between the eighth and twelfth week, the cerebrum and cerebellum begin to develop.

2. Two periods of rapid nerve development occur: between the 15th and 20th weeks of gestation and from the 30th week of gestation through the first year of extrauterine life.

3. In the first year of extrauterine life, the number of brain neurons increases rapidly.

4. Normally accounting for 12% of the body weight at birth, the brain doubles its weight by the end of the first year of extrauterine life.

5. CNS nerve myelinization, which enables progressive neuromuscular function, follows the cephalocaudal and proximodistal sequence; its rate accelerates rapidly after birth.

6. The peripheral nervous system arises from the neural crest, which originates from the neural tube during embryonic development.

B. Function

1. The neurologic system consists of three main divisions:
    a. CNS
    b. Peripheral nervous system
    c. Autonomic nervous system

2. Major CNS structures include the cerebrum, thalamus, hypo-thalamus, cerebellum, brain stem, and spinal cord.

3. The *cerebrum* is the center for consciousness, thought, memory, sensory input, and motor activity; it consists of two hemispheres (left and right) and four lobes, each with specific functions:

    a. Frontal lobe: controls voluntary muscle movements and contains motor areas, including the area for speech; also contains the centers for personality, behavioral, autonomic, and intellectual functions, and for emotional and cardiac responses.

    b. Temporal lobe: center for taste, hearing and smell and, in the brain's dominant hemisphere, the center for interpreting spoken language.

    c. Parietal lobe: coordinates and interprets sensory information from the opposite side of the body.

    d. Occipital lobe: interprets visual stimuli.

4. The *thalamus* further organizes cerebral function by transmitting impulses to and from the cerebrum. It also is responsible for primitive emotional responses, such as fear, and for distinguishing between pleasant and unpleasant stimuli.

5. Lying beneath the thalamus, the *hypothalamus* is an autonomic center that regulates blood pressure, temperature, libido, appetite, breathing, sleeping patterns, and peripheral nerve discharges associated with certain behavior and emotional expression. It also helps control pituitary secretion and stress reactions.

6. The *cerebellum,* or hindbrain, controls smooth muscle movements, coordinates sensory impulses with muscle activity, and maintains muscle tone and equilibrium.

7. The *brain stem,* which includes the mesencephalon, pons, and medulla oblongata, relays nerve impulses between the brain and spinal cord. With the thalamus and hypothalamus, it makes up the reticular formation, a nerve network that acts as an arousal mechanism.

8. The *spinal cord* forms a two-way conductor pathway between the brain stem and the peripheral nervous system. It is also the reflex center for motor activities that do not involve brain control.

9. Consisting of 31 pairs of spinal nerves and their intricate branches, the *peripheral nervous system* connects the CNS to remote body regions and conducts signals to and from these areas and the spinal cord.

10. The *autonomic nervous system* regulates body functions such as digestion, respiration, and cardiovascular function.

II. Nervous system overview

A. Assessment

1. Neurologic assessment of children must be based on the developmental level of the child and should attempt to determine if problems are acute or chronic, diffuse or focal, or stable or progressive.

2. The history should focus on:

    a. Complete developmental history

    b. Any learning problems, clumsiness, coordination problems

    c. Febrile seizures, any other seizure activity

    d. Headaches, fainting, dizziness, head trauma

    e. Tremors and tics

    f. Memory loss, speech problems, unusual habits

    g. Sensory and motor problems

    h. Recent infections or ingestion of possible toxins

3. The neurologic pediatric physical examination includes:

    a. General: general appearance, affect, interactions, speech

    b. Developmental: cognitive, psychosocial, gross and fine motor

    c. Mental status: level of consciousness (LOC), orientation, reasoning ability, memory

    d. Head circumference and fontanel assessment of infants

    e. Cranial nerve function

    f. Sensory status: vision, hearing, taste, tactile, olfactory

    g. Motor function: muscle tone and strength, posture

    h. Cerebellar status: balance and coordination

    i. Reflexes: infantile (Table 16-1), later reflexes (*e.g.*, parachute); deep tendon reflexes, superficial reflexes (also see Fig. 16-1)

4. In children with acute neurologic problems, neurologic checks may be performed every 4 or more hours. This assessment includes:

    a. Vital signs: blood pressure, pulse, respiration, and temperature

    b. LOC: may use Pediatric Coma Scale, which assesses eye opening, verbal response, and motor response

    c. Eyes: pupil size, equality and reaction to light; extraocular movements; corneal reflexes; visual disturbances

    d. Motor and sensory function: tone and movement in response to command, tactile or painful stimuli

    e. Reflexes

    f. Head circumference in infants

TABLE 16-1.
Neonatal Reflexes

REFLEX	NORMAL DURATION
Babinski	Subsides by age 1 year
Landau	Subsides by age 4–6 months
Moro	Diminishes by age 4 months; subsides by age 7 months
Palmar grasp	Diminishes by age 4 months
Perez	Subsides by age 4–6 months
Plantar grasp	Diminishes by age 4 months
Prone crawl	Subsides by age 1–2 months
Rooting and sucking	Diminishes by age 5–6 months; subsides by age 1 year
Startle	Diminishes by age 4 months
Stepping	Subsides by age 1–2 months
Swallowing	Persists for life
Tongue extrusion	Subsides by age 4 months
Tonic neck (fencing)	Diminishes by age 4 months
Trunk incurvation (Galant)	Subsides by age 4 weeks

B.   Laboratory studies and diagnostic tests
  1.   Imaging studies include:
      a.   Computed tomographic (CT) scan
      b.   Magnetic resonance imaging (MRI)
      c.   Skull series
      d.   Electroencephalography (EEG)
      e.   Isotope brain scan
      f.   Electromyography
      g.   Myelography
  2.   Other studies include:
      a.   Lumbar puncture
      b.   Subdural or ventricular taps
      c.   Blood and urine studies
C.   Psychosocial implications
  1.   Many of the specialized tests for neurologic function can be threatening to children; visual pictures of the machinery and explanations about the need to remain still during the scans are helpful to schoolagers; doll and puppet play are helpful for preschoolers.
  2.   Allow young children to have transitional objects with them during procedures.
  3.   Neurologic deficits impede development and may cause significant psychosocial stress for the child and the family.

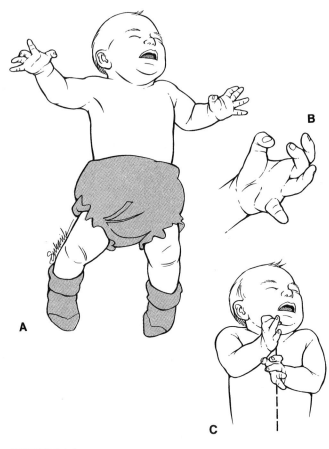

FIGURE 16-1.
(A) An easily identified infantile reflex is the startle (or Moro) reflex in which the infant throws its arms out. (B) In the Moro reflex, the infant's hand assumes a classic "C" position. (C) During the startle reflex, the infant's arms return toward the body's midline. The startle reflex is never lost; however, the Moro reflex with the hand in a "C" position is indicative of a neurologic problem in an older child.

III. Increased intracranial pressure (ICP)

   A. Description: excessive pressure within the rigid cranial vault that disrupts neurologic function.

   B. Etiology and incidence

   1. Increased ICP can result from any alteration that increases tissue or fluid volume within the cranium, including:

   a. Tumors or other space-occupying lesions

   b. Accumulation of cerebrospinal fluid (CSF) in the ventricular system

   c. Intracranial bleeding

   d. Edema of the cerebral tissues

  2. Conditions that produce increased ICP include:

   a. Craniocerebral trauma

   b. Hydrocephalus

   c. Brain tumor

   d. Meningitis

   e. Encephalitis

   f. Intracerebral hemorrhage

C. **Pathophysiology and management**

  1. Normally, ICP remains relatively constant (within its normally fluctuating range) through a system of compensatory alterations among the cranium's contents: brain tissue, meninges, CSF, and blood. Any increase in the volume of one component must be accompanied by a corresponding reduction in one or more of the others.

  2. After cranial sutures fuse and close, only two mechanisms can compensate for increasing intracranial volume: displacement of CSF to the spinal subarachnoid space and increased CSF absorption.

  3. An intracranial volume increase that exceeds the ability of the mechanisms to compensate produces signs and symptoms of increased ICP.

  4. As ICP rises, it can trigger a cycle of decreasing perfusion, increasing edema, and further increased ICP. Unchecked, this cycle can result in complete loss of cerebral arterial perfusion and brain cell death.

  5. Brain stem compression secondary to herniation can cause life-threatening deterioration of vital functions.

D. **Clinical assessment findings**

  1. **Early signs and symptoms of increased ICP usually are subtle. Children with open fontanels and sutures compensate by widening these spaces, but the compensation is limited.**

  2. Manifestations in infants and young children include:

   a. **Tense, bulging anterior fontanel**

   b. **High-pitched cry**

   c. **Increased occipital frontal circumference**

   d. **"Setting sun" sign**

   e. **Macewen's sign ("cracked pot") in infants**

   f. Irritability and restlessness

   g. Change in feeding habits

   h. Crying with cuddling and rocking

3. Manifestations in older children include:
   a. **Headache**
   b. **Vomiting, usually projectile**
   c. **Cognitive, personality, and behavioral changes**
   d. **Diplopia, blurred vision**
   e. Anorexia and nausea
   f. Seizures
4. Late manifestations of extremely high increased ICP include:
   a. Decreased LOC ranging from lethargy to coma
   b. Decreased motor response to commands
   c. Decreased sensation to painful stimuli
   d. Decreased pupil size and reactivity
   e. Decerebrate or decorticate posturing
   f. Papilledema
   g. Cheyne-Stokes respirations

E. **Diagnostic assessment findings**
   1. ICP is measured by various devices ranging from a noninvasive transducer to the more commonly used invasive devices, such as an epidural transducer and an intraventricular catheter transducer. Normal pressure ranges are from 0 to 15 mm Hg under normal conditions.
   2. Diagnostic studies will be used to determine the underlying cause.

F. **Nursing diagnoses**
   1. Altered tissue perfusion
   2. Ineffective airway clearance
   3. Anxiety
   4. Risk for injury
   5. Pain
   6. Altered nutrition: less than body requirements
   7. Sensory and perceptual alterations
   8. Altered family processes
   9. Altered thought processes
   10. Knowledge deficit
   11. Altered role performance
   12. Fluid volume deficit

G. **Planning and implementation**
   1. Because treatment of increased ICP focuses on reducing intracranial volume and treating the underlying disorder, assist in reducing intra-abdominal and intrathoracic pressure, which contribute to ICP, by elevating the head of the bed 15 to 45 degrees.

   2. **Assess for early changes in ICP by monitoring vital signs (increased systolic blood pressure, wide pulse pressure,**

and bradycardia indicate increased ICP), LOC, respiratory status, motor activity, behavior, and pupil size and reactivity.

3. If appropriate, use transducer to monitor ICP.

4. As prescribed, assist with treatments and supportive measures such as hyperventilation, mechanical ventilation, and hypothermia.

5. Prevent overhydration and underhydration for adequate cerebral perfusion pressure; monitor intake and output (I&O) and impose fluid restrictions if prescribed.

6. Help the child avoid positions or activities that increase ICP, such as neck vein compression, flexion or extension of the neck, turning the head from side to side, painful or stressful stimuli, and respiratory suctioning or percussion.

7. Promote normal bowel elimination to prevent intra-abdominal pressure increase from straining at stool.

8. Prevent weight loss by providing adequate nutrition in small frequent feedings, by administering intravenous (IV) nutrients if prescribed, or, possibly, through a gastrostomy tube if child remains unconscious or not sufficiently alert to take foods by mouth.

9. Promote normal growth and development without overstimulating the child.

10. Prevent skin breakdown by placing the child on a sheepskin or other resilient mattress appliance.

11. As appropriate, prepare the child for surgery to relieve the increased ICP; procedures may include subdural tap, ventriculotomy, epidural evacuation, placement of ventricular shunt, decompressive craniectomy, or tumor resection.

12. Administer medications as prescribed, which may include:
    a. Osmotic diuretics, such as mannitol or urea
    b. Corticosteroids

13. Provide child and family teaching:
    a. Talk about increased ICP and its underlying cause, if known.
    b. Explain all treatments, procedures, and follow-up care (including rationales).

H. Evaluation

1. The child exhibits decreased ICP and resolution of signs and symptoms.

2. The parents verbalize an understanding of follow-up care.

IV. **Seizure disorders**

A. Description: disturbance in normal brain function resulting from abnormal electrical discharge in the brain, which can cause loss of consciousness, uncontrolled body movements, and changes in behaviors and sensation and in the autonomic system.

B. **Etiology and incidence**

1. There are may underlying possible causes such as prenatal or perinatal hypoxia, infections, congenital malformations, metabolic disturbances, lead poisoning, head injuries, drug abuse, alcohol misuse, tumors, medications, and toxins.

 2. **Most seizures are idiopathic.**

3. There is some evidence of a genetic etiologic factor in which the seizure threshold is lowered in affected persons.

4. Seizures are more common before age 2 years than at any other time.

5. Up to 5% of all children experience at least one seizure by adolescence; chronic seizures or epilepsy, affect 1% to 2% of all children.

C. **Pathophysiology and management**

1. Seizures result from overly active and hypersensitive neurons in the brain that trigger excessive electrical discharges, causing a seizure.

2. The location of the abnormal cells and the pattern of discharges determine the clinical manifestations.

3. The two categories of seizures are *generalized* and *partial.*

    a. **Generalized seizures involve both hemispheres of the brain, are bilateral and symmetric, and may or may not involve prodromal syndromes.**

    b. **Partial or focal seizures involve a limited area of the cerebral cortex; these may be simple or complex.**

4. Treatment interventions include:

    a. Anticonvulsant medications, such as phenobarbital, phenytoin, diazepam, and carbamazepine, with dosage adjusted as the child grows

    b. Surgery (*e.g.*, to remove the offending area of involvement, which can range from a small area to a lobe to a complete hemisphere) without causing further deficit, if seizures cannot be controlled by medications

    c. **Diet, such as a ketogenic diet (high-fat, low-carbohydrate, low-protein to induce ketosis), in children with *absence* or other kinds of seizures; this diet is very difficult to maintain**

D. **Clinical assessment findings**

1. Generalized

    a. **Tonic-clonic (grand mal): tonic—rigidity, extension of extremities, fixed jaw, respiratory cessation, di-**

lated pupils; clonic—rhythmic jerking of extremities, autonomic symptoms, possible incontinence
  b. Tonic
  c. Clonic
  d. Minor motor, atonic—sudden loss of muscle tone followed by postictal confusion
  e. Minor motor, myoclonic—generalized short muscle contractions, each child exhibiting movements that are characteristic for him or her
  f. Infantile spasm—brief flexion of the neck, trunk, or legs
  g. **Absence seizure (petite mal): brief periods of unconsciousness, may have tonic or atonic phase or automatisms (lip smacking)**
2. Partial seizures
  a. Simple partial: consciousness usually maintained; may include focal motor component (abnormal movement of leg); sensory component (tingling); autonomic (sweating) or psychic (déjà vu, anger).
  b. Complex: begins as simple and progresses to unconsciousness. Seizures may also be unclassified, as are neonatal seizures. *Status epilepticus* involves recurrent, continuous, generalized seizure activity with the danger of cardiac arrest and brain damage. Some children also experience an aura prior to the seizures.

E. Diagnostic assessment findings
  1. EEG is performed to document abnormal activity.
  2. Complete blood count (CBC) and blood chemistries obtained.
  3. Once child is on anticonvulsant medications, blood tests may be ordered to monitor serum levels of medications.
  4. Other testing may be done to determine underlying cause.

F. Nursing diagnoses
  1. Risk for injury
  2. Body image disturbance
  3. Altered family processes
  4. Knowledge deficit
  5. Anxiety
  6. Self-esteem disturbance
  7. Ineffective breathing pattern

G. Planning and implementation
  1. Obtain thorough history (birth trauma, medications, injuries, illnesses, family history).

  2. **Maintain safety. If necessary, have child wear helmet, pad the bed's side rails, and have oxygen and suction equipment at bedside.**

3. **During seizure:** *Do not* **restrain child and** *do not* **place anything in his or her mouth during seizure.** *Do* **remove harmful objects from area, hyperextend neck to maintain airway, position child on side to allow secretions to flow from mouth, loosen clothing, observe time and duration of seizure.**
4. Document all seizure activity, including:
   a. Apparent trigger factor, if known or suspected
   b. Behavior before the seizure; aura
   c. Time seizure began and ended
   d. Clinical manifestations of the seizure
   e. Postseizure behavior and symptoms
5. Help prevent seizures by preventing the child's exposure to known precipitants (*e.g.*, emotional stress, blinking lights).
6. Minimize the child's anxiety by staying with him or her during attacks, providing reassurance, and explaining all procedures and treatments. Allow the child to participate in normal activities as much as possible.

7. **Administer anticonvulsant medications, which may include:**
   a. **Phenobarbital (check mental status, maintain safety precautions owing to sedation, monitor levels as ordered)**
   b. **Phenytonin (provide mouth care, observe gums for inflammation, monitor levels as prescribed, monitor CBC and liver function test values)**
   c. **Diazepam (monitor blood pressure; supervise ambulation and raise the bed's side rails for safety because of sedation; prevent constipation, if used over long term; monitor CBC and liver function tests)**
   d. **Carbamazepine (monitor for bone marrow depression: frequent infections, bleeding, anemia, monitor CBC)**
8. Help promote normal growth and development by encouraging age-appropriate activities.
9. Provide child and family teaching, covering:
   a. The nature of the disorder and its possible triggers
   b. Prodromal signs to watch for and steps to take if they occur
   c. Seizure precaution measures
   d. Diagnostic tests and procedures and their rationales
   e. Medication (dosage schedule and side effects)
   f. The importance of not discontinuing medication and of not switching to a different brand of the same medication
   g. The need for periodic reevaluation of medication effec-

     h.   Other treatments such as surgery or diet
     i.   The importance of encouraging as normal a lifestyle as possible
     j.   Any activity restrictions placed on the child by the physician
     k.   The need to share information about the child's special needs with significant others, such a teachers and school nurses
     l.   Follow-up care
     m.   Adolescent needs, such as information about drugs and alcohol, peer pressure, dating, getting a driver's license

H.   Evaluation
    1.   The child's seizure are well controlled.
    2.   Parents verbalize an understanding of the treatment plan, seizure prevention, and the need for continual monitoring.
    3.   The child and parents demonstrate the ability to cope with seizure activity.
    4.   The child exhibits a good self-concept, participates in normal activity to the greatest extent possible, and complies with imposed activity limitations.

V. Neural tube defects (NTDs)
  A. **Description: a group of related defects of the CNS involving the cranium or spinal cord and varying from mildly to severely disabling; may be cystic or noncystic; includes spina bifida, meningocele, and myelomeningocele.**
  B. **Etiology and incidence**
    1.   Heredity and environmental factors have been implicated.
    2.   **Recently, NTDs have been associated with the interaction of genetic predisposition and folic acid deficiency.**
    3.   The cystic defect occurs in 0.2 to 4.2 per 1000 births.
  C. **Pathophysiology and management**
    1.   During the third to fourth week of gestation, the neural plate closes to form the neural tube that eventually forms the spinal cord and brain. The vertebral column develops along with the spinal cord.
    2.   NTDs result from malformations of the neural tube during embryonic development.
    3.   There are different types of NTDs:
       a.   *Anencephaly:* This is a severe defect involving absence of the entire brain or cerebral hemispheres; the brain stem and cerebellum may be intact. Total anencephaly is incompatible with life; many anencephalics are aborted or stillborn; living infants usually survive only a few hours.

      b.   *Encephalocele:* Meningeal and cerebral tissue protrudes in a sac through a defect in the skull, with the occiput being the most common site; when possible, the brain is placed back in the skull; many infants have hydrocephalus; in mild forms there is little or no residual neurologic impairment.

      c.   *Spina bifida (SB):* A defective closure of the vertebral column, SB is the most common defect of the CNS. SB may occur anywhere but usually occurs in the lumbosacral area. The three principal types of spina bifida are *spina bifida occulta, meningocele,* and *myelomeningocele.*

4. Diagnosis is made on the basis on clinical examination; if the sac transluminates, it usually is meningocele.

5. No treatment is indicated for spina bifida occulta unless there is neurologic damage; if sinus is present, it may need to be closed.

6. Meningocele requires closure as soon after birth as possible; child should be monitored for hydrocephalus, meningitis, and spinal cord dysfunction.

7. Myelomeningocele requires a multidisciplinary approach (neurology, neurosurgery, pediatrics, urology, orthopedics, rehabilitation, nursing). There is no cure. Closure is performed within 24 hours to minimize infection and prevent further damage to the spinal cord and roots; skin grafting may be necessary; shunting is performed for hydrocephalus; antibiotics are initiated to prevent infection. Child will need correction of musculoskeletal deformities, management of urologic problems, and bowel control.

D. **Clinical assessment findings**

1. **Manifestations vary with the degree of the defect; the defect is readily apparent on inspection; the degree of neurologic dysfunction is directly related to the anatomic level of the defect and thus to the nerves involved; sensory disturbances usually parallel motor dysfunction.**

2. Spina bifida occulta: The spinal cord usually is not affected; external signs may include dimpling of the skin, nevi or hair tufts over a dermal sinus; it may go undetected and most children do not display any neurologic signs; if they do occur, there usually is motor or sensory deficit of the lower extremities and involvement of the urinary and bladder sphincter.

3. Meningocele: Sac containing meninges and CSF protrudes outside vertebrae; usually in the lumbosacral area. The spinal cord is not involved and therefore there is usually little to no neurologic involvement.

4. Myelomeningocele: This disorder is similar to meningocele,

but the spinal cord and accompanying nerve roots are involved. The most severe, most common, and usually a lumbosacral defect, myelomeningocele involves sensorimotor deficits, urinary and bowel problems and, possibly, in utero joint deformities such as congenital dislocation of the hip (CDH) and club foot.

E. Diagnostic assessment findings

1.   Ultrasonography, CT, MRI, and myelography

2.   **Prenatal detection by alpha-fetoprotein (AFP)**

F. Nursing diagnoses

1.   Risk for injury
2.   Risk for infection
3.   Sensory and perceptual alterations
4.   Bowel incontinence
5.   Constipation
6.   Altered urinary elimination
7.   Impaired skin integrity
8.   Altered family processes
9.   Impaired physical mobility
10. Self-esteem disturbance
11. Body image disturbance
12. Altered growth and development
13. Knowledge deficit

G. Planning and implementation

1.   The following interventions focus on myelomeningocele.

2.   **Help prevent infection by applying sterile, moist soaks to the lesion (possible with antibacterial agent added). Avoid placing a diaper or other covering directly over lesion to prevent fecal contamination.**

3.   Prevent trauma to the sac by placing the infant prone in an isolette or warmer.

4.   Position the infant in low Trendelenburg's position while prone to reduce the pressure of CSF in the sac.

5.   Help prevent hip subluxation by maintaining legs in abduction with a pad between the knees and the feet in a neutral position with a roll under the ankles.

6.   **Promote parent-infant relationship by encouraging parental participation with feeding, cuddling, and stimulation.**

7.   Monitor vital signs, measure head circumference, assess neurologic status, including signs of ICP (see section III, D).

8.   Help prevent skin breakdown by padding bony prominences and by placing the child in a side-lying position (postoperatively), if allowed.

9. Encourage parents to verbalize their fears.
10. Encourage parents to contact the Spinal Bifida Association of America.
11. Assist with the associated problems for the growing child:

   ♬ a. **Assess urologic status and assist with self-catheteriza-tion.**
   b. **Administer medication as prescribed to improve bladder continence (oxybutynin chloride, propanthe-line); maintain urinary diversion if child has had this procedure.**
   c. **Assist with fecal contenence.**
   d. **Promote mobility.**
   e. **Carefully monitor skin because child may have de-creased sensation in areas distal to the lesion, creat-ing an increased chance for pressure sores.**

12. Provide child and family teaching:
   a. Explain the essentials of infant care. Emphasize infection prevention and recognition of early signs and symptoms of infection and increased ICP.
   b. Explain and demonstrate bladder and bowel manage-ment and skin care.
   c. Discuss the effects of immobilization and how to deal with them.
   d. Discuss the need for lifelong care.
   e. Encourage normalcy, as possible.

13. Carefully assess the family's ability to care for the child and refer them for further assistance if needed.

H. Evaluation
1. The child's vital signs, ICP, and neurologic status are within acceptable ranges.
2. The child is free of trauma, infection, and skin breakdown.
3. The child displays neutral alignment of legs and hips.
4. Parents demonstrate ability to care for child.
5. Parents verbalize an understanding of the disorder and its im-plications, treatment, and prognosis; the need for follow-up care; and the need to allow the child to live as normal a life as possible.

VI. Hydrocephalus
   A. Description: a condition caused by an imbalance in the produc-tion and absorption of CSF in the ventricular system; when pro-duction exceeds absorption, CSF accumulates, usually under pressure, producing dilation of the ventricles.
   B. Etiology and incidence
   1. Hydrocephalus occurs with a number of anomalies such as NTDs.

2. It occurs in 5.8 per 10,000 births.
3. Hydrocephalus occurring within the first 2 years of life usually is the result of developmental defects such as spina bifida.
4. Hydrocephalus occurring in older children usually results from space-occupying lesions, hemorrhage, intracranial infections, or dormant developmental defects.

C. **Pathophysiology and management**

1. The primary site of CSF formation is believed to be the choroid plexuses of the lateral ventricles. CSF flows from the lateral ventricles through the foramen of Monro to the third ventricle, then through the aqueduct of Sylvius into the fourth ventricle through the foramen of Luschka and the midline foramen of Magendie into the cisterna magna. From there it flows to the cerebral and cerebellar subarachnoid spaces where it is absorbed (how it is absorbed is not clear).
2. Causes of hydrocephalus are varied but result in either impaired absorption of CSF within the arachnoid space *(communicating hydrocephalus)* or obstruction to the flow of CSF through the ventricular system *(noncommunicating hydrocephalus)*.
3. Most cases of noncommunicating hydrocephalus are the result of developmental malformations; others may be caused by neoplasms, infection, and trauma. Obstruction to the normal flow can occur at any point in the CSF pathway to produce increased pressure and dilation of the pathways proximal to the site of obstruction.
4. Noncommunicating hydrocephalus can result from meningitis, prenatal maternal infections, meningeal malignancy (secondary to leukemia or lymphoma), arachnoid cyst, and tuberculosis.
5. Treatment aims to relieve hydrocephalus and possible complications and to manage problems related to difficulties in psychomotor development.
6. **Treatment is surgical by direct removal of the obstruction and insertion of shunts to provide primary drainage of the CSF to an extracranial compartment, usually the peritoneum. Shunts consist of a ventricular catheter, a flush pump, a unidirectional flow valve, and a distal catheter. The major complications of shunts are infections and malfunction; others include subdural hematoma caused by a too rapid reduction of CSF, peritonitis, abdominal abscess, perforation of organs, fistulas, hernias, and ileus.**

D. **Clinical assessment findings**

1. Infants: Head grows at abnormal rate; signs and symptoms include bulging fontanel; tense anterior fontanel, often bulging and nonpulsatile; dilated scalp veins; Macewen's sign (cracked

pot); frontal bossing; setting sun sign; sluggish and unequal pupils; irritability and lethargy with varying LOC; abnormal infantile reflexes; possible cranial nerve damage.

2. Children: Possible signs of ICP, headache on awakening with improvement following emesis; papilledema; strabismus; ataxia, irritability, lethargy, apathy, and confusion.

E. **Diagnostic assessment findings**

1. Varying degrees of localized fluid accumulation on cranial translumination
2. Evidence of fluid accumulation on CT scan or MRI
3. Widened sutures and fontanels and erosion of intracranial bones seen on skull radiograph

F. **Nursing diagnoses**

1. Risk for infection
2. Risk for injury
3. Ineffective airway clearance
4. Anxiety
5. Pain
6. Altered nutrition: less than body requirements
7. Altered family processes
8. Fluid volume deficit
9. Altered role performance
10. Altered growth and development
11. Sensory and perceptual alterations
12. Impaired skin integrity
13. Altered thought processes

G. **Planning and implementation**

1. Preoperative
   a. Assess head circumference, fontanels, cranial sutures, and LOC; check also for irritability, altered feeding habits, and high-pitched cry.
   b. Firmly support head and neck when holding the child.
   c. Provide skin care for head, placing sheepskin under it.
   d. Give small, frequent feedings to decrease risk of vomiting.
   e. Encourage bonding.
2. Postoperative
   a. Assess for signs of increased ICP; check head circumference daily; check anterior fontanel for size and fullness; check behavior.
   b. In addition to routine postoperative care, monitor for increased ICP.
   c. Test patency of shunt, as prescribed, by depressing shunt valve with forefinger quickly and firmly; if valve is difficult to depress, it may be blocked, requiring immediate

medical attention (some valves require a physician's order for pumping).

d. Position child on side opposite shunt to facilitate draining.

e. Observe dressings for bloody and clear drainage (presence of glucose in drainage indicates CSF).

f. Usually, keep child flat in bed for 24 hours, keeping in mind that a sudden elevation of the head of the bed may cause fluid to drain too rapidly from the shunt, shrinking the ventricle, causing cortex to pull away from the meninges, and resulting in subdural hematoma.

g. Monitor I&O carefully; fluids may need to be restricted; feedings depend on child's tolerance of shunt; many children with ventriculoperitoneal shunts have constipation, which is regulated by diet.

h. Administer antibiotics as prescribed, IV or intraventricularly; monitor for infection.

i. Administer acetazolamide, as prescribed, to decrease CSF production.

j. Administer osmotic diuretic as prescribed to reduce increased ICP.

3. Encourage child to participate in age-appropriate activities as tolerated; encourage parents to provide as normal a lifestyle as possible without contact sports.

4. Provide child and family teaching:

a. Cover the nature of the condition and its underlying cause, if known.

b. Describe all tests and procedures, and their rationales.

c. Explain how to recognize signs and symptoms of increased ICP.

d. Add that hydrocephalus is a lifelong condition and that constant follow-up care is essential.

H. Evaluation

1. The child is free of infection, injury, and skin breakdown.

2. Parents verbalize an understanding of home care and signs and symptoms of increased ICP.

3. Parents verbalize an understanding of the need to avoid overprotecting the child and encourage activity as tolerated.

VII. **Reye's syndrome**

A. **Description: an acute, multisystem disorder that follows a mild viral infection, usually influenza or varicella.**

B. **Etiology and incidence**

1. Reye's syndrome usually is seen in children between ages 5 and 15 years. It is of unknown etiology; however, a relation-

ship has been established between the syndrome and aspirin taken during a viral illness.

2. In recent years, there has been a decline in the number of cases reported: a 91% decrease in children under age 5 years and a 75% decrease in children over age 5.

C. **Pathophysiology and management**

1. The disorder is characterized by encephalopathy and fatty degeneration of the liver.

2. Cell mitochondria are injured and become large and swollen causing cerebral edema and fatty infiltration of the liver, kidneys, and heart.

3. Hyperammonemia results from a reduction in the enzyme that converts ammonia to urea.

4. The most important aspect of treatment is early diagnosis and agressive treatment.

5. Management of increased ICP and fluid and electrolyte imbalance is a primary concern; children are treated in the intensive care setting, and an arterial line and a central venous line are inserted to monitor hemodynamic status.

6. Fluids may be restricted and the child may need mechanical ventilation.

7. A drug-induced coma may result when phenobarbital or pentobarbital with pancuronium (Pavulon) is given to paralyze skeletal muscles; hypoglycemia is controlled with hypertonic glucose and saline solution; vitamin K may be given to correct abnormal clotting.

D. **Clinical assessment findings**

1. **Although Reye's syndrome progresses in stages, deterioration can occur in 24 to 48 hours.**

2. Stage I: vomiting, lethargy, confusion, rhythmic slowing of EEG, liver dysfunction.

3. Stage II: disorientation, combativeness, hyperventilation, hallucinations, appropriate responses to painful stimuli, liver dysfunction.

4. Stage III: coma, decorticate rigidity, hyperventilation, preservation of pupillary and ocular reflexes.

5. Stage IV: deepened coma, decerebrate rigidity, loss of oculocephalic reflexes, large fixed pupils, evidence of brain stem dysfunction.

6: Stage V: seizures, flaccidity, respiratory arrest, loss of deep tendon reflexes.

E. **Diagnostic assessment findings**

1. Elevated alanine aminotransferase (ALT; formerly SGOT), as-

partate aminotransferase (AST; formerly SGPT), and lactic de-
hydrogenase (LDH) levels.

   2. Elevated ammonia levels and prolonged prothrombin time.
   3. In children with hypoglycemia, an acid-base imbalance with
       both respiratory alkalosis and metabolic acidosis.
   4. Liver biopsy establishes a definitive diagnosis.

F. Nursing diagnoses

   1. Risk for injury
   2. Risk for aspiration
   3. Altered body temperature
   4. Anxiety
   5. Sensory and perceptual alterations
   6. Altered family processes
   7. Ineffective breathing pattern
   8. Pain

G. Planning and implementation

   1. **Monitor for increased ICP by taking regular arterial and
       venous pressures, monitoring blood gas levels, and check-
       ing neurologic status.**
   2. *Keep in mind that the priority intervention is prevention and
       early identification; do not give aspirin to children with viral in-
       fections.*
   3. Maintain airway (usually on ventilator).
   4. Control increased ICP (see section III, G) and seizures (see
       section IV, G).
   5. Control hyperthermia with acetaminophen, tepid baths, and
       hypothermia blanket.
   6. Children may also have indwelling urinary catheter; monitor
       I&O and institute proper technique to prevent infection.
   7. Children may also have nasogastric tube to prevent compres-
       sion; monitor output for amount and character.
   8. Because the child who is in a drug-induced coma is totally de-
       pendent on caregivers, satisfy all biologic needs; provide sen-
       sory stimulation; ensure adequate nutritional intake, usually in-
       travenously or by nasogastric tube until child can take food
       orally.
   9. Support family members; allow them to express their concerns
       and provide information on the disease process and treatment.
       Parents may feel guilty if they administered aspirin to the child.

H. Evaluation

   1. The child is free of injury and further infection.
   2. The child receives adequate nutrition.
   3. The child receives adequate sensory stimulation.
   4. The child recovers with little or no neurologic deficit.

VIII. Brain tumors

A. Description: intracranial space-occupying lesions.

B. Etiology and incidence

1. **Most common childhood solid tumor; second most common childhood cancer**
2. Most commonly seen in the 5- to 10-year-old group
3. Classified according to histology and location: two thirds of tumors are *infratentorial* (below the tentorium), which includes the cerebellum, fourth ventricle, and brain stem; one-third are *supratentorial* (above the tentorium). Most tumors are gliomas, originating from the glial cells, the supporting structural cells of the CNS.

C. Pathophysiology and management

1. Tumor or tumors enlarge and obstruct the circulation of CSF resulting in increased ICP. As the tumor grows, it exerts pressure on nervous system components.
2. Surgery, and possibly radiation, may be needed, especially if the tumor cannot be excised. If the tumor is a glioma or medulloblastoma, chemotherapy may be used with steroids administered to decrease cerebral edema. Supportive therapy is indicated as well.

D. Clinical assessment findings

1. **Characteristic findings usually are related to location of the tumor.**
2. **Most common symptom is headache, usually intermittent and most common after the child wakes up, but also occurs with sneezing, coughing, and straining during a bowel movement.**
3. Usually vomiting is projectile and occurs in the morning.
4. Other characteristic signs and symptoms: ataxia, hypotonia, and decreased reflexes are commonly reported in cerebellar tumors.
5. Children may also display behavior changes, changes in dexterity, weakness, spasticity, paralysis, and slurred speech with cerebral involvement.
6. Seizures, increased blood pressure, decreased pulse, and visual problems may also be seen.

E. Diagnostic assessment findings

1. CT scan and MRI may detect lesion.
2. Angiography may determine the source of the tumor's blood supply.

F. Nursing diagnoses

1. Sensory and perceptual alterations

  2. Risk for injury
  3. Pain
  4. Altered family processes
  5. Anxiety
  6. Anticipatory grieving

G. **Planning and implementation**

 1. Preoperative

  a. Prepare family and child for head shaving, bandaging, the intensive care unit (ICU) and monitoring, facial edema, and headache.

 2. Postoperative

  a. Monitor vital signs and neurologic status frequently during the first 24 to 48 hours after surgery.

  b. Position child to prevent pressure on operative site.

  c. Elevate head to decrease edema and promote venous drainage from the cranial vault.

  d. Provide eye care to prevent corneal irritation.

  e. Monitor for cerebral edema and increased ICP.

  f. Provide analgesia for headaches.

  g. Observe for seizure activity; child may receive anticonvulsant medications.

  h. Monitor incision for signs of infection.

  i. Prepare family for procedures and treatments, and for radiation and chemotherapy, if needed.

  j. Support family who may need to address death and dying issues or deficits created by tumor.

 3. Encourage child and family to verbalize their fears.

H. **Evaluation**

 1. The child recovers and returns to optimal function.

 2. The child remains free of infection and other complications.

 3. The child and family verbalize their feelings.

 4. The family helps devise a realistic discharge plan.

IX. Head injury

A. **Description: anything from a mild bump to severe damage to the head.**

B. **Etiology and incidence**

 1. **Head injury is one of the most common causes of disability and death in children.**

 2. Head injury usually is caused by motor vehicle accidents, abuse, falls, and birth trauma, with the etiology related to the child's age.

C. **Pathophysiology and management**

 1. Pathophysiology and management are directly related to the force of the impact.

2. Intracranial contents are damaged when the force is too great to be absorbed by the skull.

☀ 3. **Types of head traumas include:**
   a. **Skull fractures**
   b. **Brain injury**
   c. **Hematomas**

4. Therapeutic interventions depend on symptoms, which must be closely observed and monitored. Surgical evacuation of hematomas may be needed and may be facililtated by burr holes for evacuation and relief of increased ICP.

D. Clinical assessment findings

1. Skull fractures: Type, extent, and accompanying symptoms depend on the velocity, force, and mass of the object; on the area of skull involved; and on the age of the child. Fracture types include:

   ☀ a. **Linear: resembles a thin line; usually no other signs than those found on x-ray film; child is observed for neurologic changes; fracture heals on its own.**
   b. **Comminuted: "cracked eggshell" appearance, may also be classified as depressed.**
   c. **Depressed: skull indented at point of impact, which may cause compression, shifting of brain tissue, and intercranial damage; symptoms depend on area damaged.**
   d. **Basal: linear fracture through base of skull; classic signs are "raccoon eyes," and a "battle sign" (bruising behind ear from bleeding into mastoid sinus); possible CSF leak into ears or nose.**

2. Brain injury: signs and symptoms depend on location and severity; posttraumatic syndromes (seizures, hydrocephalus, focal neurological deficits) and metabolic complications (diabetes insipidus, hyponatremia or hypernatremia, hyperglycemic hyperosmolar states) may occur; all of these may occur up to 2 years after the injury.

3. Hematomas: *epidural* (between the skull and the dura) and *subdural* (between dura and arachnoid layer) are most common types.
   a. Epidural: rapid onset, life-threatening, characterized by rapid deterioration, headache, seizures, coma, brain herniation with compression of the brain stem.
   b. Subdural: occurs within 48 hours of injury, characterized by headache, agitation, confusion, drowsiness, decrease LOC, and increased ICP; chronic subdurals may also occur.

    4. General minor characteristics of head trauma:
        a. May or may not involve loss of consciousness
        b. Transient confusion
        c. Listlessness and irritability
        d. Pallor and vomiting
    5. Signs of progression
        a. Altered mental status
        b. Increasing agitation
        c. Development of focal signs
        d. Marked changes in vital signs
        e. Reflexes hyporesponsive, hyperresponsive, or nonexistant

E. Diagnostic assessment findings
    1. Fractures may be visualized by radiography.
    2. Brain injuries and hematomas are viewed by CT or MRI.
    3. Complete blood count, blood chemistries, toxicology screening and urinalysis.

F. Nursing diagnoses
    1. Risk for injury
    2. Altered tissue perfusion
    3. Ineffective breathing pattern
    4. Sensory and perceptual alterations
    5. Risk for infection
    6. Anticipatory grieving
    7. Altered health maintenance

G. Planning and implementation
    1. Promote prevention, especially of falls. Urge pediatric clients to wear bike helmets, seat belts, and practice safe driving.
    2. Perform neurologic assessments of cerebral functioning (alertness, orientation, memory, speech); vital signs (check for increased blood pressure, decreased pulse); pupils; motor and sensory function (testing must be appropriate for developmental stage).

    3. Assess for other injuries, especially cervical. Raise head of bed to 30 degrees if there is no cervical injury.
    4. Monitor for complications, which can develop rapidly; monitor vital signs and neurologic status frequently; check for increased ICP; check for drainage from nose and ears (CSF, blood).
    5. Utilize planning and intervention strategies for increased ICP (see section III, G).
    6. Provide child and family teaching:
        a. Cover posttraumatic syndrome and signs and symptoms of same (see section IX, E).
        b. Teach that seizures may occur for up to 2 years after injury.

        c.   Explain that child may also have extensive damage requiring rehabilitation.

        d.   Explain all tests and procedures.

    7.   Encourage child and family to verbalize their concerns and refer them to the National Head Injury Foundation, if needed.

H.   Evaluation

    1.   Child remains free of further injury.

    2.   Child returns to an optimal level of functioning.

    3.   Child has minimal or no complications from injury.

    4.   Child and family verbalize home care, follow-up, and prevention methods.

X.   **Mental retardation (MR)**

    A.   Description: part of a broad category of developmental disability and defined by the American Association of Mental Deficiency as ". . . significantly subaverage, general intellectual functioning existing concurrently with deficits in adaptive behavior and manifested during the developmental period (18 years of age)."

    B.   Etiology and incidence

        1.   A diagnosis of MR cannot be made on the basis of intellectual ability alone; there must be both intellectual and adaptive (personal independence and social responsibility) impairment.

        2.   **Causes are genetic, biochemical, viral, and developmental: infection and intoxication, trauma or physical agent (lack of oxygen), metabolic disturbance, nutrition, gross postnatal brain disease (neurofibromatosis, tuberous sclerosis), chromosomal abnormalities, prematurity, low birth weight, autism, and environmental deprivation.**

        3.   Associated factors include maternal lifestyles (poor nutrition, smoking, substance abuse). Chromosomal disorders account for 20% to 25% of MR, with most related to Down's syndrome; 25% specific disorders; 10% to 20% cerebral palsy, microcephaly, or infantile spasms.

    C.   Pathophysiology and management

        1.   Pathophysiology and management and prognosis depend on cause; early diagnosis and prompt treatment may be particularly important in cases involving an identifiable and possibly correctable cause, such as phenylketonuria (PKU), malnutrition, or child abuse.

        2.   Diagnosis usually is made after period of suspicion; may be made at birth from recognition of specific syndromes such as Down's syndrome. Diagnosis and classification are based on standard IQ test scores.

        3.   The treatment goal is to promote optimal development.

Preventive measures include regular prenatal care, support for high-risk infants, rubella immunization, genetic counseling, education, and injury reduction.

D. **Clinical assessment findings**

1. Findings vary depending on the classification or degree of retardation.

2. **Mild (50 to 70 IQ)**
    a. Preschool: often not noted as retarded, but slow to walk, talk, and feed self.
    b. Schoolage: can acquire practical skills, and learn to read and do arithmetic to 6th grade level with special education classes; achieves mental age of 8 to 12 years.
    c. Adult: can usually achieve social and vocational skills; may need occasional guidance; may handle marriage but not childrearing.

3. **Moderate (35 to 55 IQ)**
    a. Preschool: noticeable delays, especially in speech.
    b. Schoolage: can learn simple communication, health and safety habits, simple manual skills; mental age of 3 to 7 years.
    c. Adult: can perform simple tasks under sheltered conditions; can travel alone to familiar places; usually needs help with self- maintenance.

4. **Severe (20 to 40 IQ)**
    a. Preschool: marked motor delay; little to no communication skills; may respond to training in elementary self-help such as feeding.
    b. Schoolage: usually walks with disability; some understanding of speech and response; can respond to habit training; mental age of toddler.
    c. Adult: can conform to daily routines and repetitive activities; needs constant direction and supervision in protective environment.

5. **Profound (below 20 IQ)**
    a. Preschool: gross retardation; capacity for function in sensorimotor areas; needs total care.
    b. Schoolage: obvious delays in all areas; shows basic emotional response; may respond to skillful training in use of legs, hands, and jaws; needs close supervision; mental age of young infant.
    c. Adult: may walk; needs complete custodial care; has primitive speech; usually benefits from regular physical activity.

E. **Nursing diagnoses**
1. Impaired verbal communication
2. Altered family processes
3. Altered growth and development
4. Altered health maintenance
5. Altered role performance
6. Self-care deficits
7. Risk for impaired skin integrity
8. Impaired social interaction
9. Social isolation

F. **Planning and implementation**
1. Support the family at time of initial diagnosis by actively listening to their feelings and concerns and assessing their composite strengths.
2. Facilitate the child's self-care abilities by encouraging the parents to enroll the child in an early stimulation program, establishing a self-feeding program, initiating independent toileting, and establishing an independent grooming program (all developmentally appropriate).
3. Promote optimal development by encouraging self-care goals and emphasizing the universal needs of children, such as play, social interaction, and parental limit setting.
4. Promote anticipatory guidance and problem solving by encouraging discussion regarding physical maturation and sexual behaviors.
5. Assist family in planning for the child's future needs (alternative to home care, especially as the parents near old age); refer them to community agencies.
6. Provide child and family teaching:
   a. Identify normal developmental milestones and appropriate stimulating activities, including play and socialization.
   b. Discuss the need for patience with the child's slow attainment of developmental milestones.
   c. Inform parents about stimulation, safety, and motivation.
   d. Supply information regarding normal speech development and how to accentuate nonverbal cues, such as facial expressions and body language, to help cue speech development.
   e. Explain the need for discipline that is simple, consistent, and appropriate to the child's development.
   f. Review an adolescent's need for simple, practical sexual information that includes anatomy, physical development, and conception.
   g. Demonstrate ways to foster learning other that verbal ex-

planation because the child is better able to deal with concrete objects than abstract concepts.

    h.   Point out the importance of positive self-esteem, built by accomplishing small successes, in motivating the child to accomplish other tasks.

G. Evaluation

1. The child participates in self-care activities appropriate for his or her abilities.
2. The child and the family are actively involved in early intervention programs and appropriate special education programs.
3. Parents verbalize understanding of appropriate discipline and recreational and social activities.
4. Family members express feelings and concerns regarding the child's limited abilities.
5. Family members verbalize realistic goals for the care of the child.
6. The family demonstrates acceptance of the child.

XI. Down's syndrome

A. Description: most common chromosomal abnormality, formerly called mongolism.

B. Etiology and incidence

1. Occurs more in whites than other groups.
2. Cause unknown; multiple theories; concept of multiple causality most accepted.
3. Cytogenetics of the disorder well established; approximately 92% to 95% of cases attributed to an extra chromosome 21, hence the name *trisomy 21*.
4. Children with Down's syndrome are born to parents of all ages; there is a higher incidence among mothers over age 35, but most are born to mothers under age 35 (80%).

C. Pathophysiology and management

1. About 4% of cases may be caused by translocation of chromosomes 15 and 21 or 22; this usually is hereditary and has no bearing on age. From 1% to 3% of persons demonstrate mosaicism (cells with both normal and abnormal chromosomes).
2. The degree of cognitive and physical impairment is related to the percentage of cells with the abnormal chromosome makeup.
3. Diagnosis is made by physical examination and chromosomal analysis.
4. Although there is no cure, surgery may be used to correct congenital defects and some cosmetic surgeries may "normalize" the child's appearance. Behavior modification may be recommended for dealing with negative behaviors.

D. **Clinical assessment findings**
1. Most common findings include separated sagittal suture, oblique palpebral fissures, small nose, depressed nasal bridge, high-arched palate, skin excess and laxity, wide space between big and second toe, plantar crease between big and second toe, hyperextensible and lax joints, muscle weakness.
2. Other common findings include small penis; short, broad hands (transverse [simian] palmar crease); protruding tongue; small ears; Brushfield spots; dry skin.
3. Associated problems and features:
   a. Intelligence varies from severely retarded to low-normal.
   b. Social development may be 2 to 3 years beyond mental age; temperament range is similar to normal children, with a trend toward the easy child.
   c. Congenital anomalies: 30% to 40% have congenital heart disease, especially septal defects, renal agenesis, duodenal atresia, Hirschsprung's disease, tracheoesophageal fistula, and skeletal deformities.
   d. Sensory problems include strabismus, nystagmus, myopia, hyperopia, excessive tearing and cataracts, conductive hearing loss.
   e. Other physical disorders include respiratory infections, leukemia, thyroid disfunction.
4. Growth is reduced, with rapid weight gain.
5. Sexual development may be delayed, incomplete, or both. Male genitalia and secondary characteristics are underdeveloped. Breast development is mild to moderate with menarche at appropriate age. Women may be fertile; men are infertile.

E. **Nursing diagnoses**
Same as for MR, plus diagnoses relevant to the associated problems and features, especially:
1. Impaired physical mobility (hypertonicity)
2. Risk for injury (hypertonicity)
3. Impaired gas exchange (decreased muscle tone compromises respiratory expansion)
4. Risk for infection
5. Infant feeding pattern is ineffective (protruding tongue)
6. Constipation
7. Impaired skin integrity

F. **Planning and implementation**
1. Implement the same as for MR plus planning and intervention strategies for the associated problems and features.
2. Encourage genetic counseling.
3. Explain hypertonicity and joint hyperextensibility to parents,

and that the child's resultant lack of clinging is physiologic and not a sign of detachment.

4. Clear nose with bulb syringe; use cool mist vaporizer; perform chest physiotherapy when needed; provide good hand washing and avoid exposing child to infection.
5. When feeding, use small, straight-handled spoon to push food to the side and back of mouth.
6. Encourage fluids and foods rich in fiber.
7. Provide good skin care.

G. Evaluation

1. Implement the same as for MR plus evaluation of goals relevant to the associated problems and features.
2. Parents will verbalize understanding of child's hypertonicity and hyperextensibility.
3. The child will remain free of infection.
4. The child will maintain adequate nutrition.
5. The child will have normal bowel elimination.
6. The child's skin will remain intact.

Bibliography

Alfaro-LeFevre, R., et al. (1992). *Drug Handbook: A Nursing Process Approach.* Redwood City, CA: Addison-Wesley.

Betz, C.L., Hunsberger, M.M., and Wright, S. (1994). *Family Centered Nursing Care of Children,* 2nd ed. Philadelphia: W.B. Saunders.

Castiglia, P.T. and Harbin, R.B. (1993). *Child Health Care: Process and Practice.* Philadelphia: J.B. Lippincott.

Finke, L.M., et al. (1993). National workshop: Implementation of practices with severely mentally and emotionally disturbed children and adolescents. *Journal of Child and Adolescent Psychiatric Mental Health Nursing, 6,* 31.

Hauser, W.A. (1994). The prevalence and incidence of convulsive disorders in children. *Epilepsia, 35,* 51.

Jackson, D.B. and Saunders, R.B. (1993). *Child Health Nursing: A Comprehensive Approach to the Care of Children and Their Families.* Philadelphia: J.B. Lippincott.

Louis, P.T. (1994). Reye's syndrome. In Oski, F.A., et al (Eds.). *Principles and Practice of Pediatrics,* 2nd ed. Philadelphia: J.B. Lippincott.

Sizer, F. and Whitney, E. (1994). *Nutrition Concepts and Controversies,* 6th ed. Minneapolis/St. Paul: West Publishing.

Wong, D.L. (1993). *Whaley and Wong's Essentials of Pediatric Nursing,* 4th ed. St. Louis: C.V. Mosby.

Wong, D.L. (1995). *Whaley and Wong's Nursing Care of infants and Children,* 5th ed. St. Louis: C.V. Mosby.

STUDY QUESTIONS

1. When performing assessment of a newborn, the pediatric nurse would expect to note all of the following infantile reflexes, except:
   a. Moro
   b. Grasp
   c. Rooting
   d. Parachute

2. When caring for a child with increased intracranial pressure, the nurse understands that the rationale for elevating the head of the bed 15 to 45 degrees includes all of the following except:
   a. To let the child see better without lifting the head
   b. To help alleviate headache
   c. To reduce intra-abdominal pressure
   d. To increase intrathoracic pressure

3. Early clinical manifestations of increased intracranial pressure in older children include:
   a. Macewen's sign
   b. Setting sun sign
   c. Papilledema
   d. Diplopia

4. Which of the following is not a priority nursing objective for a child with a seizure disorder?
   a. Teach the family about anticonvulsant drug therapy
   b. Assess for signs and symptoms of increased ICP
   c. Ensure safety and protection from injury
   d. Observe and record all seizures

5. When preparing parents to address their child's unique psychological needs related to epilepsy, the nurse should point out to the parents that the child may experience additional stress related to all of the following except:
   a. Poor self-image
   b. Dependency
   c. Feeling different from peers
   d. Cognitive delays

6. Which of the following is the most useful tool in diagnosing seizure disorder?
   a. Electroencephalography
   b. Lumbar puncture
   c. Brain scan
   d. Skull radiographs

7. Which of the following definitions most accurately describes meningocele?
   a. Complete exposure of the spinal cord and meninges
   b. Herniation of spinal cord and meninges into a sac
   c. Sac formation containing meninges and spinal fluid
   d. Spinal cord tumor containing nerve roots

8. The primary reason for surgical repair of a myelomeningocele is to:
   a. Correct the neurologic defect
   b. Prevent hydrocephalus
   c. Prevent epilepsy
   d. Decrease the risk of infection

9. Adolescents with seizure disorders need teaching and counseling on all of the following except:
   a. Obtaining a driver's license
   b. Increased risk for infections
   c. Drug and alcohol use
   d. Peer pressure

10. The development of Reye's syndrome has been associated with the use of aspirin and:
    a. Influenza
    b. Meningitis
    c. Encephalitis
    d. Strep throat

11. Characteristics of brain tumors in children include all of the following except:
    a. Headache after awakening
    b. Projectile vomiting
    c. Behavioral changes
    d. Decreased blood pressure

12. Signs of mild mental retardation include:
    a. Lateness in walking
    b. Mental age of a toddler
    c. Noticeable developmental delays
    d. Very obvious developmental delays

13. Clinical manifestations of Down's syndrome include:
    a. Large nose
    b. Small tongue
    c. Oblique palpebral fissures
    d. Low-arched palate

14. The American Association of Mental Deficiency's definition of mental retardation stresses:
    a. No responsiveness to contact
    b. Deficits in adaptive behavior with intellectual impairment
    c. Cognitive impairment occurring after age 22 years
    d. IQ level must be below 50

ANSWER KEY

1. *Correct response: d*
   The parachute reflex appears at approximately 9 months of age.
   a, b, and c. All are infantile reflexes that are present at birth and that subside at approximately age 3 months.
   Knowledge/Health Promotion/ Assessment

2. *Correct response: d*
   Head elevation decreases intrathoracic pressure.
   a, b, and c. All are appropriate rationales for increasing the elevation of the head of the bed in a child with increased intracranial pressure.
   Application/Safe Care/Implementation

3. *Correct response: d*
   Diplopia is an early sign of increased intracranial pressure in an older child.
   a and b. Macewen's sign (cracked pot sign) and the setting sun appearance of the eyes are noted in infants with increased intracranial pressure.
   c. Papilledema is a late sign of increased intracranial pressure.
   Application/Physiologic/Assessment

4. *Correct response: b*
   Signs and symptoms of increased intracranial pressure are not associated with seizure activity.
   a. Improper administration of and incomplete compliance with anticonvulsant therapy can lead to status epilepticus.
   c. Safety is always a priority in the care of a child with a seizure disorder; seizures may occur at any given time.
   d. Careful observation and documentation of seizures provide valuable information to aid prevention and treatment.
   Application/Safe Care/Planning

5. *Correct response: d*
   Children with seizure disorders do not necessarily have cognitive delays.

a, b, and c. All of these factors can put additional stress on a child trying to understand and manage chronic illness.
Comprehension/Health Promotion/ Planning

6. *Correct response: a*
   The electroencephalogram detects abnormal electrical activity in the brain. The pattern of various spikes can help a physician diagnose specific seizure disorders.
   b. Lumbar puncture confirms problems related to cerebral spinal fluid infection or trauma.
   c. Brain scans confirm space-occupying lesions.
   d. Skull radiographs can detect fractures and structural abnormalities.
   Knowledge/Physiologic/Assessment

7. *Correct response: c*
   Meningocele is a sac formation containing meninges and cerebrospinal fluid (CSF).
   a. Meningocele does not involve complete exposure of the spinal cord and meninges; this is a massive defect that is incompatible with life.
   b. Myelomeningocele is a herniation of the spinal cord, meninges, and CSF into a sac that protrudes through a defect in the vertebral arch.
   d. Tumor formation is not associated with this defect.
   Knowledge/Physiologic/Assessment

8. *Correct response: d*
   Surgical closure decreases the risk of infection stemming from damage to the fragile sac, which can lead to meningitis.
   a. The neurologic deficit cannot be corrected; however, some surgeons believe that early surgery reduces the risk of stretching spinal nerves and preventing further damage.

b. Surgical repair does not help relieve hydrocephalus; in fact, some researchers believe that repair exaggerates the Arnold-Chiari malformation and decreases the absorptive surface for CSF, leading to more rapid development of hydrocephalus.

c. Surgical repair of the sac does not prevent epilepsy, which is impairment of the brain neuron tissue.

Knowledge/Physiologic/Analysis

9. *Correct response: b*
Adolescents with seizure disorders are at no greater risk for infections than other adolescents.

a. Obtaining a driver's license may be influenced by the adolescent's seizure history.

c. Drug and alcohol use may interfere with or create side effects from anticonvulsant medications.

d. Peer pressure may put the child at risk for increased risk-taking behaviors that may exacerbate seizure activity.

*Application/Health Promotion/
Implementation*

10. *Correct response: a*
Reye's syndrome has been associated with the ingestion of aspirin in children with viral infections such as influenza.

b. The is no association with meningitis and the development of Reye's syndrome.

c. Encephalitis is a component of Reye's syndrome.

d. There is no association with bacterial infections such as strep throat.

*Comprehension/Health Promotion/
Evaluation*

11. *Correct response: d*
Children with brain tumors may demonstrate signs of increased intracranial pressure such as increased blood pressure.

a, b, and c. All are characteristic signs of brain tumor in children.

Analysis/Physiologic/Assessment

12. *Correct response: a*
Mild mental retardation is minimally noticeable in young children, with one of the signs being a delay in achieving developmental milestones.

b. Severe mental retardation is marked by the mental age of a toddler.

c. Children with moderate mental retardation have noticeable developmental delays.

d. Profound mental retardation is marked by very obvious and severe developmental delays.

Comprehension/Psychosocial/Assessment

13. *Correct response: c*
Oblique palpebral fissure is another term for the "mongolian slant" of the eyes of children with Down's syndrome.

a. Children with Down's syndrome have small noses with a wide nasal bridge.

b. Children with Down's syndrome have large protruding tongues.

d. Children with Down's syndrome tend to have high-arched palates.

Comprehensive/Physiologic/Assessment

14. *Correct response: b*
The definition states that besides subaverage functioning, the child must exhibit deficits in adaptive behavior.

a. An early behavioral sign suggestive of cognitive impairment but not part of the definition.

c. The definition states that cognitive impairment or compromise must occur before age 18 years.

d. IQ 70 or below is considered significant subaverage intellectual functioning.

Knowledge/Psychosocial/Assessment

Endocrine Dysfunction

I. Essential concepts: endocrine system structures and function

A. Development

1. Most endocrine glands and structures develop during the first trimester of gestation.

2. The thyroid develops in three stages between the seventh and fourteenth week of gestation.

3. The parathyroid is recognizable between 5 and 7 weeks of gestation.

4. The pancreas forms from two different cells that fuse to form a single organ at the seventh week of gestation; insulin can be detected in beta cells several weeks later.

5. The pituitary originates from fusion of two ectodermal processes. The primordia of anterior and posterior segments can be seen by the fourth week of gestation, and the gland takes its permanent shape and location in the sella turcica between the third and fourth month.

6. The adrenal gland reaches its maximal size by the fourth month of gestation. The medulla arises from the ectoderm via the neural crest; the cortex, from the lateral plate of the embryonic mesoderm. Both corticosterone and aldosterone are secreted in utero.

B. Function

1. The endocrine system consists of:
    a. Cells that transmit chemical signals via hormones
    b. Target cells or end organs that receive the chemical messages
    c. An environment through which the chemical is transported (lymph, blood, extracellular fluids)

2. The endocrine glands are as follows:
    a. *Pituitary gland* consists of two portions:
        (1) Anterior (adenohypophysis): secretes somatotropic hormone (STH), growth hormone (GH), thyrotropin (thyroid-stimulating hormone [TSH]), adrenocorticotropic hormone (ACTH), gonadotropins, follicle-stimulating hormone (FSH), luteinizing hormone (LH), prolactin, and melanocyte-stimulating hormone (MSH).
        (2) Posterior (neurohypophysis) that secretes antidiuretic hormone (ADH) and oxytocin.
    b. *Thyroid gland:* secretes thyroxine (T4), triiodothyronine (T3), and thyrocalcitonin.
    c. *Parathyroid gland:* secretes parathyroid hormone (PTH).
    d. *Adrenal glands* consists of two portions
        (1) Adrenal cortex: secretes mineralocorticoids (aldosterone), sex hormones (androgens, estrogens, progesterone), and glucocorticoids (cortisol, corticosterone).
        (2) Adrenal medulla: secretes epinephrine and norepinephrine.
    e. The *islets of Langerhans of the pancreas:* secrete insulin (beta-cells), glucagon (alpha-cells), and somatostatin.
    f. *Ovaries:* secrete estrogen and progesterone.
    g. *Testes:* secrete testosterone.

3. The endocrine system regulates energy production, growth, fluid and electrolyte balance, response to stress, and sexual reproduction.

4. Hormonal regulation is based on a negative feedback system.

5. The anterior pituitary or "master gland" is primarily responsible for stimulation and inhibition of target glandular secretions.
6. Most endocrine disorders are chronic in nature and require ongoing care related to health maintenance, education, development, and psychosocial needs.

II. Endocrine system overview

A. Assessment

1. Health history should focus on family history of endocrine disorders, prenatal history, history of chronic childhood disease, and growth and development patterns.
2. Many endocrine disorders present with alterations in weight, height, or sexual development, either alone or in combination.
3. Other common presenting signs and symptoms include:
   a. Neurologic symptoms, such as blurred vision, faintness, nervousness, confusion
   b. Changes in facial features, hair, or skin
   c. Polydipsia or polyuria

B. Laboratory studies and diagnostic tests

1. Important blood chemistry studies include thyroid function tests and hormone, calcium, phosphorus, alkaline phosphatase, and electrolyte levels.
2. Urine studies in endocrine assessment evaluate sodium, calcium, phosphorus, and glucose levels and specific gravity.
3. Radiographic studies are done to evaluate bone age and density, as well as soft tissue calcification.
4. Genetic studies may detect enzyme deficiencies (*e.g.*, congenital adrenal hypoplasia).

C. Psychosocial implications

1. Preparing a child for invasive procedures and tests requires sensitivity to the child's developmental needs.
2. Parents and children need the opportunity to express their concerns and fears before and after diagnosis and throughout the course of treatment.
3. The nurse should realistically reinforce the parents' and child's expectations of treatment and prospects for improvement.
4. A young child may interpret therapy, such as daily or weekly hormonal injections, as punishment for wrongdoing; this child needs clear communication to help him or her distinguish between disease treatment and disciplinary measures.
5. Injections may be a source of fearful fantasies and may enhance a child's body mutilation anxieties.

III. Hypopituitarism

A. Description: a condition resulting from diminished or deficient secretion of pituitary hormones, usually growth hormone (GH).

B. **Etiology and incidence**

1. Hypopituitarism may be caused by several conditions, including developmental defects, destructive lesions such as tumors or trauma, certain hereditary disorders, or functional disorders such as anorexia nervosa or psychosocial dwarfism.

2. The most common organic cause is a tumor in the pituitary or hypothalamic region, especially craniopharyngiomas.

3. More than half the cases are idiopathic and related to GH deficiency.

C. **Pathophysiology and management**

1. GH deficiency produces varied effects, depending on the degree of dysfunction, including:

   a. Decreased synthesis of somatomedin, resulting in decreased linear growth.

   b. Inhibited transport of protein-building amino acids into cells and increased protein catabolism, leading to decreased muscle mass, thin hair, poor skin quality, and delayed growth.

   ·c. Decreased fat catabolism and increased glucose uptake in muscles, resulting in excessive subcutaneous fat and hypoglycemia.

2. Associated deficiencies of other hormones, such as ACTH, TSH, LH, and FSH, produce effects related to the functions of these hormones.

3. A complete diagnostic evaluation includes family history (midparental height is an important prognosticator of the child's ultimate height), a history of the child's growth patterns and previous health status (to rule out prenatal maternal disorders that affect growth and to check for evidence of chronic illness in the child), physical examination with accurate measurements, psychosocial evaluation, and radiographic and endocrine studies.

4. Treatment of GH deficiency resulting from organic etiology is directed at correcting the underlying cause (*e.g.*, a tumor).

5. The definitive treatment for children with functional GH deficiency is GH replacement therapy, which succeeds about 80% of the time. A biosynthetic GH agent prepared by recombinant DNA technology is the therapy of choice. Other hormone deficiencies also require replacement.

6. Early diagnosis and treatment is crucial for children to achieve their genetic growth potential.

D. **Clinical assessment findings**

1. The chief presenting complaint is short stature.

2. Children generally grow during the first year, then follow a slow curve below the third percentile. Progressive growth slowing

suggests idiopathic hypopituitarism, whereas sudden slowing suggests a tumor.

3. Partial GH deficiency presents with less dramatic growth retardation.

4. Height increase may be slower than weight gain and child may even become obese.

5. Skeletal proportions are normal, but children appear younger than chronologic age.

6. Premature aging is common later in life.

7. Primary teeth usually appear when expected, but secondary tooth eruption is delayed.

8. Sexual development usually is delayed, but normal.

9. Most children have normal intelligence, but appear precocious, and emotional problems are common. Academic problems also are common as many of these children are not encouraged to perform at their chronologic age.

E. Diagnostic assessment findings

1. Bone age is younger than chronologic age but is closely related to height age, with the degree depending on duration of hormone deficiency.

2. Definitive diagnosis is made based on absence or subnormal reserves of pituitary GH. Became GH levels are normally low in children, GH secretions should be stimulated (followed by testing to assess serum levels of GH). Definitive diagnosis is based on radioimmunoassay of serum GH levels stimulated pharmacologically with two or more agents, which include insulin and levodopa; a GH level under 10 ng/mL after two tests confirms diagnosis.

3. Hypoglycemia

F. Nursing diagnoses

1. Body image disturbance
2. Family coping: potential for growth
3. Altered growth and development
4. Risk for injury
5. Knowledge deficit
6. Altered nutrition: more than body requirements
7. Self-esteem disturbance
8. Impaired social interaction

G. Planning and implementation

1. Identify children with growth problems (the primary nursing intervention).

2. Help parents promote their child's normal growth and development by teaching them about age-related developmental milestones and encouraging them to notify their primary care provider of abnormalities.

3. Prepare child for radiographic and endocrine studies; explain that endocrine studies may require multiple venipunctures or drawing of blood. Describe a heparin lock device as needed.

4. Monitor for early signs and symptoms of hypoglycemia, particularly during provocative tests for GH. If hypoglycemia occurs, elevate the child's blood glucose level rapidly by giving him or her orange juice.

5. Administer GH replacement therapy as prescribed; monitor for adverse reactions stemming from antibody production. Optimal dosing usually is achieved when GH is given at bedtime because physiologic release is more normally stimulated by pituitary release of GH during the first 45 to 90 minutes of sleep.

6. Assess for GH overdose:
   a. Acute overdose marked by initial hypoglycemia followed by hyperglycemia.
   b. Chronic overdose marked by signs and symptoms of acromegaly (overgrowth).

7. Implement meal planning to ensure that the child receives adequate nutrition for optimal growth.

8. Help promote the child's self-esteem and a positive self-image by encouraging him or her to express feelings and concerns and to focus on personal strengths and assets.

9. Encourage parents to emphasize the child's positive aspects and abilities, rather then dwell on the child's size.

10. Promote child's social adjustment by encouraging interpersonal relationships with peers and involvement with special peer counseling groups.

11. Promote functional family coping by referring parents and child to a support group composed of parents and children with similar disabilities.

12. Provide child and family teaching, covering:
   a. Diagnosis and nature of the disorder
   b. GH administration, including dosage schedule, administration techniques, what to do if a dose is missed, and adverse reactions
   c. Realistic expectations for the child's growth, based on age, personal abilities and strengths, and the effectiveness of GH replacement therapy
   d. The importance of continual medical supervisionand compliance with drug therapy and follow-up visits

H. Evaluation

1. The child demonstrates a positive response to GH therapy, manifested by a height increase of 3 inches to 5 inches during the first year of therapy and less dramatic but measurable increases in subsequent years.

2. Parents report normal growth and developmental milestones for their child.
3. The child and the parents verbalize an understanding of the signs and symptoms of hypoglycemia and the appropriate actions to take should they occur.
4. The child and parents voice an understanding of diet planning and food selection.
5. The child interacts appropriately with his or her peer group.
6. The child verbalizes his or her feelings or concerns as well as personal strengths and assets.
7. Parents identify family strengths and available community support systems.
8. The child and parents express an understanding that GH deficiency is a chronic problem and that therapeutic care is necessary until young adulthood.

IV. Cushing's syndrome

A. Description: a cluster of clinical abnormalities resulting from excessive levels of adrenocortical hormones, particularly cortisol, and to a lesser extent, related corticosteroids, androgens, and aldosterone.

B. Etiology and incidence

1. The cause can fall into one of four general categories:
   a. Pituitary with adrenal hyperplasia, usually from excessive ACTH
   b. Adrenal with hypersecretion of glucocorticoids, usually from adrenocortical neoplasms
   c. Ectopic with autonomous secretion of ACTH, usually from extrapituitary neoplasms
   d. Iatrogenic, usually from administration of large amounts of corticosteroids
2. Cushing's syndrome is uncommon in children but when it occurs, it is usually iatrogenic, reversible after gradual removal of the corticosteroids.

C. Pathophysiology and management

1. Ineffectiveness of the normal feedback mechanisms that control adrenocortical function results in excessive secretion of cortisol from the adrenal cortex despite adequate levels in circulation.
2. Clinical manifestations are the direct result of hormone excess (glucocortocoids, mineralocorticoids, and sex hormones); the predominant hormone excess—most commonly, glucocorticoids—determines the predominant manifestations.
3. Depending on the underlying cause, treatment may involve surgical removal or irradiation of adrenal or pituitary tumors, or adrenalectomy to resect hyperplastic tumors.

4. A child undergoing one of these treatments requires life-long hormone replacement as prescribed therapy; specific agents depend on the nature of the procedure and on the particular deficiencies.

D. **Clinical assessment findings**
   1. Centripetal fat distribution: truncal obesity, fat pads on supraclavicular and neck areas ("buffalo hump")
   2. Rounded or "moon" face, with reddened, oily skin
   3. Muscle wasting, thin extremities, pendulous abdomens
   4. Fragile, thin skin and subcutaneous tissue; acne, excessive bruising, petechiae
   5. Reddish, purple abdominal striae

 6. **Increased susceptibility to infection, poor wound healing**
   7. Elevated blood pressure
   8. Compression fractures of vertebrae, kyphosis, backache
   9. Retarded linear growth
   10. Irritability, insomnia, euphoria or depression, frank psychosis
   11. Precocious puberty in children
   12. Virilization in adolescent girls, marked by hirsutism, voice deepening, clitoral enlargement, breast atrophy, amenorrhea
   13. Loss of libido, impotence, and gynecomastia in adolescent boys

E. **Diagnostic assessment findings**
   1. Excessive plasma cortisol level
   2. Hyperglycemia, glycosuria, latent or overt diabetes
   3. Hypokalemia
   4. Hypocalcemia and alkalosis
   5. Elevated urine levels of 17-hydroxy-corticosteroid and 17-ketosteroid
   6. Decreased ACTH production on dexamethasone (cortisone) suppression test, helping to establish a more definitive diagnosis
   7. Identification of adrenal tumor on computed tomographic (CT) scan, ultrasonography, or angiography
   8. Location of pituitary tumor on CT scan of the head

F. **Nursing diagnoses**
   1. Risk for infection
   2. Activity intolerance
   3. Body image disturbance
   4. Ineffective individual coping
   5. Ineffective family coping
   6. Risk for injury
   7. Self-esteem disturbance
   8. Fluid volume excess
   9. Risk for impaired skin integrity

G.   Planning and implementation

1.   Prevent infection by practicing good hand washing and limiting the child's exposure to persons with infections.

2.   Help maintain skin integrity by providing and promoting good hygiene and skin care.

3.   In collaboration with dietitian and physician, implement meal planning to ensure good nutrition. Provide a high-protein, low-sodium diet with potassium supplements.

4.   Promote adequate rest to prevent fatigue.

5.   Administer prescribed medications, which may include:

   a.   Cortical hormone replacement therapy for a child with bi-lateral adrenalectomy.

   b.   GH, thyroid extract, antidiuretic hormone, gonadotropin, and steroid replacement for a child who has had a pituitary tumor removed.

6.   If Cushing's syndrome results from necessary steroid therapy, inform the child and family that the medication should never be abruptly stopped or a dose missed; either of these actions can precipitate an adrenal crisis. Reinforce this information as necessary. Explain that cushingoid symptoms caused by steroid therapy may be relieved by consulting with the physician who may recommend administering the steroids on an alternate-day basis and in the early morning.

7.   Monitor vital signs for cardiac irregularities and hypertension.

8.   Promote the child's positive self-image by encouraging him or her to vent fears and concerns and to identify personal assets and strengths.

9.   Provide child and family teaching, covering:

   a.   Diagnosis and nature of the disorder

   b.   Purpose of treatment and procedures

   c.   Reason for surgery, and its benefits and disadvantages

   d.   Dosage schedule, administration techniques, and side effects for all prescribed hormone replacements

   e.   Signs of acute adrenal insufficiency during the withdrawal of corticosteroid therapy

H.   Evaluation

1.   The child remains free of infection.

2.   The child and family verbalize understanding of meal planning and select appropriate foods.

3.   The child engages in activities appropriate to developmental level and condition.

4.   The child's skin remains intact and free of irritation or breakdown.

5.   The child maintains adequate fluid balance.

6.   The child and family voice feelings and concerns.

7. Family members identify individual family strengths and support systems.
8. The child and family state an understanding of each prescribed replacement hormone describing its action, dosage, administration, and possible adverse effects.
9. The child and family verbalize an understanding that Cushing's syndrome is a chronic illness that requires continual therapeutic management.

V. Diabetes mellitus (DM)

A. Description: results from either a relative (non—insulin-dependent [NIDDM], type-II) or and absolute (insulin-dependent [IDDM], type-I) deficiency of pancreatic insulin resulting in chronic high blood glucose levels and problems with fat and carbohydrate metabolism. The following information refers to insulin-dependent diabetes mellitus.

B. Etiology and incidence
1. IDDM is the most common endocrine disease of childhood, with a prevalence rate of about 20 per 100,00 children and adolescents. The peak incidence occurs between ages 10 and 15.
2. The etiology is unclear. Genetics play an important role in predisposition, but the diseases is not considered a genetic disorder.
3. There is some evidence that environmental factors, such as viruses, play a role in the cause.
4. There is also strong evidence to support an autoimmune response that somehow involves pancreatic beta cell destruction.

C. Pathophysiology and management
1. Insulin is needed to support carbohydrate, protein, and fat metabolism, primarily to facilitate entry of these substances into cells.
2. Destruction of 90% or more of the pancreatic beta cells results in a clinically significant drop in insulin secretion.
3. This loss of insulin, the major anabolic hormone, leads to a catabolic state characterized by decreased glucose use and increased glucose production, eventually resulting in *hyperglycemia.*
4. In a state of insulin deficiency, glucagon, epinephrine, growth hormone (GH), and cortisol levels increase, stimulating lipolysis, fatty acid release, and ketone production.
5. Persistent blood glucose concentration above 180 mg/dL (the renal threshold) results in glycosuria, leading to osmotic diuresis with polyuria and polydypsia.
6. **Excessive ketone production can cause *diabetic ketoacidosis (DKA),* an acutely life-threatening condition characterized by marked hyperglycemia, metabolic acidosis, dehydration,**

and altered level of consciousness ranging from lethargy to coma.

7. The *Somogyi effect*, a unique phenomenon in children late in the course of the disease, involves a temporary decrease in blood glucose level followed by rebound hyperglycemia.

8. Treatment measures in acute care involve restoring homeostasis through intravenous (IV) fluid infusion; continuous, regular low-dose insulin; and electrolyte replacement.

9. The goals of long-term therapy focus on restoring glycemic control through medication, exercise, and diet.

D. **Clinical assessment findings**

1. **The classic symptoms of diabetes mellitus are polydypsia, polyuria, polyphagia, and fatigue.**

2. Other symptoms include weight loss, dry skin, and blurred vision.

E. **Diagnostic assessment findings**

1. Fasting blood glucose level above 120 mg/dL

2. Random blood glucose level above 200 mg/dL

3. Glycosuria

4. In DKA: hyperglycemia, acidosis, glycosuria, and ketonuria

F. **Nursing diagnoses**

1. Acute care:
   a. Fluid volume deficit
   b. Risk for injury
   c. Impaired skin integrity
   d. Ineffective breathing pattern (metabolic acidosis)

2. Long-term care:
   a. Activity intolerance
   b. Ineffective individual coping
   c. Altered family processes
   d. Fluid volume deficit
   e. Risk for infection
   f. Knowledge deficit
   g. Altered nutrition: less than body requirements
   h. Powerlessness
   i. Impaired skin integrity

G. **Planning and implementation**

1. Acute care:
   a. Promote adequate fluid volume by maintaining accurate and careful records of IV fluid infusion, blood glucose level, intake and output (I&O), and urine specific gravity.
   b. Monitor electrolytes and cardiac status for signs of hypokalemia.

      c.   Administer continuous infusion of low-dose regular in-sulin, as prescribed.

      d.   Help prevent hypotension and convulsions by closely monitoring vital signs, cardiac status, and blood glucose levels.

      e.   Assess neurologic status by monitoring vital signs and noting any changes in level of consciousness.

      f.   Help maintain skin integrity by turning the child frequently and encouraging regular ambulation.

      g.   Protect the child from physical injury by keeping the bed's side rails up and padding hard surfaces that may cause pressure and injury to soft tissue and extremities.

2. Long-term care:

      a.   Assess child's and family's unique learning needs based on age, educational background, capacity to learn, and personal experience.

      b.   Assess child's and family's emotional and psychological state. Initial diagnosis may trigger shock and denial, which will hinder learning; acceptance of the disease is an important first step in learning to cope with long-term management.

      c.   Create a positive learning environment: comfortable temperature; quiet, unhurried atmosphere; sufficient supplemental educational materials.

      d.   Focus client and family teaching on survival skills:

         (1) Describe the disease process.

         (2) Explain urine and blood glucose testing.

         (3) Teach insulin administration and explain insulin therapy.

         (4) Identify signs and symptoms of hypoglycemia and hyperglycemia.

         (5) Cover meal planning (adequate intake for age, constant menus, complex carbohydrates, consistent eating times, and understanding the exchange list), skin care, and special problems.

         (6) Limit teaching sessions to no longer than 15 or 20 minutes, and teach one survival skill at a time.

         (7) Organize teaching to present simple information first and proceed to the more complex.

         (8) Evaluate how well the child and family understand the information by having them perform return demonstrations and provide verbal explanations.

      e.   Refer the family to an organization that can assist the family in coping with diabetes, such as the Juvenile Diabetes Foundation International.

      f.   Promote a sense of self-esteem in the child by encouraging him or her to express feelings and concerns and to identify personal strengths and positive aspects of his or her situation.

H.   Evaluation

1. The child maintains adequate fluid balance and desirable body weight.
2. The child maintains normal cardiac functioning.
3. The child remains injury free.
4. The child maintains skin integrity.
5. The child and family members verbalize understanding of the disease process, essential skills, and necessary follow-up care.
6. The child and family demonstrate proper insulin administration technique.
7. The child and family verbalize an understanding of the exchange diet and proper nutritional management.
8. The child maintains peer relationships that he or she had before diagnosis.
9. The child becomes involved in peer support groups.
10. Family members can identify family strengths and incorporate child's needs into family lifestyle.
11. The child and family members verbalize that diabetes mellitus is a chronic illness that requires ongoing therapeutic management.

Bibliography

Betz, C.L., Hunsberger, M.M., and Wright, S. (1994). *Family Centered Nursing Care of Children*, 2nd ed. Philadelphia: W.B. Saunders.

Brenchley, S. (1993). Children with diabetes: Current dietary advice. *Professional Care of Mother and Child, 3,* 52.

Castiglia, P.T. and Harbin, R.B. (1993). *Child Health Care: Process and Practice.* Philadelphia: J.B. Lippincott.

Hirsch, I.B. and Farkas-Hirsch, R. (1993). Type I diabetes and insulin therapy. *Nursing Clinics of North America, 28,* 9.

Jackson, D.B. and Saunders, R.B. (1993). *Child Health Nursing: A Comprehensive Approach to the Care of Children and Their Families.* Philadelphia: J.B. Lippincott.

Sizer, F. and Whitney, E. (1994). *Nutrition Concepts and Controversies,* 6th ed. Minneapolis/St. Paul: West Publishing.

Wong, D.L. (1993). *Whaley and Wong's Essentials of Pediatric Nursing,* 4th ed. St. Louis: C.V. Mosby.

Wong, D.L. (1995). *Whaley and Wong's Nursing Care of Infants and Children,* 5th ed. St. Louis: C.V. Mosby.

STUDY QUESTIONS

1. Hypofunction of which hormone causes poor linear growth and insulin sensitivity?
   a. Antidiuretic hormone
   b. Melanocyte-stimulating hormone
   c. Parathyroid hormone
   d. Growth hormone

2. Short stature may result from:
   a. Anterior pituitary gland hypofunction
   b. Posterior pituitary gland hyperfunction
   c. Parathyroid gland hyperfunction
   d. Thyroid gland hyperfunction

3. A 12-year-old girl is diagnosed with type I (IDDM) diabetes mellitus; she asks the nurse why she cannot take a pill instead of shots, like her grandfather does. Which of the following would be the nurse's best reply?
   a. "The pills only correct fat and protein metabolism, not carbohydrate metabolism."
   b. "If you have a Somogyi effect, you can switch to using the pills."
   c. "The pills only work on the adult pancreas, you can switch when you're 18."
   d. "The pills only add to existing insulin; your body does not make insulin so you need to replace insulin by injection replacement."

4. Which of the following phrases best describes hypothyroidism?"
   a. Normal growth for the first 5 years, followed by progressive linear growth retardation.
   b. Growth retardation in which height and weight are equally affected.
   c. Linear growth retardation with skeletal proportions normal for chronologic age.
   d. A completely normal growth pattern, but with the onset of precocious puberty.

5. A 6-year-old boy is admitted to the hospital with height measured below the third percentile and weight at the fortieth percentile. His admitting diagnosis is idiopathic hypopituitarism. One of the nurse's first actions should be to:
   a. Place him in a room with a 2-year-old boy.
   b. Arrange for a tutor for his precocious intellectual ability.
   c. Plan for a dietician to assess his caloric needs.
   d. Suggest orthodontic referral for underdeveloped jaw.

6. The father of a 6-year-old boy with idiopathic hypopituitarism shares with the nurse the child's desire to play baseball; however, the mother feels that the child will get hurt because he is so much smaller than the other children. In planning anticipatory guidance for these parents, the nurse should keep in mind:
   a. Children with idiopathic hypopituitarism have very fragile bones making them more prone to fractures.
   b. Activity could aggravate insulin sensitivity, causing hyperglycemia.
   c. Activity would aggravate the child's joints, already over tasked by obesity.
   d. The child should be allowed to participate as he can to foster healthy self-esteem.

7. Which of the following endocrine malfunctions commonly results in Cushing's syndrome?
   a. Hyperfunction of the anterior pituitary
   b. Hypofunction of the anterior pituitary
   c. Hyperfunction of the posterior pituitary
   d. Hypofunction of the posterior pituitary

8. When caring for a child with Cushing's syndrome, which of the following nursing interventions would be most important?

a. Handling the child carefully to prevent bruising

b. Monitoring for signs and symptoms of hypoglycemia

c. Observing for signs and symptoms of metabolic acidosis

d. Monitoring vital signs for hypotension and tachycardia

9. Diabetic ketoacidosis (DKA) results from an excessive accumulation of:

a. Glucose from carbohydrate metabolism

b. Ketone bodies from fat metabolism

c. Potassium from cell death

d. Sodium bicarbonate from renal compensation

10. Which of the following is a primary nursing action in the care of a child who is admitted to the intensive care unit for DKA?

a. Restrict fluids to prevent aggravating cerebral edema

b. Administer intravenous NPH insulin in high doses

c. Monitor child for hypertension

d. Monitor child for cardiac irregularities

11. When preparing a child with IDDM for discharge, the nurse discusses symptoms of hypoglycemia. Which of the following actions should the nurse instruct the parents to take when the child displays such symptoms?

a. Give the child nothing by mouth.

b. Give the child a simple sugar, such as candy.

c. Give the child a complex sugar, such as milk.

d. Do nothing until they contact the physician.

For additional questions, see
Lippincott's Self-Study Series Software
Available at your bookstore

ANSWER KEY

1. **Correct response: d**
   Growth hormone (GH) stimulates protein anabolism, promoting bone and soft tissue growth.
   a. Hypofunction of antidiuretic hormone (ADH) causes diabetes insipidus, marked by dehydration and hypernatremia.
   b. Hypofunction of melanocyte-stimulating hormone causes diminished or absent skin pigmentation.
   c. Hypofunction of parathyroid hormone causes hypocalcemia, marked by tetany, convulsions, and muscle spasms.
   Comprehensive/Physiologic/Assessment

2. **Correct response: a**
   Short stature usually results from diminished or deficient growth hormone, which is released from the anterior pituitary gland.
   b. Posterior pituitary hyperfunction results in increased secretion of antidiuretic hormone (ADH) or oxytocin, leading to a syndrome of inappropriate ADH secretion (SIADH), marked by fluid retention and hyponatremia.
   c. Parathyroid hypofunction leads to hypocalcemia.
   d. Thyroid hyperfunction causes increased secretion of T4, T3, and thyrocalcitonin, resulting in Grave's disease, marked by accelerated linear growth and early epiphyseal closure.
   Knowledge/Physiologic/Analysis

3. **Correct response: d**
   Oral hypoglycemic agents are only indicated for clients with some functioning beta cells, as in type II diabetes (NIDDM). Type I (IDDM) has no functioning beta cells.
   a. Oral hypoglycemics do not correct metabolism.
   b. A child with IDDM cannot substitute a hypoglycemic agent for insulin. The Somogyi effect is only a temporary physiologic reflex that decreases blood glucose level followed by rebound hyperglycemia.
   c. This is an inaccurate statement.
   Application/Health Promotion/Implementation

4. **Correct response: c**
   Although linear growth retardation occurs in hypopituitarism, delayed epiphyseal maturation allows for normal skeletal proportions.
   a. Normal growth may occur for the first year, followed by linear growth thereafter.
   b. Height is affected more profoundly than weight, contributing to obesity.
   d. The child with hypopituitarism commonly experiences delayed sexual maturation.
   Knowledge/Physiologic/Assessment

5. **Correct response: c**
   Because the child's weight is excessive for his height, he needs dietary assessment and planning to lose weight.
   a. Placing the child in a room with a toddler could contribute to poor self-esteem.
   b. Arranging for a school teacher to instruct him is an appropriate action, but the rationale is incorrect. Children with hypopituitarism often appear intellectually precocious because of the disparity between their size and their cognitive ability; they are usually of normal intelligence.
   d. This is not normally a problem with hypopituitarism.
   Application/Health Promotion/Planning

6. **Correct response: d**
   Engaging in peer group activities can help foster a sense of belonging and a positive self-concept. T-ball is a good sport to choose because physical stature is not an important consideration in the

ability to participate, unlike some other sports such as basketball and football.

a. Hypopituitarism does not affect calcium and phosphorus homeostasis and demineralization of bone.

b. Physical activity without adequate carbohydrate intake can cause hypoglycemia, not hyperglycemia, although this rarely occurs.

c. Moderate physical activity increases caloric use and reduces weight without undue strain on weight-bearing joints.

Comprehension/Psychosocial/Planning

7. *Correct response: a*
Cushing's syndrome is caused by excessive circulating cortisol, which can result from hypersecretion of ACTH by the anterior pituitary.

b. Hypofunction of the anterior pituitary with respect to ACTH causes a low ACTH concentration in the blood, inhibiting adrenal cortex secretion of glucocorticoid and resulting in Addison's disease.

c. Hyperfunction of the posterior pituitary can lead to SIADH.

d. Hypofunction of the posterior pituitary causes diabetes insipidus.

Knowledge/Physiologic/Analysis

8. *Correct response: a*
Cushing's syndrome causes capillary fragility, resulting in easy bruising and calcium excretion, resulting in osteoporosis.

b. Cushing's syndrome causes hyperglycemia not hypoglycemia.

c. Cushing's syndrome causes increased excretion of potassium and hydrogen ions, resulting in alkalosis.

d. Cushing's syndrome causes increased water and sodium retention, and hypokalemia, resulting in a sluggish and irregular heart beat.

Analysis/Physiologic/Implementation

9. *Correct response: b*
Inability to use glucose causes lipolysis, fatty acid oxidation, and release of ke-

tones, resulting in metabolic acidosis and coma.

a. Inability to use glucose, not impaired carbohydrate metabolism, is the primary mechanism in diabetes mellitus.

c. Potassium depletion, not potassium excess, occurs in DKA.

d. Sodium bicarbonate administration is a treatment for DKA.

Comprehension/Physiologic/Assessment

10. *Correct response: d*
Total body potassium depletion, particularly as fluid volume deficit is corrected, leaves the child vulnerable to cardiac arrest. The nurse should monitor the cardiac cycle for prolonged QT interval, low T wave, and depressed ST segment, which indicate weakened heart muscle and potential irregular heart beat.

a. Intravenous fluids should be given to correct dehydration.

b. Regular insulin is the only insulin that can be given intravenously, NPH is an intermediate-acting insulin; continuous low-dose infusion of a rapid-acting insulin is preferred.

c. Hypertension is more likely to occur owing to dehydration.

Application/Physiologic/Implementation

11. *Correct response: b*
Giving a little sugar temporarily corrects low serum glucose level. Simple sugar is converted to glucose more quickly than a complex sugar.

a. A hyperglycemic child needs fluids to prevent dehydration.

c. Complex sugars are absorbed more slowly and do not provide an immediate response.

d. Immediate action is necessary to prevent complications of hypoglycemia.

Analysis/Health Promotion/Evaluation

Children With Cancer

18

I. Essential concepts of cancer in children

A. General information

1. Cancer is the leading cause of death from disease in children ages 3 to 15 years. In the United States, the occurrence in this age group is approximately 12.9 per 100,000 Caucasian children and 10.1 per 100,000 African-American children.

2. There are changing incidences for various cancers throughout childhood. In all groups, leukemia is the most common, followed by brain tumors and lymphomas.

345

3.   The prognosis for childhood cancer has improved over the years. Now, more than 65% of children treated in major cancer centers survive more than 5 years.

4.   Cure criteria include: cessation of therapy; continuous freedom from clinical and laboratory evidence of cancer, and minimal or no risk of relapse, as determined by previous experience with the disease. Time that must elapse ranges from 2 to 5 years.

B.   Characteristics of cancers

1.   Types of malignant cells

a.   Embryonal: arise from embryonic tissue, such as blastomas.

b.   Lymphomas: arise from the lymphatic system.

c.   Leukemias: arise from blood-forming organs.

d.   Sarcomas: derived from connective and supportive tissue, such as bone.

e.   Carcinomas: derived from epithelial cells.

f.   Adenocarcinomas: carcinoma of glandular tissue, such as breast.

2.   Properties of tumor cells

a.   Growth rate usually is rapid.

b.   Anaplasia is the loss of differentiation and organization of cells for a specific function.

c.   Invasion: Cancer cells invade adjacent tissue and replace normal cells.

d.   Metastasis: Cancer cells spread to distant sites (by the blood or lymphatic system or by iatrogenic methods, such as biopsy) to form colonies of malignant growth.

e.   Competition: Cancer cells compete with normal cells for essential nutrients.

f.   Expansion: Unrestricted growth of cancer cells compresses adjacent tissue and causes organ damage.

C.   Staging

1.   Various staging criteria and terminology are used, depending on the specific tumor or treatment center, to describe and classify the extent of malignant neoplasms and their metastases. The staging systems are used to guide therapy and evaluate progress.

II.   Overview of cancer in children

A.   Assessment

1.   Specific clinical findings vary depending on particular body system involved.

2.   The cardinal signs and symptoms of cancer in children are:

a.   Fever, night sweats

b.   Persistent, localized pain or limping

c.   Tendency to bruise easily

d.   Palpable mass

      e.   Sudden changes in behavior, gait, balance, vision
      f.   Sudden, unexplained weight loss and anorexia
      g.   Unexplained paleness and fatigue

B.   **Laboratory studies and diagnostic tests**
1. Complete blood count, urinalysis, and blood chemistries
2. Peripheral blood smears to determine cell type and maturity
3. A 24-hour urinalysis to detect homovanillic acid, vanillylmandelic acid, and catecholamine
4. Bone marrow aspiration or biopsy for definitive diagnosis of leukemia
5. Lumbar puncture to analyze cerebrospinal fluid (CSF) for leukemic cells
6. Imaging techniques (computed tomography [CT], ultrasonography, magnetic resonance imaging [MRI]) to detect solid tumors

C.   **Therapeutic modes**
1. Several *protocols,* or *treatment plans,* exist for managing cancer in children.
2. Protocols may include surgery, chemotherapy, radiotherapy, immunotherapy, and bone marrow transplantation (BMT).
3. Supportive therapy is needed when serious damage occurs to normal cells as the result of cancer treatment.
4. Complications that may occur from therapy include oncologic emergencies, such as acute tumor lysis syndrome, obstruction, superior vena cava syndrome, and infections.

D.   **Psychosocial implications**
1. A child and his or her family need to adjust to living with the various phases of a life-threatening illness.
2. The child's reaction largely depends on his or her age, the information the child is given, and the physical impact of the disease on his or her energy level and coping skills (see Chapter 8, section I)

III. Leukemia

A.   **Description: a proliferation of abnormal white blood cells.**
1. Several different types of leukemia exist; each type is based on the morphology of the cells and the course of the disease; each type has a different prognosis and different characteristics.
2. Most leukemia in children is acute (97%), involving a proliferation of very immature white blood cells or blasts. Acute leukemia has a short history of symptoms and, without treatment, a rapidly declining course leading to death in 3 to 6 months.
3. **The most common leukemia in children is acute lymphocytic leukemia (ALL), occurring 85% to 90% of the time.**

ALL results from malignant changes in lymphocytes or their precursors.

4. Acute nonlymphocytic leukemia (ANLL) is less common in children. It includes abnormal cells of the myeloid (granulocytic or monocytic classification).

5. Chronic leukemia runs a more gradual course of about 2 years. Chronic granulocytic leukemia (CGL), the only type of chronic leukemia in children, is very rare.

B. Etiology and incidence

1. **Leukemia is the most common cancer found in children; about one third of all children with cancer have leukemia.**

2. Leukemia may be diagnosed at any age but has a peak onset between ages 3 and 5 years.

3. The etiology is unknown; a few cases in adults have been linked to environmental factors such as chemicals and radiation.

4. Several genetic diseases have been associated with increased incidences of leukemia, including Down's syndrome and Fanconi's hypoplastic anemia.

C. Pathophysiology and management

1. Malignant leukemia cells arise from precursor cells in blood-forming elements.

2. These cells can accumulate and crowd out normal bone marrow elements, spill into peripheral blood, and eventually invade all body organs and tissues.

3. Replacement of normal hematopoietic elements by leukemic cells results in bone marrow suppression, marked by decreased production of red blood cells (RBCs), normal white blood cells (WBCs), and platelets.

4. Bone marrow suppression results in anemia from deceased RBC production, predisposition to infection due to neutropenia, and bleeding tendencies due to thrombocytopenia, puts the child at risk of death from infection or hemorrhage.

5. Infiltration of reticuloendothelial organs (spleen, liver, lymph glands) causes marked enlargement and, eventually, fibrosis.

6. Leukemic infiltration of the central nervous system (CNS) results in increased intracranial pressure (ICP) and other effects depending on the specific areas involved.

7. Other possible sites of long-term infiltration include the kidneys, testes, prostate, ovaries, gastrointestinal (GI) tract, and lungs.

8. The hypermetabolic leukemic cells eventually deprive all body cells of nutrients necessary for survival. Uncontrolled growth of leukemic cells can actually result in metabolic starvation.

9. Leukemia treatment commonly involves a combination of chemotherapy and radiation therapy, provided at four levels:

a. **Remission induction to reduce the number of cancer cells:** Chemotherapy includes vincristine, prednisone, and L-asparaginase, with or without another drug such as doxorubicin or daunorubicin.

 b. **Sanctuary to treat cancer cells not reached by remission induction (gonads, CNS):** CNS treatment usually consists of intrathecal administration of medications with methotrexate used most frequently; other medications include cytosine arabinoside, hydrocortisone sodium succinate, and other agents. Radiation also may be applied to the brain or spinal cord. The testis, the second most common site of metastasis, may be treated with radiation; prepubertal boys are monitored closely for development and may require androgen replacement therapy; sterility may also occur.

 c. **Maintenance to decrease the risk of reoccurrence:** Therapy often includes daily oral mercaptopurine, weekly methotrexate, and monthly vincristine and prednisone.

 d. **Reinduction, if exacerbation occurs:** Antineoplastic agents or bone marrow transplant may be used. The prognosis becomes worse with each relapse.

10. Bone marrow transplantation (BMT), when successful, destroys leukemic cells and replenishes bone marrow with healthy cells. Bone marrow transplants are not recommended for first remissions of ALL owing to the success of chemotherapy. However, they may be used in ANLL for first remissions owing to the poor prognosis of this disorder. The selection process of a suitable donor and the potential complications in transplantation are related to the human leucocyte antigen (HLA) system complex. The importance of HLA matching is to prevent graft-versus-host disease. There are three types of BMTs:
    a. Allogenic: refers to tissue from a histocompatible donor, usually a sibling, but may also involve an unmatched donor.
    b. Autologous: refers to tissue that is collected from the child's own tissue, frozen, and sometimes processed to remove undesired cells.
    c. Syngeneic: refers to tissue that is identical to the child's tissue and which comes from an identical twin.

D. **Clinical assessment findings**
  1. Anemia from RBC suppression: fatigue, pallor, tachycardia
  2. Bleeding from platelet suppression: petechiae, purpura, hematuria, epistaxis, tarry stools

3. Immunosuppression from WBC suppression: fever, infection, poor wound healing
4. Symptoms from reticuloendothelial involvement: hepatospleno-megaly (HSM), bone pain, lymphadenopathy
5. CNS symptoms, if CNS metastasis: headache, meningeal irritation, signs of increased ICP
6. General symptoms: weight loss, anorexia, vomiting

E. **Diagnostic assessment findings**
   1. Complete blood count (CBC) may reveal normal, decreased, or increased WBC count with immature cells (blasts); decreased RBCs; and decreased platelets.
   2. **Diagnosis is confirmed with bone marrow aspiration, showing extensive replacement of normal bone marrow elements by leukemic cells.**
   3. Lumbar puncture is performed to assess abnormal cell migration to CNS.

F. **Nursing diagnoses**
   1. Risk for infection
   2. Risk for injury
   3. Risk for impaired skin integrity
   4. Altered oral mucous membranes
   5. Altered nutrition: less than body requirements
   6. Fluid volume deficit
   7. Fear
   8. Anxiety
   9. Self-esteem disturbance
   10. Body image disturbance
   11. Pain
   12. Altered health maintenance
   13. Altered growth and development
   14. Altered family processes
   15. Anticipatory grieving
   16. Fatigue
   17. Activity intolerance

G. **Planning and implementation**
   1. Set realistic goals depending on the type of therapy prescribed:
      a. Curative: goal is complete disease eradication.
      b. Adjuvant: goal is eradication of disease and subclinical micro metastases with systemic adjuvant modalities.
      c. Palliative: goal is not to cure but to provide quality survival with symptom control.
   2. Prepare the child for diagnostic tests and treatments by:
      a. Assessing child's level of understanding
      b. Addressing specific fears and misunderstandings

      c.   Providing information appropriate to the child's age and developmental level
      d.   Specifying exactly what he or she will see, smell, hear, and feel, rather than merely what will happen

3.   Help prevent complications related to bone marrow suppression, such as infection, bleeding, and anemia.

4.   Prepare the child and family for BMT if the procedure is scheduled.

5.   Promote optimal nutrition to maintain and rebuild healthy tissue. Serve small, frequent meals in a pleasant, relaxed environment, and involve the child in food selection, as appropriate.

6.   For a child receiving blood transfusions, assess for transfusion reaction.

7.   Promote adequate rest by providing a calm, quiet, environment and by scheduling nursing care and procedures to ensure periods of rest.

8.   Minimize risk of infection secondary to diagnosis and chemotherapy:
      a.   Help child avoid contact with others who have infections.
      b.   Monitor child's temperature every 4 hours.
      c.   Practice proper hand washing.
      d.   Avoid live plants and flowers and uncooked fruits and vegetables, which may contain pathogens.

9.   Prevent injury secondary to thrombocytopenia from diagnosis and chemotherapy:
      a.   Handle child gently.
      b.   Avoid administering aspirin and alcohol.
      c.   Minimize injections; when necessary, apply pressure to sites for 3 to 5 minutes to stop bleeding.
      d.   Avoid taking rectal temperatures.
      e.   Monitor hemoglobin and hematocrit values regularly.
      f.   Monitor for hemorrhagic bleeding and report same; check oral mucosa, skin, urine, and stools; check for sudden headaches, which may signify intracranial bleeding.

10.   Minimize nausea and vomiting, secondary to chemotherapy:
      a.   Administer antiemetics 30 minutes before chemotherapy begins.
      b.   Continue antiemetics as prescribed, as needed after chemotherapy is completed.

11.   Minimize discomfort from stomatitis secondary to chemotherapy:
      a.   Assess mouth frequently.
      b.   Assist the client to use toothettes or a soft toothbrush.

      c.   Avoid potential irritants such as a firm toothbrush, commercial mouthwash, lemon-glycerin swabs.

      d.   Give mouth care every 2 hours.

      e.   Offer cool, soothing, bland foods and liquids.

12. Minimize body image disturbance related to alopecia:

      a.   Reassure client that hair loss is temporary; inform client that new hair may have different texture from the hair he or she lost.

      b.   Encourage use of hats, scarves, and wigs.

      c.   Avoid use of hair chemicals, such as permanent wave solutions, when hair grows back.

      d.   Encourage child to voice feelings.

13. Minimize other side effects of specific chemotherapeutic agents:

      a.   Vincristine (neurotoxicity): Assess for problems such as foot drop, depression, ataxia, and vision changes.

      b.   Methotrexate (nephrotoxicity): Monitor intake and output (I&O), urine, and blood urea nitrogen (BUN), and creatinine levels.

      c.   L-asparaginase (hepatotoxicity): Assess for lethargy, confusion, and anaphylaxis; monitor liver function study results.

      d.   Daunorubicin and doxorubicin (cardiotoxicity): Observe for changes in heart rate and rhythm.

      e.   Prednisone (multiple side effects): Observe for moon face, fluid retention, mood changes, gastric irritation, and increased susceptibility to infection.

14. Support the child and family by encouraging verbalization of concerns, fostering family support systems, and utilizing appropriate resources.

15. Provide death and dying counseling as appropriate and use appropriate resources and personnel, including clergy.

16. Encourage normal growth and development by fostering activities appropriate for the child's age and condition.

17. Provide child and family teaching, covering:

      a.   Diagnosis and nature of the disorder

      b.   All treatments and other procedures

      c.   Side effects of treatments and medications

      d.   All aspects of home care, including the importance of follow-up care and how to monitor the child for signs of recurrent disease

H. Evaluation

    1. The child experiences partial or total remission of the disorder.

    2. The child remains free of infection, injury, and pain.

3. The child retains food and fluid and is well nourished.
4. The child and family cope with the illness, its implications and treatments.
5. The child has positive self-esteem and body image, and experiences life as normally as possible.

IV. Wilms' tumor (nephroblastoma)

A. Description: a malignant neoplasm of the kidney; the most common intra-abdominal tumor in children; the most curable solid tumor in children.

B. Etiology and incidence
1. Wilms' tumor occurs most often in young children but may occur in adolescents.
2. Usually it is unilateral and occurs with other abnormalities such as an absent iris or genitourinary problems.
3. The median age at diagnosis is between 2 and 3 years.
4. Siblings of children with Wilms' tumor have a higher risk of developing the disorder than the general population.

C. Pathophysiology and management
1. The tumor originates from immature renoblast cells located in the renal parenchyma.
2. It is well encapsulated in early stages but may later extend into lymph nodes and the renal vein or vena cava and metastasize to the lungs and other sites.
3. Wilms' tumors are classified into five stages:
   a. Stage I: tumor is confined to one kidney.
   b. Stage II: tumor extends beyond kidney.
   c. Stage III: tumor has residual nonhematogenous tumor cells confined to the abdomen.
   d. Stage IV: tumor is characterized by distant metastases involving lung, liver, bone, or brain.
   e. Stage V: tumor involves both kidneys.
4. Treatment typically involves surgery, a nephrectomy, with removal of regional nodes and any resectable regional tumor.
5. Chemotherapy may be effective at all stages; radiation may be used as well, but not for stages I and II.

D. Clinical assessment findings
1. There may be no symptoms.
2. Characteristics may include a firm, nontender upper quadrant mass, fever, abdominal pain, hematuria, hypertension (due to secretion of excess renin from the tumor), and anorexia.

E. Diagnostic assessment findings
1. Blood studies may show anemia secondary to bleeding from the tumor.
2. Intravenous pyelography (IVP) may disclose mass.

3. Other studies (*e.g.*, imaging or scans) may show evidence of metastasis.

F. Nursing diagnoses
1. Risk for infection
2. Risk for injury
3. Altered tissue perfusion
4. Constipation
5. Altered nutrition: less than body requirements
6. Fluid volume deficit
7. Fear
8. Anxiety
9. Body image disturbance
10. Pain
11. Altered health maintenance
12. Altered family processes
13. Grieving

G. Planning and implementation
1. Prepare the child for diagnostic tests and treatments by:
   a. Assessing the child's level of understanding.
   b. Addressing specific fears and misconceptions.
   c. Providing information appropriate to the child's age and developmental level.
   d. Explaining what he or she will see, hear, smell, and feel rather than merely specifying what will happen.

2. **Help prevent rupture of an encapsulated tumor by avoiding abdominal palpation and by promoting careful bathing and handling.**

3. Monitor bowel sounds and assess for signs and symptoms of intestinal obstruction resulting from abdominal surgery, vincristine-induced adynamic ileus, and radiation-induced edema.

4. Help prevent infection by maintaining scrupulous hand washing and limiting the child's exposure to persons with infections. Monitor for evidence of infections.

5. Help prevent postoperative pulmonary complications by providing frequent position changes and by encouraging coughing and deep-breathing exercises and ambulation.

6. Provide child and family teaching, covering:
   a. Diagnosis and nature of the disorder
   b. Surgery and other treatments
   c. Side effects of chemotherapy and radiation treatment

7. If child receives chemotherapy, follow plan described above for child with leukemia (section III, H.9 through H.14).

8. Support child and family by encouraging verbalization of concerns, fostering family support systems, and utilizing appropriate resources.

9. Provide death and dying counseling, when appropriate, and utilize appropriate resources and personnel, including clergy.
10. Encourage normal growth and development by fostering activities that are appropriate for the child's age and condition.
11. Provide child and family teaching, covering:
    a. Diagnosis and nature of the disorder
    b. All treatments, surgeries and other procedures
    c. Side effects of treatments and medications
    d. All aspects of home care, including the importance of follow-up care

H. Evaluation
1. The child experiences partial or total remission of the disorder.
2. The child remains free of infection, injury, and pain.
3. The child remains well nourished.
4. The child and family cope with the illness, its implications and treatments.
5. The child has positive self-esteem and body image, and experiences life as normally as possible.

V. Brain tumors
A. Description: tumor arising from cells anywhere in the cranium; types include astrocytoma, medulloblastoma, brainstem glioma, and ependymoma.
B. Etiology and incidence
1. CNS tumors account for about 20% of all childhood cancers.
2. About half are infratentorial (below the tentorium cerebelli), occurring primarily in the cerebellum or brain stem.
3. The others are supratentorial and occur mainly in the cerebrum.

C. Pathophysiology and management
1. Tumors arise from anywhere in the cranium, glial cells, nerve cells, neuroepithelium, cranial nerves, blood vessels, pineal gland, and hypophysis.
2. Specific cells may be involved to provide a histologic classification.
3. Treatment may involve surgery, chemotherapy, radiation, or all three.

D. Clinical assessment findings
1. Recurrent and progressive headache
2. Severe, morning vomiting that becomes projectile
3. Loss of balance and coordination
4. Behavioral changes such as irritability, lethargy
5. Failure to thrive
6. Cranial nerve neuropathy
7. Signs of increased ICP
8. Seizures

E. **Diagnostic assessment findings**
1. MRI permits early diagnosis of brain tumors.
2. CT permits direct visualization of the brain parenchyma, ventricles, and surrounding subarachnoid space.
3. Angiography provides information about the tumor's blood supply.
4. Definitive diagnosis is made by biopsy during surgery.

F. **Nursing diagnoses**
1. Anxiety
2. Ineffective individual coping
3. Risk for injury
4. Risk for infection
5. Pain
6. Risk for peripheral neurovascular dysfunction
7. Sensory and perceptual alterations

G. **Planning and implementation**
1. Assess for signs and symptoms of brain tumor when the diagnosis has not yet been established in a child who is suspected of having a brain tumor.
2. Prepare the family for diagnostic and operative procedures.
3. Set realistic goals depending on the type of therapy prescribed:
   a. Curative: The goal is complete disease eradication.
   b. Adjuvant: The goal is eradication of disease and subclinical micrometastases with systemic adjuvant modalities.
   c. Palliative: The goal is not to cure but to provide quality survival with symptom control.
4. Prepare the child for diagnostic tests and treatments by:
   a. Assessing child's level of understanding
   b. Addressing specific fears and misunderstandings
   c. Providing information appropriate to the child's age and developmental level
   d. Specifying what he or she will see, smell, hear, and feel, rather than merely what will happen
5. Prevent postoperative complications by monitoring vital signs, positioning, fluid regulation, and medication.
6. Monitor for signs of increased ICP and intervene as appropriate (see Chapter 16, section III).
7. Monitor for seizure activity, and intervene as appropriate (See Chapter 16, section IV).
8. If the child receives chemotherapy, follow the planning and interventions suggested in this chapter for the child with leukemia receiving chemotherapy.
9. Provide child and family support by encouraging verbalization of concerns, fostering family support systems, and utilizing appropriate resources.

10. Provide death and dying counseling as appropriate and utilize appropriate resources and personnel, including clergy.
11. Encourage normal growth and development by fostering activities appropriate for the child's age and condition.
12. Provide child and family teaching, covering:
    a. Diagnosis and nature of the disorder
    b. All treatments and other procedures
    c. Side effects of treatments and medications
    d. All aspects of home care, including the importance of follow-up care and how to monitor the child for signs of exacerbation

H. Evaluation

1. The child experiences partial or total remission of the disorder.
2. The child remains free of infection, injury, and pain.
3. The child retains food and fluid and is well nourished.
4. The child and family cope with the illness and its implications and treatments.
5. The child maintains positive self-esteem and body image and experiences life as normally as possible.

Bibliography

Alfaro-LeFevre, R., et al. (1992). *Drug Handbook: A Nursing Process Approach.* Redwood City, CA: Addison-Wesley.

Betz, C.L., Hunsberger, M.M., and Wright, S. (1994). *Family Centered Nursing Care of Children,* 2nd ed. Philadelphia: W.B. Saunders.

Castiglia, P.T. and Harbin, R.B. (1993). *Child Health Care: Process and Practice.* Philadelphia: J.B. Lippincott.

Jackson, D.B. and Saunders, R.B. (1993). *Child Health Nursing: A Comprehensive Approach to the Care of Children and Their Families.* Philadelphia: J.B. Lippincott.

Ritchie, M.A. (1992). Psychosocial functioning of adolescents with cancer: A developmental perspective. *Oncology Nursing Forum, 19,* 1497.

Ruccione, K. (1992). Wilms' tumor: A paradigm, a parallel and a puzzle. *Seminars in Oncology Nursing, 8,* 241.

Sizer, F. and Whitney, E. (1994). *Nutrition Concepts and Controversies,* 6th ed. Minneapolis/St. Paul: West Publishing.

Wong, D.L. (1993). *Whaley and Wong's Essentials of Pediatric Nursing,* 4th ed. St. Louis: C.V. Mosby.

Wong, D.L. (1995). *Whaley and Wong's Nursing Care of Infants and Children,* 5th ed. St. Louis: C.V. Mosby.

STUDY QUESTIONS

1. What is the most common form of childhood cancer?
   a. Lymphoma
   b. Brain tumors
   c. Leukemia
   d. Osteosarcoma

2. A 4-year-old child with leukemia is admitted to the hospital because of pneumonia. Which of the following is the most likely cause of this?
   a. Anemia
   b. Leukopenia
   c. Thrombocytopenia
   d. Eosinophilia

3. A child is suspected of having leukemia. The nurse should prepare the parents for which of the following tests that would confirm this diagnosis?
   a. Lumbar puncture
   b. Bone marrow aspiration
   c. Complete blood count
   d. Blood culture

4. An appropriate nursing diagnosis for a child who is receiving chemotherapy is:
   a. Ineffective breathing pattern
   b. Constipation
   c. Altered skin integrity
   d. Altered oral mucous membrane

5. In caring for a child with leukemia, which of the following goals should be considered primary?
   a. Meeting developmental needs
   b. Promoting adequate nutrition
   c. Preventing infection
   d. Promoting diversional activities

6. What is the treatment goal of intrathecal methotrexate in managing leukemia?
   a. Sanctuary therapy
   b. Bone marrow suppression
   c. Induction remission
   d. Palliative treatment

7. What is the most common presenting manifestation of Wilms' tumor?
   a. Hematuria
   b. Pain on voiding
   c. Nausea and vomiting
   d. Abdominal mass

8. When caring for a child awaiting surgery for a Wilms' tumor, which of the following nursing actions would be most important?
   a. Handle the child with care, particularly during bathing.
   b. Place the child on low blood count precautions and isolation.
   c. Monitor bowel sounds for vincristine-induced ileus.
   d. Place child in high Fowler's position to facilitate breathing.

9. Which of the following nursing interventions can help prevent or reduce nausea and vomiting during chemotherapy?
   a. Providing a high-fiber diet
   b. Administering allopurinol 30 minutes before chemotherapy
   c. Encouraging increased fluid intake
   d. Administering antiemetic 30 minutes before chemotherapy

10. A 4-year-old boy is about to be discharged after undergoing surgery and follow-up treatment for a Wilms' tumor. Which of the following points would be a vital part of the teaching program for the child's parents?
    a. Allowing him to resume activity, including contact sports
    b. Monitoring signs and symptoms of urinary tract infection
    c. Making arrangements for a return visit in 6 months
    d. Arranging for hospice care because Wilms' tumor is fatal

ANSWER KEY

1. **Correct response: c**
   Leukemia accounts for approximately one third of all childhood cancers.
   a. Lymphoma accounts for about 12% of all childhood cancers.
   b. Brain tumors account for about 19%, but they are the most common form of solid tumor cancer in childhood.
   d. Bone cancers account for 5% with osteosarcoma being the most common type.
   Knowledge/Health Promotion/ Assessment

2. **Correct response: b**
   The decrease in functioning white blood cells in leukemia causes the increased risk for infection in children with leukemia.
   a. Anemia would result in fatigue.
   c. Thrombocytopenia, decreased platelet count, would result in bleeding.
   d. An increased eosinophil count is not related to leukemia.
   Comprehension/Physiologic/Analysis (Dx)

3. **Correct response: b**
   A bone marrow aspiration is performed to confirm the diagnosis of leukemia through the examination of abnormal cells in the bone marrow.
   a. A lumbar puncture is performed to detect spread into the CNS, but it is not used to confirm the diagnosis.
   c. An abnormal CBC may suggest leukemia, but it is not used to confirm the diagnosis.
   d. A blood culture may be performed if infection is suspected.
   Comprehensive/Physiologic/Planning

4. **Correct response: d**
   Chemotherapy destroys rapidly growing cells, including those in the GI tract, resulting in stomatitis, an inflammatory condition of the mouth.
   a. In general, there should not be an effect on the respiratory system related to chemotherapy.
   b. Because chemotherapy affects the GI tract, the child would have diarrhea, not constipation.
   c. In general, skin integrity should not be affected by chemotherapy.
   Application/Physiologic/Analysis (Dx)

5. **Correct response: c**
   The child is at high risk for infection due to immunosuppression from both the disease and the treatment, and infection is the primary cause of death in leukemia.
   a, b, and d. All are important goals; however, they are not the primary goal in caring for a child with leukemia.
   Analysis/Safe Care/Planning

6. **Correct response: a**
   Sanctuary therapy involves administering intrathecal medications to attack leukemic cells in the CNS.
   b. Bone marrow suppression is a side effect of chemotherapy, not a specific goal of intrathecal therapy, especially with methotrexate.
   c. Initial induction of remission is accomplished by oral prednisone and intravenous chemotherapy.
   d. The goal of palliative therapy is to improve the patient's quality of life rather than to effect a cure.
   Comprehension/Physiologic/Analysis (Dx)

7. **Correct response: d**
   The most common sign of Wilms' tumor is a painless palpable mass, sometimes marked by an increase in abdominal girth.
   a. Gross hematuria is uncommon; microscopic hematuria may be present.
   b. Pain on voiding is not associated with Wilms' tumor.
   c. Tumor encroachment should not cause abdominal obstruction and resulting nausea and vomiting.
   Comprehension/Physiologic/Assessment

8. *Correct response: a*

Handling the child carefully is essential to prevent rupture of an encapsulated tumor.

b. The child usually does not undergo myelosuppression before surgery. In fact, the child may be suffering from polycythemia due to increased production of erythropoietin.

c. Vincristine is administered postoperatively.

d. Respiratory difficulty is not a common problem with Wilms' tumor.

Application/Safe Care/Implementation

9. *Correct response: d*

Antiemetics counteract nausea most effectively when given before administration of an agent that causes nausea. Antiemetics also work best when given on a continuous basis rather than as needed.

a. A high-fiber diet does nothing to reduce nausea and vomiting.

b. Allopurinol, a xanthine-oxidase inhibitor, is thought to prevent renal damage due to large releases of uric acid during chemotherapy; it has no antiemetic properties.

c. High fluid intake during periods of nausea exaggerates the symptoms and cause vomiting.

Application/Physiologic/Planning

10. *Correct response: b*

Urinary tract infections pose a threat to the remaining kidney.

a. Rough play and contact sports should be discouraged because of the residual effect of radiation to the abdomen and because the child needs to protect his or her lone kidney.

c. Six months is too late; children receive chemotherapy for 6 to 15 months after surgery.

d. Wilms' tumor is the most curable solid tumor of childhood; prognosis is usually favorable.

Application/Safe Care/Planning

COMPREHENSIVE TEST—QUESTIONS

1. Children with cleft palate are prone to frequent episodes of otitis media owing to which of the following?
   a. Lowered resistance due to malnutrition
   b. Ineffective functioning of the eustachian tubes
   c. Plugging of the eustachian tubes with food particles
   d. Constant associated congenital defects of the middle ear

2. What is the approximate healing time for a fractured femur in a 3-week-old infant?
   a. 2 to 4 weeks
   b. 4 to 6 weeks
   c. 8 to 10 weeks
   d. 10 to 16 weeks

3. Which of the following phases of cancer treatment involves treatment of the central nervous system and the gonads?
   a. Remission induction
   b. Sanctuary
   c. Maintenance
   d. Reinduction

4. A disorder that results in pathologic fractures and which usually is characterized by blue sclera is:
   a. Osteomyelitis
   b. Osteogenesis imperfecta
   c. Osteosarcoma
   d. Osteoarthritis

5. Which of the following assessments would suggest the possibility that a child has developed an infection under a cast?
   a. Cold toes
   b. Absent pedal pulses
   c. "Hot spots" on the cast
   d. Cyanotic extremities

6. Initial nursing implementations for a 3-month-old infant with a serum lead level of 90 mcg/dL are directed primarily toward:

   a. Monitoring neurologic status due to possible encephalopathy
   b. Initiating comfort measures to relieve bone pain
   c. Teaching parents about lead sources to stop child's pica
   d. Including dietary sources of iron to correct anemia

7. A child is placed on lead chelation therapy with edathamil calcium-disodium (CaNa2EDTA) and dimercaprol (BAL). Which of the following potential side effects should the nurse watch for?
   a. Seizures
   b. Muscular atrophy
   c. Depression
   d. Increased appetite

8. Which of the following characteristics would be expected in a healthy 3-month-old infant?
   a. A strong Moro reflex
   b. A strong parachute reflex
   c. Rolling from front to back
   d. Lifting head and chest when prone

9. A child's birth weight usually triples by the end of the first:
   a. 4 months
   b. 7 months
   c. 9 months
   d. 12 months

10. Which of the following best describes parallel play between two toddlers?
    a. Sharing crayons to color separate pictures
    b. Playing a board game with a nurse
    c. Sitting near each other playing with separate dolls
    d. Sharing their dolls with two different nurses

11. The best way to examine a toddler is:
    a. From head to toe
    b. Distally to proximally
    c. Starting with the abdomen
    d. From least to most intrusive

12. Which of the following would best soothe a colicky infant?
   a. Shaking
   b. Swaddling
   c. An extra feeding
   d. Withholding feeding

13. When performing a well-child care examination on a 12-year-old girl, the nurse should check for:
   a. Hip dislocation
   b. Transient synovitis
   c. Scoliosis
   d. Tibial torsion

14. In caring for a child after surgery for cleft lip repair, the nurse should watch for which of the following immediate postoperative complications?
   a. Bleeding and respiratory difficulty
   b. Scarring problems and infection
   c. Infection and respiratory distress
   d. Bleeding and infection

15. Which of the following organisms is responsible for the development of rheumatic fever?
   a. *Streptococcus pneumonia*
   b. *Haemophilus influenzae*
   c. Group A beta-hemolytic streptococcus
   d. *Staphylococcus aureus*

16. Nursing actions for a child with rheumatic fever should include all of the following except:
   a. Providing adequate rest periods
   b. Isolating the child to prevent disease transmission
   c. Ensuring compliance with medication therapy
   d. Providing adequate nutrition

17. Early characteristics of plumbism include:
   a. Diarrhea, blurred vision, and headache
   b. Dizziness, fever, and chills
   c. Anorexia, abdominal cramps, and vomiting
   d. Developmental delay, seizures, and coma

18. Which acid-base disorder is likely to develop secondary to diarrhea in a 6-month-old child?
   a. Metabolic acidosis
   b. Metabolic alkalosis
   c. Respiratory acidosis
   d. Respiratory alkalosis

19. Which of the following nursing interventions is a priority in caring for a 4-month-old with acute gastroenteritis?
   a. Initiating respiratory isolation
   b. Obtaining daily weights
   c. Administering antiemetics
   d. Monitoring CBC results

20. Which of the following assessments would you expect to note in an infant who has lost 11% of his body weight owing to dehydration?
   a. Pallor
   b. Decreased pulse
   c. Bulging fontanel
   d. Marked oliguria

21. The priority nursing goal for a child with acute lymphocytic leukemia is:
   a. Decrease the risk of infection.
   b. Encourage intake of iron-rich foods.
   c. Discuss death and dying.
   d. Discourage injections.

22. A child receiving chemotherapy is also receiving allopurinol because:
   a. It prevents acid formation.
   b. It prevents hyperuricemia.
   c. It aids in tumor disintegration.
   d. It protects the liver.

23. On average, the adolescent growth spurt begins:
   a. Earlier for boys than for girls
   b. Earlier for girls than boys
   c. The same time for both sexes
   d. Between ages 7 and 8

24. The most common gastrointestinal complication that may be noted in children with cystic fibrosis is:
   a. Meconium ileus
   b. Ulcerative colitis
   c. Rectal prolapse
   d. Diverticulitis

25. When should chest physical therapy be given to children with cystic fibrosis?
   a. Before meals and at bedtime
   b. Immediately after meals
   c. Immediately on arising
   d. Never; it is contraindicated

26. Why do children with cystic fibrosis receive Pancrease?
   a. To soften their stools
   b. To aid in fat digestion
   c. To prevent diabetes
   d. To treat their pneumonia

27. One of the rationales for ordering a croupette for children with acute laryngotracheobronchitis is:
   a. It provides 100% oxygen.
   b. It liquefies secretions.
   c. It warms the respiratory tract.
   d. It provides reverse isolation.

28. Which of the following must be monitored preoperatively before a child has a tonsil- and adenoidectomy?
   a. Bleeding and clotting times
   b. Urinalysis
   c. Serum electrolyte levels
   d. Differential count

29. Which of the following is true of status asthmaticus?
   a. It is highly contagious.
   b. It is difficult to control.
   c. It indicates the presence of emphysema.
   d. It is always fatal.

30. To treat congenital hip dysplasia, which position should be maintained?
   a. Extended and abducted
   b. Extended and adducted
   c. Flexed and abducted
   d. Flexed and adducted

31. What type of immunity does tetanus toxoid give?
   a. Artificial active
   b. Artificial passive
   c. Natural passive
   d. Natural active

32. The nurse knows that a mother understands home care instructions following the administration of a diphtheria, tetanus, and pertussis injection when the mother states feedback regarding:
   a. Instructions on how to reduce fever
   b. Explanation of dietary restrictions
   c. Explanation of subsequent rash
   d. Instructions for subsequent diarrhea

33. During a home health examination, a community health nurse notes multiple bruises and burns on an 18-month-old child. What should the nurse do?
   a. Report the child's condition to protective services immediately.
   b. Schedule a follow-up visit to check for more bruises.
   c. Notify the child's physician immediately.
   d. Nothing, this is normal in a toddler.

34. To evaluate the effectiveness of theophylline (Slo-bid) therapy for treating asthma, the nurse should watch for:
   a. Vomiting and lethargy
   b. Nausea and dyspnea
   c. Diarrhea and wheezing
   d. Improved color and respirations

35. Which of the following assessment findings would be noted in a 6-week-old with pyloric stenosis?
   a. Projectile vomiting
   b. Choking cough after feedings
   c. Currant jelly stools
   d. Abdominal distention

36. A cerebral vascular accident that results from congenital heart disease is most likely due to:
   a. Polycythemia
   b. Cardiomyopathy
   c. Endocarditis
   d. Low blood pressure

37. Symptoms of congestive heart failure in a 9-month-old child with congenital heart disease include:
   a. Bradycardia and cyanosis
   b. Dyspnea and bradycardia

c. Strong peripheral pulses and edema

d. Tachycardia and hepatomegaly

38. A 4-year-old's intense psychosexual preoccupations can lead to which of the following fears during hospitalization?

a. Loss of control

b. Fear of the dark

c. Fear of castration

d. Fear of separation

39. When a 7-year-old child is hospitalized and thus separated from peers and schoolwork, the child may develop feelings of:

a. Inferiority

b. Guilt

c. Shame and doubt

d. Role diffusion

40. Adults who commit child sexual abuse usually are:

a. Strangers to the child

b. Known to the child

c. Dependent on drugs

d. Sociopathic personalities

41. The head-to-tail direction of growth is called:

a. Proximodistal

b. Sequential

c. Specific

d. Cephalocaudal

42. A hospitalized 8-year-old boy states "I'm real brave, I'm not afraid of anything; I'm the toughest one here!" This is an example of:

a. Reaction formation

b. Repression

c. Sublimation

d. Regression

43. At which age is a child most likely to personify death as the bogeyman?

a. 3 to 5 years

b. 5 to 6 years

c. 7 to 9 years

d. 9 to 11 years

44. An 18-month-old girl cries inconsolably when her mother leaves her to go to the admissions office. What stage of separation anxiety is the child exhibiting?

a. Protest

b. Despair

c. Detachment

d. Denial

45. The mother of a hospitalized child calls the student nurse and states "You idiot, you have no idea how to care for my sick child!" This is an example of:

a. Displacement

b. Projection

c. Repression

d. Psychosis

46. The most overwhelming adverse influence on health in children is which of the following?

a. Race

b. Customs

c. Low socioeconomic status

d. Genetic constitution

47. In caring for a family with a different cultural background, which of the following would be an appropriate goal?

a. Strive to keep background from influencing health needs.

b. Discourage continuation of cultural practices in the hospital.

c. Gently attempt to change family's cultural beliefs,

d. Adapt family's cultural practices to health needs as necessary.

48. Appropriate nursing interventions to promote parenting skills include all of the following except:

a. Teaching normal growth and development

b. Reinforcing the child's individuality

c. Acting as a surrogate parent

d. Encouraging realistic parenting roles

49. Which of the following adolescents would most likely be allowed to give his or her own consent for examination and treatment?

a. A 14-year-old with strep throat

b. A 15-year-old requesting a school physical

c. A 16-year-old with a sexually transmitted disease

d. A 17-year-old with a broken arm

50. Which of the following is a possible complication of oxygen therapy in a premature infant?

a. Bronchopulmonary dysplasia

b. Necrotizing enterocolitis

c. Congestive heart failure

d. Meconium aspiration syndrome

51. Which of the following structural defects are found in tetralogy of Fallot?

a. Pulmonary stenosis, ventricular septal defect, overriding aorta, hypertrophy of the left ventricle

b. Pulmonary stenosis, ventricular septal defect, overriding aorta, hypertrophy of the right ventricle

c. Aortic stenosis, ventricular septal defect, overriding aorta, hypertrophy of the right ventricle

d. Aortic stenosis, ventricular septal defect, overriding aorta, hypertrophy of the left ventricle

52. Which position may a child with tetralogy of Fallot assume as a compensatory mechanism?

a. Low Fowler's

b. Prone

c. Supine

d. Squatting

53. Which of the following should the nurse expect to note as a frequent complication for a child with congenital heart disease?

a. Susceptibility to respiratory infection

b. Bleeding tendencies

c. Frequent vomiting and diarrhea

d. Seizure disorder

54. Therapeutic management for a child with thalassemia major primarily includes which of the following?

a. Oxygen therapy

b. Adequate hydration

c. Supplemental iron

d. Frequent blood transfusions

55. A 9-year-old girl is admitted to the hospital with a diagnosis of rheumatic fever. Which of the following is most likely to be noted in her history?

a. She was treated for strep throat 3 weeks ago.

b. She was born with a congenital heart defect.

c. She had chicken pox 1 month ago.

d. She had an untreated fever and sore throat 2 weeks ago.

56. An infant with bronchiolitis is put on nothing by mouth status and is placed on intravenous fluids. What is the most likely reason for this?

a. Tachypnea

b. Irritability

c. Fever

d. Tachycardia

57. Hemorrhage after a tonsil- and adenoidectomy may occur 5 to 10 days postoperatively owing to:

a. Infection

b. Tissue soughing

c. Secretions

d. Increased vascularity

58. In which season is sudden infant death syndrome most likely to occur?

a. Summer

b. Spring

c. Fall

d. Winter

59. The complete blood count of a child with iron deficiency anemia is likely to demonstrate all of the following except:

a. Low hemoglobin

b. Low hematocrit

c. Elevated mean corpuscular volume

d. Elevated total iron-binding capacity (TIBC)

60. The treatment of iron deficiency anemia in infants and children will most likely include:

a. Oral iron supplements

b. Parenteral iron

c. Intravenous iron

d. Blood transfusions

61. A hemorrhagic disorder in which the number of circulating platelets is reduced because of antiplatelet antibody is:
    a. Idiopathic thrombocytopenic purpura
    b. Hemophilia A
    c. Hemophilia B
    d. Thalassemia minor

62. The condition in which the meatus is located on the ventral side of the penis is:
    a. Epispadias
    b. Hypospadias
    c. Hyperspadias
    d. Exstrophy

63. What is the most common symptom noted in children with Wilms' tumor?
    a. Abdominal pain
    b. Hematuria
    c. Hypertension
    d. Abdominal mass

64. Which statement best describes primary enuresis in a child?
    a. "He never attained dryness."
    b. "She was once bladder trained for a year."
    c. "He is dry only during the day."
    d. "She is usually incontinent during the day."

65. Enuresis may be treated with a nasal spray to reduce urinary output. This spray is called:
    a. Imipramine (Tofranil)
    b. Amoxicillin (Amoxil)
    c. Pseudoephedrine (Sudafed)
    d. Desmopressin (DDAVP).

66. A physician orders ribavirin for a child with severe bronchiolitis. Which nursing implication is appropriate for this medication?
    a. Give the medication deep intramuscularly.
    b. Give the medication directly to the croupette.
    c. Monitor the child's vital signs every 1 to 2 hours.
    d. Administer the medication with milk.

67. Which of the following nursing interventions is most appropriate for a 3-year-old boy who arrives in the emergency room with a temperature of 105 degrees, inspiratory stridor and restlessness, and who is leaning forward and drooling?
    a. Auscultate his lungs and place him in a croupette.
    b. Have him lie down and rest after encouraging fluids.
    c. Examine his throat and perform a throat culture.
    d. Notify the physician immediately and be prepared for intubation.

68. Which nursing implementation should not be included in the care plan for a child receiving an aminoglycoside?
    a. Assess the child's hearing.
    b. Increase the child's fluid intake.
    c. Assess kidney functioning.
    d. Administer medication with food.

69. A 5-year-old boy is placed on an antibiotic. Which one would be contraindicated because of his age?
    a. Tetracycline
    b. Erythromycin
    c. Penicillin
    d. Theophylline

70. A nurse caring for a child with thalassemia being given a blood transfusion should monitor the child for:
    a. Iron toxicity
    b. Anemic reaction
    c. Fluid underload
    d. Sickle cell crisis

71. How often should an adolescent in sickle cell crisis receive medication for pain?
    a. Infrequently to avoid addiction
    b. Only once at bedtime
    c. As needed, as prescribed
    d. Never, owing to depression

72. Aspirin, rectal temperatures, and intramuscular injections should be avoided in children with:
    a. Iron deficiency anemia
    b. Idiopathic thrombocytopenic purpura

c. Sickle cell anemia

d. Thalassemia

73. A child with hemophilia complains of a sudden, severe headache. He is confused, lethargic, and vomiting. The nurse should suspect:

a. Intracranial bleeding

b. Factor reaction

c. Psychogenic stress

d. AIDS

74. The teaching plan for a 13-year-old with sickle cell anemia should include all of the following except:

a. Frequent aerobic exercise

b. Avoiding infected persons

c. Well-balanced diet

d. Discussing the possibility of bed wetting

75. The nurse should suggest genetic counseling for each of the following except:

a. Sickle cell anemia

b. Thalassemia

c. Hemophilia

d. Idiopathic thrombocytopenic purpura

76. Which of the following factors predisposes the urinary tract to infection?

a. A short urethra in females

b. Frequent emptying of the bladder

c. Increased fluid intake

d. Ingestion of acidic juices

77. Which of the following is the most likely cause of acute glomerulonephritis in a schoolager?

a. Impaired reabsorption of bicarbonate ions

b. An antecedent streptococcal infection

c. Gross inability to concentrate urine

d. Vesicoureteral reflux

78. What should the nurse expect to note in the urinalysis of a child in the acute phase of poststreptococcal glomerulonephritis?

a. Bacteria and hematuria

b. Hematuria and proteinuria

c. Bacteria and increased specific gravity

d. Proteinuria and decreased specific gravity

79. Which of the following manifestations would the nurse expect to note in a child with nephrotic syndrome?

a. Hematuria and bacteriuria

b. Massive proteinuria and edema

c. Gross hematuria and fever

d. Hypertension and weight loss

80. The primary objective in caring for a child with nephrotic syndrome is:

a. Reducing excretion of urinary protein

b. Encouraging a low-protein diet

c. Controlling the development of hematuria

d. Encouraging normal development

81. Which of the following are the most common symptoms of a brain tumor in children?

a. Ataxia and seizures

b. Poor fine and gross motor control

c. Fever and irritability

d. Headache and vomiting

82. A 10-year-old fell and injured his head. The nurse notes that he has "raccoon eyes" and a "battle sign." The child most likely has:

a. Linear skull fracture

b. Basilar skull fracture

c. Epidural hematoma

d. Subdural hematoma

83. What is the most likely cause of non-communicating hydrocephalus?

a. Developmental malformation

b. Bacterial meningitis

c. Prenatal infection

d. Birth trauma

84. Which of the following phrases best describes the pathophysiology of non-communicating hydrocephalus?

a. Precursor of spina bifida occulta

b. Obstruction of cerebrospinal fluid flow in ventricular system

c. Impaired absorption of cerebrospinal fluid in subarachnoid spaces

d. Cystic formation of the cerebral hemisphere

85. Which prenatal maternal disorder may have significance in the development of myelomeningocele?
   a. Iron deficiency anemia
   b. Protein-losing enteropathy
   c. Folic acid deficiency
   d. Diabetes insipidus

86. Which of the following is most characteristic of spastic cerebral palsy?
   a. Athetosis
   b. Dyskinesia
   c. Wide-based gait
   d. Hypertonicity

87. Which of the following is a progressive degenerative disorder characterized by the absence of dystrophin?
   a. Neural tube defect
   b. Cerebral palsy
   c. Muscular dystrophy
   d. Mental retardation

88. Which one of the following clinical manifestations is characteristic of rubeola?
   a. Koplik's spots
   b. Occipital adenopathy
   c. Vesicular rash
   d. Parotid swelling

89. When is varicella no longer communicable?
   a. When crusts form
   b. In 2 to 3 weeks
   c. After the coryza subsides
   d. During the prodromal phase

90. What is the most dangerous complication of rubella?
   a. Arthralgia
   b. Pyrexia
   c. Purpura
   d. Teratogenic effects

91. A 4-month-old infant's diagnosis of HIV infection was most likely confirmed by:
   a. ELISA
   b. Western blot
   c. HIV culture
   d. CD4 count

92. A whitish-gray membrane adherent to the tonsils is characteristic of:
   a. Pertussis
   b. Diphtheria
   c. Poliomyelitis
   d. Kawasaki's disease

93. A healthy 4-month-old child would receive which of the following immunizations at a well child care visit?
   a. DTP, TOPV, HB
   b. DTP, TIPV, Hib
   c. DTP, TOPV, Hib
   d. DT, TOPV, Hib

94. Which of the following is a contraindication for receiving MMR?
   a. Previous anaphylactic reaction to eggs
   b. Presence of HIV disease
   c. Concurrent administration of DTP
   d. Administration of immunoglobulins 12 months ago

95. Which child would most likely receive Acelimmune (acellular pertussis)?
   a. A healthy 2-month-old
   b. An immunosuppressed 2-month-old
   c. An immunosuppressed 6-month-old
   d. A healthy 4-year-old

96. All of the following manifestations are characteristic in all clients with cerebral palsy except:
   a. Delayed gross motor development
   b. Decreasing cognitive functioning
   c. Abnormal muscle performance
   d. Altered muscle tone

97. Which is characteristic of a preschooler with mild mental retardation?
   a. Slow to feed self
   b. Lack of speech
   c. Marked motor delays
   d. Inability to walk

98. Characteristics of Down's syndrome include:
   a. Small tongue
   b. Transverse palmar crease
   c. Large nose
   d. Restricted joint movement

99. Gower's sign is a prominent characteristic in the early stages of:
   a. Cerebral palsy

b. Spina bifida
c. Muscular dystrophy
d. Down's syndrome

100. Which of the following statements is true about the immunizations that should be given to a child with AIDS?
   a. She should not receive MMR.
   b. He should receive TIPV.
   c. She should receive all immunizations as scheduled.
   d. He should not receive any immunizations.

101. Unilateral or bilateral parotid enlargement is noted in which of the following:
   a. Diphtheria
   b. Poliomyelitis
   c. Mumps
   d. Pertussis

102. Which of the following nursing diagnoses takes priority for a child in a fresh hip spica cast?
   a. Risk for infection
   b. Risk for injury
   c. Risk for impaired skin integrity
   d. Altered tissue perfusion

103. Which of the following should not be taught to the parents of a child with a Denis-Browne splint or bar?
   a. Protect feet with socks.
   b. Reposition shoes on bar as needed.
   c. Check feet for swelling.
   d. Cut out toes of shoes for growth.

104. The nurse can best assist parents to prevent rheumatic fever by teaching them to:
   a. Avoid all exposure to strep infections.
   b. Treat all sore throats with antibiotics.
   c. Identify early signs and symptoms of rheumatic fever.
   d. Use prescribed treatment for streptococcal infections.

105. A toddler cries and clings to his mother as she attempts to leave the hospital. The mother asks the nurse what she should do. The nurse should respond:
   a. "Don't worry, he'll stop crying as soon as you leave."
   b. "It's probably better if you didn't visit that often."
   c. "I'll stay with him while you leave."
   d. "Try to sneak away while he is playing."

106. A 15-year-old boy with a full leg cast is screaming in unrelenting pain and his pale right foot signifies compartment syndrome. What should the nurse do first?
   a. Medicate him with acetaminophen.
   b. Notify the physician immediately.
   c. Release the traction.
   d. Monitor him every 5 minutes.

107. A child was placed in a Pavlik harness for bilateral congenital hip dysplasia (congenital dislocated hip). Which of the following should be included in parent teaching?
   a. Remove the harness during baths.
   b. Turn the child only three times a day.
   c. Have the child lie only on the affected side.
   d. Check the child's skin for breakdown.

For additional questions, see
***Lippincott's Self-Study Series* Software**
Available at your bookstore

Answer Sheet for Comprehensive Exam

With a pencil, blacken the circle under the option you have chosen for your correct answer.

	A	B	C	D		A	B	C	D		A	B	C	D
1.	○	○	○	○	21.	○	○	○	○	41.	○	○	○	○
2.	○	○	○	○	22.	○	○	○	○	42.	○	○	○	○
3.	○	○	○	○	23.	○	○	○	○	43.	○	○	○	○
4.	○	○	○	○	24.	○	○	○	○	44.	○	○	○	○
5.	○	○	○	○	25.	○	○	○	○	45.	○	○	○	○
6.	○	○	○	○	26.	○	○	○	○	46.	○	○	○	○
7.	○	○	○	○	27.	○	○	○	○	47.	○	○	○	○
8.	○	○	○	○	28.	○	○	○	○	48.	○	○	○	○
9.	○	○	○	○	29.	○	○	○	○	49.	○	○	○	○
10.	○	○	○	○	30.	○	○	○	○	50.	○	○	○	○
11.	○	○	○	○	31.	○	○	○	○	51.	○	○	○	○
12.	○	○	○	○	32.	○	○	○	○	52.	○	○	○	○
13.	○	○	○	○	33.	○	○	○	○	53.	○	○	○	○
14.	○	○	○	○	34.	○	○	○	○	54.	○	○	○	○
15.	○	○	○	○	35.	○	○	○	○	55.	○	○	○	○
16.	○	○	○	○	36.	○	○	○	○	56.	○	○	○	○
17.	○	○	○	○	37.	○	○	○	○	57.	○	○	○	○
18.	○	○	○	○	38.	○	○	○	○	58.	○	○	○	○
19.	○	○	○	○	39.	○	○	○	○	59.	○	○	○	○
20.	○	○	○	○	40.	○	○	○	○	60.	○	○	○	○

	A	B	C	D			A	B	C	D			A	B	C	D
61.	○	○	○	○		77.	○	○	○	○		93.	○	○	○	○
62.	○	○	○	○		78.	○	○	○	○		94.	○	○	○	○
63.	○	○	○	○		79.	○	○	○	○		95.	○	○	○	○
64.	○	○	○	○		80.	○	○	○	○		96.	○	○	○	○
65.	○	○	○	○		81.	○	○	○	○		97.	○	○	○	○
66.	○	○	○	○		82.	○	○	○	○		98.	○	○	○	○
67.	○	○	○	○		83.	○	○	○	○		99.	○	○	○	○
68.	○	○	○	○		84.	○	○	○	○		100.	○	○	○	○
69.	○	○	○	○		85.	○	○	○	○		101.	○	○	○	○
70.	○	○	○	○		86.	○	○	○	○		102.	○	○	○	○
71.	○	○	○	○		87.	○	○	○	○		103.	○	○	○	○
72.	○	○	○	○		88.	○	○	○	○		104.	○	○	○	○
73.	○	○	○	○		89.	○	○	○	○		105.	○	○	○	○
74.	○	○	○	○		90.	○	○	○	○		106.	○	○	○	○
75.	○	○	○	○		91.	○	○	○	○		107.	○	○	○	○
76.	○	○	○	○		92.	○	○	○	○						

COMPREHENSIVE TEST—ANSWERS

1. *Correct response: b*
   Children with cleft palate may have ineffective functioning of their eustachian tubes creating frequent bouts of otitis media.
   a. Most children with cleft palate remain well nourished owing to the institution of proper feeding techniques.
   c. Food does not pass through the cleft and into the eustachian tubes.
   d. There is no association between cleft palate and congenital ear deformities.
   Analysis/Physiologic/Assessment

2. *Correct response: a*
   The healing time for a femoral fracture in a small infant is 2 to 4 weeks.
   b. Children tend to heal in 4 to 6 weeks.
   c. Adolescents tend to heal in 8 to 10 weeks.
   d. Adults tend to heal in 10 to 16 weeks.
   Knowledge/Physiologic/Planning

3. *Correct response: b*
   The sanctuary phase of cancer therapy involves the use of treatments that will affect areas that are not affected by remission induction therapy because the medications do not cross their barriers.
   a. Remission induction is the first phase of therapy that is used to induce remission.
   c. Maintenance therapy is begun after the nadir or remission induction is resolved and is used to keep the child in remission.
   d. Reinduction therapy involves the reinitiation of treatment when exacerbation occurs; a different protocol may be utilized.
   Knowledge/Physiologic/Implementation

4. *Correct response: b*
   Osteogenesis imperfecta is a congenital disorder that results in pathologic fractures and is usually characterized by blue sclera.
   a. Osteomyelitis is an infection of the bone.
   c. Osteogenesis imperfecta is a cancer of the bone that may result in a fracture but is not associated with blue sclera.
   d. Osteoarthritis is a degenerative disorder.
   Comprehension/Physiologic/Analysis (Dx)

5. *Correct response: c*
   Hot spots on the cast are areas of warmth that radiate from inflamed tissue below the cast, which usually signifies infection.
   a, b and d. Cold toes, absent pulses, and cyanosis may all indicate neurovascular compromise.
   Application/Safe Care/Assessment

6. *Correct response: a*
   A lead level greater than 70 mcg/dL is indicative of the possibility of lead encephalopathy; therefore the child's neurologic status must be carefully monitored.
   b. Bone pain is unusual in lead poisoning.
   c. Teaching the parents how to decrease or stop pica to stop lead ingestion is important but not primary.
   d. Iron-rich foods are important to decrease anemia, but this is not primary.
   Application/Safe Care/Implementation

7. *Correct response: a*
   Side effects of lead chelators include seizure activity.
   b, c and d. These are not associated with BAL and CaNa2EDTA.
   Application/Safe Care/Implementation

8. *Correct response: d*

A 3-month-old infant should be able to lift the head and chest when prone.

  a. The Moro reflex should diminish or subside by 3 months.

  b. The parachute reflex appears at 9 months.

  c. Rolling front to back usually is accomplished at about 5 months.

Comprehension/Health Promotion/ Assessment

9. *Correct response: d*

A child's birth weight usually triples by 12 months.

  a. The child's birth weight usually doubles by 4 months.

  b and c. There are no set parameters at these ages.

Comprehensive/Health Promotion/ Assessment

10. *Correct response: c*

Toddlers engaging in parallel play will play near but not with each other.

  a, b and d. All are examples of cooperative play.

Comprehensive/Health Promotion/Planning

11. *Correct response: d*

The best way to examine a small child is to go from the least intrusive to the most intrusive.

  a. The head examination is intrusive.

  b. Distal to proximal is inappropriate at any age.

  c. The abdominal examination is intrusive.

Application/Health Promotion/ Assessment

12. *Correct response: b*

Swaddling has a soothing effect on some infants with colic.

  a. Shaking is *never* appropriate and may result in shaken baby syndrome, which could lead to brain damage or death.

  c and d. Neither of these has been proved to help infants with colic.

Application/Physiologic/Implementation

13. *Correct response: c*

Idiopathic scoliosis is most likely to occur in adolescent females during their growth spurt.

  a. Congenital hip dysplasia should be noted in infancy.

  b. Transient synovitis usually is seen in preschoolers.

  d. Tibial torsion should be noted during infancy.

Application/Health Promotion/ Assessment

14. *Correct response: a*

Postoperative bleeding and respiratory distress, secondary to anesthesia or edema, are the primary complications in a child immediately after cleft lip repair.

  b. Scarring and infection are likely to occur later in the postoperative course.

  c and d. Infection is likely to occur later.

Application/Safe Care/Implementation

15. *Correct response: c*

Rheumatic fever results as a delayed reaction to inadequately treated group A beta-hemolytic streptococcal infection.

  a. *Streptococcus pneumonia* does not result in rheumatic fever.

  b. *Haemophilus influenzae*, depending on strain, is responsible for illnesses such as otitis media, epiglottitis, and meningitis.

  d. *Staphylococcus aureus* is responsible for a number of pyrogenic infections but it does not result in rheumatic fever.

Knowledge/Physiologic/Analysis (Dx)

16. *Correct response: b*

Rheumatic fever is not contagious and therefore does not require isolation.

  a. The child will need adequate rest periods, especially if carditis is present.

  c. Adherence to medication therapy is needed to promote recovery and

to prevent relapse of streptococcal infection.
d. Adequate nutrition is needed to promote recovery.

Application/Physiologic/Implementation

17. **Correct response: c**
Anorexia, abdominal cramps, and vomiting are all early signs of plumbism, another name for lead poisoning.
   a. Plumbism may present with constipation; blurred vision and headache may be later signs, associated with encephalopathy.
   b. Dizziness may be a later sign associated with encephalopathy, but fever and chills are not associated with lead poisoning.
   d. Mild developmental and behavioral changes may be noted in early plumbism; however, seizures and coma accompany encephalopathy.

Application/Physiologic/Assessment

18. **Correct response: a**
Metabolic acidosis may result from a loss of base that would occur in diarrhea, and a 6-month-old has an immature homeostatic regulation system.
   b. Metabolic alkalosis is produced by a gain in base or a loss of acid (as in vomiting).
   c. Respiratory acidosis results from diminished or inadequate pulmonary ventilation, leading to elevated PCO_2 level.
   d. Respiratory alkalosis results from an increase in the rate and depth of respiration leading to decreased PCO_2 level.

Comprehensive/Physiologic/Analysis (Dx)

19. **Correct response: b**
The best way to monitor hydration status is by monitoring daily weights.
   a. Enteric, not strict, precautions usually are used for diarrhea.
   c. A 4-month-old usually is too young for antiemetics.

d. Monitoring the CBC would be helpful to note hydration status by monitoring the hematocrit, but it would not be a primary method.

Application/Physiologic/Implementation

20. **Correct response: d**
Severe dehydration (loss of more than 10% of body weight) would result in marked oliguria.
   a. Pallor would be noted in mild dehydration (<5% loss).
   b. The pulse increases as the child becomes more dehydrated and "shocky."
   c. The fontanel becomes depressed in dehydration.

Analysis/Physiologic/Assessment

21. **Correct response: a**
Acute lymphocytic leukemia (ALL) causes leukopenia, resulting in immunosuppression and increasing the risk of infection, a leading cause of death in children with ALL; therefore, the priority nursing intervention would be to decrease the risk of infection.
   b. Iron-rich foods help with anemia, but dietary iron is not the primary intervention.
   c. The prognosis of ALL usually is good, although death and dying may still be an issue in need of discussion. However, it is still not the primary intervention.
   d. Injections should be discouraged owing to increased risk from bleeding due to thrombocytopenia; however, injection issues are not primary.

Application/Safe Care/Planning

22. **Correct response: b**
Allopurinol is given in conjunction with chemotherapy to prevent kidney damage due to hyperuricemia from cell breakdown.
   a. Allopurinol does not prevent acid formation.

c. Allopurinol does not aid in tumor disintegration.

d. Allopurinol does not protect the liver and may actually alter liver function study results.

Knowledge/Physiologic/Planning

23. Correct response: b
Girls begin puberty between the ages of 8 and 14 years.
a, c and d. Boys begin puberty between the ages of 9 and 16 years.

Knowledge/Health Promotion/ Evaluation

24. Correct response: c
Rectal prolapse is the most common GI complication in cystic fibrosis.
a. Meconium ileus is the earliest manifestation of cystic fibrosis.
b. There is no association between cystic fibrosis and ulcerative colitis.
d. Diverticulitis is not the most common GI complication in cystic fibrosis.

Knowledge/Physiologic/Analysis (Dx)

25. Correct response: a
Chest percussion and postural drainage should be given before meals to increase the ease of eating and before sleep to promote adequate rest.
b. If chest physical therapy is given after meals it may induce vomiting.
c. Many children with CF cough spontaneously on awakening.
d. Chest physiotherapy is a crucial component in the treatment of CF.

Application/Physiologic/Planning

26. Correct response: b
Pancrease is a pancreatic enzyme supplement that aids fat digestion in children who have CF and who, therefore, have thickened secretions that inhibit the release of pancreatic fat-digesting enzymes.
a. Pancrease is not given to soften stools and children with CF may have loose fatty stools from malabsorption.

c. Pancrease does not prevent diabetes mellitus.

d. Pancrease is not an antibiotic.

Comprehensive/Physiologic/Analysis (Dx)

27. Correct response: b
The moisturized air in the croupette aids in thinning secretions, thereby easing respirations.
a. Usually, it is inadvisable to have the oxygen level greater than 40%.
c. The croupette cools and soothes the respiratory tract.
d. Although the croupette does provide a bit of isolation, it is not used for this purpose.

Comprehension/Physiologic/Planning

28. Correct response: a
Bleeding and clotting times must be carefully monitored before a tonsil- and adenoidectomy because of the increased vascularity of that surgical site.
b and d. A urinalysis and a differential blood count are helpful preoperatively, and may be required; however, they are not priorities.
c. Serum electrolyte levels are seldom needed unless there are complicating factors.

Application/Physiologic/Planning

29. Correct response: b
Status asthmaticus is an acute asthmatic episode that is difficult to control.
a. Asthma is not contagious.
c. The presence of asthma does not usually indicate the presence of emphysema.
d. Status asthmaticus may be fatal, but not always.

Comprehensive/Physiologic/Analysis (Dx)

30. Correct response: c
The position used to treat congenital hip dysplasia is flexed and abducted.
a, b and d. All are inappropriate positions.

Comprehensive/Physiologic/ Implementation

31. *Correct response: a*
Tetanus toxoid provides artificial active immunity. It is man-made and it causes the body to produce its own antibodies.
  b. Artificial passive immunity is a substance that is man-made, but the antibodies are given directly to the child (tetanus immunoglobulin).
  c. Natural passive immunity results from a natural substance that gives antibodies (placental transfer).
  d. Natural active immunity results from the disease itself, whereby the person's body makes its own antibodies.
Knowledge/Health Promotion/ Analysis (Dx)

32. *Correct response: a*
The pertussis component may result in fever and the tetanus component may result in injection soreness; therefore, feedback on fever reduction instructions indicates understanding.
  b. There are no dietary restrictions for this injection.
  c. A subsequent rash is more likely to be seen 5 to 10 days after receiving the MMR vaccine.
  d. Diarrhea is unrelated to the DTP.
Application/Health Promotion/ Evaluation

33. *Correct response: a*
Multiple bruising and burns on a toddler are signs of child abuse; it is the nurse's responsibility to report the case to protective services immediately to protect the child from further harm.
  b. Additional harm may come to the child if the nurse waits for further assessment data.
  c. Notifying the physician immediately does not initiate the removal of the child from harm nor does it absolve the nurse from responsibility.
  d. These are not normal toddler injuries.
Application/Safe Care/Assessment

34. *Correct response: d*
Theophylline is administered to promote bronchodilation; therefore, the nurse would monitor its effectiveness by assessing for improved color and respiratory status.
  a. Vomiting and lethargy are signs of theophylline toxicity; dyspnea does not indicate improvement.
  b. Nausea is a side effect, or may indicate toxicity.
  c. Diarrhea may be side effect and wheezing does not indicate improvement.
Application/Physiologic/Evaluation

35. *Correct response: a*
Projectile vomiting is a key indicator of pyloric stenosis.
  b. Choking after feedings usually is seen in tracheoesophageal fistula.
  c. Currant jelly stools are indicative of intussusception.
  d. Abdominal distention is not usually noted in pyloric stenosis, but a pyloric "olive" may be palpated.
Application/Physiologic/Assessment

36. *Correct response: a*
Polycythemia results from an inadequate mechanism to compensate for decreased oxygen saturation, and the resultant increase in red blood cells may lead to clumping and emboli formation.
  b. Cardiomyopathy usually is not directly associated with emboli formation.
  c. Endocarditis may develop from infection.
  d. CVAs are more likely to be associated with high blood pressure.
Comprehensive/Physiologic/Analysis (Dx)

37. *Correct response: d*
Tachycardia and hepatomegaly are manifestations of congestive heart failure.
  a and b. The child would have tachycardia not bradycardia.
  c. The child would have weak pulses.
Comprehensive/Physiologic/Evaluation

38. *Correct response: c*

The preschool period is a time when children are preoccupied with their genitalia and the time of the Oedipal conflict.

a. A fear of loss of control is noted more often in toddlers.

b. Preschoolers do have fear of the dark but this is not related to psychosexual preoccupations.

d. Fear of separation may be noted in preschoolers, but it is seen more often in toddlers and it is not related to psychosexual preoccupations.

Comprehensive/Psychosocial/Evaluation

39. *Correct response: a*

According to Erikson, when the school-age child is stressed, he or she may develop a sense of inferiority.

b. Guilt may develop in the preschool period.

c. Shame and doubt may develop in the toddler period.

d. Role diffusion may develop in the adolescent.

Comprehensive/Psychosocial/Analysis (Dx)

40. *Correct response: b*

Adult perpetrators of child sexual abuse usually are known to the child.

a. Adult perpetrators of child sexual abuse usually are known to the child.

c. Perpetrators may have substance abuse problems, but this is not always the case.

d. Perpetrators may have personality problems, but this is not always the case.

Knowledge/Psychosocial/Planning

41. *Correct response: d*

The head-to-tail direction of growth is called cephalocaudal development.

a. Proximodistal development occurs from the center of the body to the extremities.

b. Sequential development denotes predictable sequences of growth.

c. Mass-to-specific development denotes the ability to perform simple before the complex.

Knowledge/Physiologic/Assessment

42. *Correct response: a*

The child is experiencing a reaction formation, which is the doing or saying of the opposite of how one feels. This is a common reaction to hospitalization in the school-age child.

b. Repression is the submerging of painful ideas into the unconscious.

c. Sublimation is the conversion of drives into acceptable activities.

d. Regression is the turning back to a former state.

Analysis/Psychosocial/Analysis (Dx)

43. *Correct response: c*

Seven to nine year olds are more likely to personify death.

a. Three to five year olds see death as reversible.

b. Five to six year olds see death in degrees.

d. Nine to eleven year olds defy death with daredevil behavior.

Knowledge/Psychosocial/Analysis (Dx)

44. *Correct response: a*

Protest is the initial stage of separation anxiety, and it is the stage during which the child cries inconsolably and searches for the lost parents.

b. During despair, the child demonstrates a disinterest in the environment and is very passive.

c and d. Denial and detachment are names for the same stage during which the child demonstrates a superficial adjustment.

Analysis/Psychosocial/Analysis (Dx)

45. *Correct response: b*

Projection is the defense mechanism used when a person attributes his or her own undesirable traits to another.

a. Displacement is the transfer of emotion onto an unrelated object.

c. Repression is the submerging of painful ideas into the unconscious.

d. Psychosis is a state of being out of touch with reality.

Analysis/Psychosocial/Analysis (Dx)

46. *Correct response: c*
The most overwhelming adverse influence on health in children is low socioeconomic status.
  a, b and d. All are influences on health, but none of them is the most influential.

Knowledge/Health Promotion/ Evaluation

47. *Correct response: d*
When caring for a family with a different cultural background, the nurse should adapt cultural practices to health care needs as necessary.
  a. Cultural influences are always present.
  b. Practices should be allowed as possible.
  c. The nurse should not attempt to change a family's sociocultural beliefs.

Comprehensive/Health Promotion/ Analysis (Dx)

48. *Correct response: c*
The nurse should not attempt to function as a surrogate parent.
  a, b and d. All are appropriate interventions for promoting parenting skills.

Application/Psychosocial/Implementation

49. *Correct response: c*
In most states, adolescents with sexually transmitted diseases can be evaluated and treated by their own consent.
  a, b and d. In most states, nonemergent medical interventions require parental consent for a minor unless the minor is emancipated.

Comprehension/Health Promotion/ Analysis (Dx)

50. *Correct response: a*
Bronchopulmonary dysplasia usually results in low birth weight infants who receive oxygen therapy.
  b. Necrotizing enterocolitis is an acute inflammatory bowel disorder that usually is seen in low birth weight infants and is of unknown etiology.
  c. Congestive heart failure usually results secondarily to congenital heart disease.
  d. Meconium aspiration syndrome usually results from some form of intrauterine stress.

Knowledge/Physiologic/Evaluation

51. *Correct response: b*
Tetralogy of Fallot consists of pulmonary stenosis, ventricular septal defect, overriding aorta, and hypertrophy of the right ventricle.
  a. There is hypertrophy of the right, not left, ventricle.
  c. There is pulmonic, not aortic, stenosis.
  d. There is pulmonic, not aortic, stenosis, and there is right, not left, ventricular failure.

Knowledge/Physiologic/Analysis (Dx)

52. *Correct response: d*
The child with tetralogy of Fallot may assume a squatting position to decrease venous return of blood with lower oxygen concentration from the lower extremities.
  a, b and c. Low Fowler's, prone, and supine positioning do not alleviate the problem and therefore are not utilized.

Comprehensive/Physiologic/Analysis (Dx)

53. *Correct response: a*
Children with congenital heart disease are more prone to respiratory infections.
  b, c and d. None of these are associated with congenital heart disease.

Comprehensive/Physiologic/Analysis (Dx)

54. Correct response: d
Therapy for thalassemia consists of frequent blood transfusions to replace faulty hemoglobin.
   a. Oxygen therapy is not the primary treatment modality.
   b. Adequate hydration is important, but it is more crucial in children with sickle cell anemia.
   c. Supplemental iron is contraindicated in children with thalassemia because iron toxicity would develop.
Comprehensive/Physiologic/Planning

55. Correct response: d
Rheumatic fever results from inadequately treated infections from group A beta-hemolytic streptococci.
   a. Rheumatic fever should not develop if the child has been adequately treated.
   b. Children with congenital heart disease are prone to endocarditis.
   c. There is no association between chicken pox and rheumatic fever.
Comprehensive/Physiologic/Assessment

56. Correct response: a
Children with tachypnea may be unable to suck and may aspirate; therefore, the child may be placed on intravenous fluids and NPO.
   b. Irritability alone does not interfere with fluid intake.
   c. The presence of fever may require IV fluids, but the child would not need to be NPO.
   d. Tachycardia alone does not interfere with fluid intake.
Comprehensive/Safe Care/Analysis (Dx)

57. Correct response: b
Hemorrhage may occur 5 to 10 days after a tonsil- and adenoidectomy from tissue sloughing that occurs with healing.
   a. Infection usually is not related to bleeding.
   c. Secretions do not cause bleeding.
   d. Increased vascularity most likely causes bleeding immediately postoperatively.
Knowledge/Safe Care/Analysis (Dx)

58. Correct response: d
SIDS occurs most frequently in the winter.
   a, b and c. SIDS occurs more commonly in the winter than it does in the other seasons.
Knowledge/Safe Care/Analysis (Dx)

59. Correct responses: c
Children with iron deficiency anemia have decreased, not elevated, MCV levels demonstrating microcytic anemia.
   a, b and d. Low hemoglobin and hematocrit and an elevated serum iron-binding capacity are all noted in iron deficiency anemia.
Knowledge/Physiologic/Analysis

60. Correct response: a
Most children with iron deficiency anemia may be managed with oral iron supplements.
   b and d. Parenteral iron and blood transfusions usually are not needed.
   c. Intravenous iron is not used.
Comprehensive/Physiologic/Planning

61. Correct response: a
Idiopathic thrombocytopenic purpura is a hemorrhagic disorder in which the number of circulating platelets is reduced owing to antiplatelet antibodies.
   b. Hemophilia A is a deficiency in factor VIII.
   c. Hemophilia B is a deficiency in factor IX.
   d. Thalassemia minor is the heterozygous form of thalassemia.
Knowledge/Planning/Analysis (Dx)

62. Correct response: b
The meatus is located on the ventral side of the penis in hypospadias.
   a. The meatus is located on the dorsal side of the penis in epispadias.

c. There is no hyperspadias.
d. Exstrophy of the bladder is a condition in which the bladder develops outside of the abdominal wall, in utero.

Knowledge/Physiologic/Assessment

63. *Correct response: d*
The most common presenting sign in Wilms' tumor is an abdominal mass.
a and c. Abdominal pain and hypertension may be noted as later signs.
b. There may be microscopic hematuria, but not usually frank bleeding, and it is not the most common sign.

Comprehensive/Physiologic/Analysis (Dx)

64. *Correct response: a*
Children with primary eneuresis have never attained dryness.
b. Children who have previously been bladder trained and then develop eneuresis have secondary eneuresis.
c. Dryness during the day, nocturesis, does not specifically denote primary eneuresis.
d. Daytime incontinence is not a sign of enuresis.

Comprehensive/Physiologic/Analysis (Dx)

65. *Correct response: d*
Desmopressin (DDAVP) is the nasal spray that is used to treat enuresis by reducing urinary output.
a. Imipramine is an oral antidepressant that may be used for eneuresis.
b. Amoxicillin is an antibiotic that may be used for a urinary tract infection.
c. Pseudoephedrine is a decongestant and is unrelated to enuresis.

Knowledge/Physiologic/Planning

66. *Correct response: c*
Ribavirin may cause hypotension; therefore, vital signs, including blood pressure, must be monitored frequently.

a. Ribavirin is given by aerosol means.
b. Ribavirin is given through a small particle aerosol generator and is not placed directly into the croupette reservoir.
d. Ribavirin is administered by an aerosol device and, therefore, does not need to be given with milk.

Application/Safe Care/Implementation

67. *Correct response: d*
The child is exhibiting classic signs of epiglottitis, which is always a pediatric emergency. The physician must be notified immediately and the nurse must be prepared for an emergency intubation or tracheotomy.
a. Further assessment wastes valuable time.
b. Having the child lie down causes more distress and may result in respiratory arrest.
c. Throat examination may result in laryngospasm that could be fatal.

Application/Safe Care/Implementation

68. *Correct response: d*
Most aminoglycosides are administered either IM or IV.
a. Aminoglycosides are ototoxic.
b and c. Aminoglycosides are renal toxic.

Application/Safe Care/Implementation

69. *Correct response: a*
Tetracycline may cause dental and bone problems in children under age 9.
b and c. Erythromycin and penicillin are not contraindicated in this age group.
d. Theophylline is not an antibiotic.

Analysis/Physiologic/Planning

70. *Correct response: a*
Children with thalassemia may experience iron toxicity during blood transfusions.
b, c and d. These are not associated with thalassemia.

Application/Safe Care/Planning

71. Correct response: c
Sickle cell crisis is extremely painful and adolescents should be medicated as needed, as ordered.
a. Addiction is not a priority issue in this case.
b. Bedtime-only medication is highly inadequate.
d. These children need to be medicated for pain, even if depressed, as pain may increase depression.
Application/Physiologic/Planning

72. Correct response: b
Children with idiopathic thrombocytopenic purpura are prone to excessive bleeding; therefore, any medications or treatments that may increase the risk of bleeding should be avoided. Aspirin has antiplatelet properties and idiopathic thrombocytopenic purpura results in decreased platelets.
a, c and d. No excessive bleeding is noted in these disorders.
Analysis/Safe Care/Planning

73. Correct response: a
These symptoms strongly suggest intracranial bleeding in a child with hemophilia who is at risk for same.
b. These symptoms are not associated with factor reaction.
c. Psychogenic stress would not be as sudden.
d. Although some of these symptoms may be noted in AIDS, the onset would not be as abrupt.
Analysis/Safe Care/Analysis (Dx)

74. Correct response: a
Frequent aerobic exercise may cause sickling.
b. Children with sickle cell anemia may go into sickle cell crisis when they develop infections; therefore, they should avoid contact with infected persons.
c. A well-balanced diet will help the child to remain as healthy as possible.

d. Children with sickle cell anemia are prone to bed wetting.
Application/Physiologic/Evaluation

75. Correct response: d
Idiopathic thrombocytopenic purpura is not genetic.
a. Sickle cell anemia is autosomal recessive.
b. Thalassemia major is autosomal recessive.
c. Hemophilia usually is X-linked.
Comprehensive/Health Promotion/ Implementation

76. Correct response: a
A short urethra in females decreases the distance for organisms to travel, thereby increasing the chance of developing a urinary tract infection.
b. Frequent emptying of the bladder would help to decrease urinary tract infections by avoiding sphincter stress.
c. Increased fluid intake prevents urinary tract infections by enabling the bladder to be cleared more frequently.
d. Acidic juices help to keep the urine pH acidic and thus decrease the chance of flora development.
Analysis/Health Promotion/ Analysis (Dx)

77. Correct response: b
AGN usually is associated with an antecedent infection, most commonly streptococcus.
a. There is no relationship between AGN and impaired reabsorption of bicarbonate ions.
c. The gross inability to concentrate urine usually is a sign of diabetes insipidus.
d. Vesicoureteral reflux is not associated with AGN.
Knowledge/Physiologic/Analysis (Dx)

78. Correct response: b
Urinalysis results of a child in the acute phase of AGN would show hematuria and proteinuria.

a and c. Bacteria usually are not noted.

d. The specific gravity may be elevated.

Comprehensive/Physiologic/Analysis (Dx)

79. Correct response: b
Manifestations of nephrotic syndrome include massive proteinuria and edema.

a. Hematuria and bacteriuria usually are not noted.

c. Gross hematuria and fever are not noted; fever indicates an infection.

d. The blood pressure is either normal or decreased.

Application/Physiologic/Assessment

80. Correct response: a
The primary objective in caring for a child with nephrotic syndrome is reducing the excretion of urinary protein.

b. The diet should be rich in protein.

c. There is no hematuria.

d. Normal development should be encouraged, but it is not the primary objective.

Analysis/Physiologic/Analysis (Dx)

81. Correct response: d
The most common symptoms of brain tumors in children are headache and vomiting (usually projectile).

a. Ataxia and seizures are late signs and are not noted in all children.

b. Poor fine and gross motor control may develop, but this is not typical.

c. Occurrence of fever depends on location of the tumor.

Comprehensive/Physiologic/Assessment

82. Correct response: b
"Raccoon eyes" and "battle sign" (bruising behind the ear from bleeding into the mastoid sinus) are classic signs of a basilar skull fracture.

a. Linear skull fractures usually do not trigger any symptoms.

c. An epidural hematoma is charac-

terized by rapid deterioration, including headache, seizures, coma, and brain herniation.

d. A subdural hematoma is characterized by developing agitation, lethargy, headache, and drowsiness within the first 48 hours of a head injury.

Analysis/Physiologic/Analysis (Dx)

83. Correct response: a
The most common cause of noncommunicating hydrocephalus is developmental malformation.

b, c and d. All may cause hydrocephalus, but they are not the most common cause.

Comprehensive/Physiologic/Analysis (Dx)

84. Correct response: b
Noncommunicating hydrocephalus results from obstructed CSF flow in the ventricular system.

a. Hydrocephalus is not a precursor of neural tube defects, such as spina bifida occulta, but they may occur together.

c. Communicating hydrocephalus results from impaired absorption of CSF in the subarachnoid spaces.

d. Cystic formation of the cerebral hemispheres is incompatible with life.

Comprehensive/Physiologic/Analysis (Dx)

85. Correct response: c
Folic acid deficiency has been associated with the development of neural tube defects.

a, b and d. There has been no relationship noted with these disorders.

Knowledge/Physiologic/Analysis (Dx)

86. Correct response: d
Hypertonicity is associated with spastic cerebral palsy.

a. Athetosis is associated with dyskinetic CP.

b. Dyskinesia is associated with dyskinetic CP.

c. Wide-based gait is associated with ataxic CP.

Comprehensive/Physiologic/Analysis (Dx)

87. *Correct response: c*
Muscular dystrophy is characterized by the absence of dystrophin.
   a. NTDs are central nervous system defects involving the cranium and the spinal cord.
   b. Cerebral palsy is a group of disabilities caused by injury or insult to the brain before birth, during birth, or in the first year of life.
   d. Mental retardation describes subaverage intellectual functioning accompanied by adaptive behavior deficits.

Comprehensive/Physiologic/Analysis (Dx)

88. *Correct response: a*
Koplik's spots are seen in measles.
   b. Occipital adenopathy occurs in German measles.
   c. A vesicular rash may be seen in herpes.
   d. Parotid swelling is noted in mumps.

Knowledge/Physiologic/Assessment

89. *Correct response: a*
Varicella ceases to be contagious when the crusts are formed.
   b. Two to three weeks is not specific enough.
   c and d. The child will still be contagious after the coryza subsides and during the prodromal phase.

Comprehensive/Safe Care/Planning

90. *Correct response: d*
The most dangerous complication of rubella is its teratogenic effects on the fetus.
   a and b. Arthralgia and fever may occur, but they usually are mild and self-limiting.
   c. There are no purpura.

Comprehensive/Safe Care/Analysis (Dx)

91. *Correct response: c*
An HIV culture, which can detect the presence of maternal antibodies, is used to confirm HIV in children under 18 months.
   a and b. The ELISA and Western blot tests are not helpful because of the presence of maternal antibodies.
   d. A CD4 count will not be used for confirmation, but will be needed for assessing immune status.

Comprehensive/Physiologic/Analysis (Dx)

92. *Correct response: b*
A whitish-gray membrane adherent to the tonsils is characteristic of diphtheria.
   a. Whooping cough is characteristic of pertussis.
   c. Paralysis is characteristic of poliomyelitis.
   d. Kawasaki's disease is characterized by involvement of the skin, conjunctive, and mucous membranes.

Knowledge/Physiologic/Assessment

93. *Correct response: c*
DTP, TOPV, and Hib are routinely given at the 6-month visit.
   a. HB is routinely given during the newborn period, 2 months and 6 months.
   b. TIPV is not used in healthy children.
   d. DT is not used unless the child cannot have the pertussis vaccine.

Comprehensive/Health Promotion/ Planning

94. *Correct response: a*
MMR is contraindicated in children who have had a previous serious allergic reaction to eggs because the vaccine in cultivated in eggs.
   b. Children with HIV disease may receive MMR.
   c. There is no contraindication for the concurrent administration of DTP.

d. The vaccine should be held for 3 to 4 months after the client receives immunoglobulin.

Comprehensive/Safe Care/Analysis (Dx)

95. *Correct response: d*
Acelimmune is used for children age 18 months and older to decrease the reaction to the pertussis vaccine.
a, b and c. Acelimmunne has not been approved as yet for children under age 18 months.

Comprehensive/Safe Care/Planning

96. *Correct response: b*
Decreased cognitive functioning is not noted in all children with CP; in fact, it is very possible to have CP without cognitive impairment.
a, c and d. All of these are associated with CP.

Knowledge/Physiologic/Assessment

97. *Correct response: a*
Children with mild mental retardation may be slow to perform tasks such as feeding.
b, c and d. These are noted with more severe degrees of mental retardation.

Knowledge/Physiologic/Assessment

98. *Correct response: b*
A transverse palmar crease (simian crease) is characteristic of Down's syndrome.
a. Children with Down's syndrome have large tongues.
c. Children with Down's syndrome have small noses.
d. Children with Down's syndrome have loose joints.

Knowledge/Physiologic/Assessment

99. *Correct response: c*
Gower's sign is classic in muscular dystrophy.
a, b and d. There is no association.

Comprehensive/Physiologic/Analysis (Dx)

100. *Correct response: b*
Children with HIV disease should not receive the live polio vaccine (TOPV);

therefore, they are given the inactivated form (TIPV).
a. Children with HIV do receive MMR.
c. Children with HIV do not receive all immunizations as scheduled; they receive TIPV instead of TOPV.
d. Children with HIV need to be immunized.

Analysis/Safe Care/Planning

101. *Correct response: c*
Unilateral or bilateral parotid swelling is noted in mumps.
a. Diphtheria is characterized by a whitish-gray membrane on the tonsils.
b. Poliomyelitis is characterized by paralysis.
d. Pertussis is characterized by a whooping cough.

Knowledge/Physiologic/Analysis (Dx)

102. *Correct response: d*
Altered tissue perfusion is the priority nursing diagnosis for a child in a new spica cast because of the likelihood that neurovascular complications may develop.
a, b and c. All are appropriate diagnoses, but they are not the priority.

Application/Safe Care/Analysis (Dx)

103. *Correct response: b*
The shoes of the Denis-Browne splint (or bar) should not be repositioned by the parents.
a, c and d. All are appropriate items to teach the parents.

Application/Safe Care/Evaluation

104. *Correct response: d*
Rheumatic fever can best be prevented by using prescribed treatment for streptococcal infections.
a. It is almost impossible to avoid contact with all streptococcal infections.
b. Not all sore throats are caused by streptococcal infection; a rapid

strep test or a culture must be obtained for verification.

c. Identification of the early signs of a disease is not prevention.

Comprehensive/Health Promotion/ Implementation

105. Correct response: c
Staying with a toddler who is experiencing separation anxiety is an appropriate intervention for both the child and the parent.

a. The child will not stop crying when the mother leaves.

b. Visiting should be encouraged.

d. The parent should never sneak away; this could injure the child's sense of trust.

Application/Psychosocial/Implementation

106. Correct response: b
Compartment syndrome is an emergent situation and the physician needs to be notified immediately.

a. Acetaminophen (Tylenol) will be ineffective and the physician should be contacted first.

c. There is no indication to release traction.

d. In an emergent situation, monitoring every 5 minutes will create disastrous consequences and complications.

Application/Safe Care/Implementation

107. Correct response: d
Children in a Pavlik harness must be assessed for skin breakdown.

a. The harness usually is not removed and the child is sponge bathed around it.

b. The child needs to be turned at least every 4 hours.

c. The child needs to be turned frequently.

Application/Physiologic/Evaluation

Index

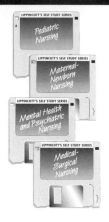
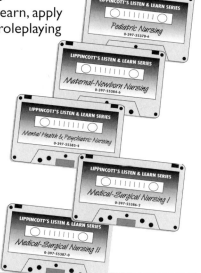
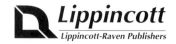